Psychosocial issues in palliative care

SECOND EDITION

Mari Lloyd-Williams

Professor/Director,

Academic Palliative and Supportive Care Studies Group,

University of Liverpool

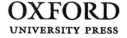

OXFORD

UNIVERSITY PRESS

OXFORD
UNIVERSITY PRESS

Great Clarendon Street, Oxford OX2 6DP

Oxford University Press is a department of the University of Oxford.
It furthers the University's objective of excellence in research, scholarship,
and education by publishing worldwide in

Oxford New York

Auckland Cape Town Dar es Salaam Hong Kong Karachi
Kuala Lumpur Madrid Melbourne Mexico City Nairobi
New Delhi Shanghai Taipei Toronto

With offices in

Argentina Austria Brazil Chile Czech Republic France Greece
Guatemala Hungary Italy Japan Poland Portugal Singapore
South Korea Switzerland Thailand Turkey Ukraine Vietnam

Published in the United States by Oxford University Press Inc., New York
in the UK and in certain other countries

Published in the United States
by Oxford University Press Inc., New York

A catalogue record for this book is available from the British Library
Library of Congress Cataloging in Publication Data
Data available

Typeset by Cepha Imaging Private Ltd., Bangalore, India
Printed in the United Kingdom by
Biddles Ltd., King's Lynn,
Norfolk

ISBN 978–0–19–921642–0

10 9 8 7 6 5 4 3 2 1

Foreword

David W. Kissane

The healing art of medicine is at the core of the psychosocial approaches we undertake within palliative care. Here we meet a person with a serious and invariably fatal illness, sometimes alone and alienated from their community, at other times comforted and supported by their family and friends. We have the opportunity to get to know these people, understand and respond to their distress, acknowledge their suffering and accompany them on their journey. We may not be able to cure, but we can comfort and care for them during these dire times. We can honour them and through the respect we convey, affirm the value and worth of their lives as people who share our common humanity. Whatever their concern&emdash;symptom burden, grief at loss of independence, fear of becoming a burden, sense of loss of control, feelings of vulnerability and frailty&emdash;we respond with compassion and clinical skill. Our competence as physicians is paramount. This skill remains fundamental to our ability to heal. And healers we must be.

Our medical literature struggles to describe the psychology of dying well. The classics do better, exemplified by Leo Tolstoy's *The death of Ivan Ilyich*! The existential challenges that we all must meet in our dying have been grappled with philosophically, but have not been transformed into a typology that can be readily taught and used clinically. Professor Mari Lloyd-Williams responds to this deficit with this second edition. Together with members of the Academic Palliative and Supportive Care Studies Group, which she Directs at the University of Liverpool, she enlists internationally regarded scholars and clinicians to better define the psychosocial issues in palliative care. They set forth an approach to make us better healers, quintessentially responding to the suffering of our patients. The prescription of medication is the easy part; joining with our patients, understanding their uniqueness, as Anatole Broyard described eloquently, surveying their essence as well as their flesh—herein lies the art.

The scene for this book is set by Rod McLeod from New Zealand who outlines different models of palliative care and makes overt why psychosocial care is so important. Approaches to psychosocial assessment are presented, with due attention to the social, emotional, cognitive, cultural, sexual, and ethical contexts. While recognizing the importance of the dignity and autonomy of the person, virtue ethics is seen as underpinning palliative care provision, as this theory recognizes the internal goods that the caring doctor brings to the clinical encounter. Kindness, generosity, respect for others, honesty, compassion, prudence, fairness, and competence&emdash;these virtuous practices create the integrity of the professional role. This lays a solid foundation from which to consider care provision.

How wonderful to see a chapter on communication from the late Peter Maguire, with the adroit support of Cathy Heaven. Maguire's masterful scholarship highlighted facilitative and inhibitory behaviours with respect to communication skills. A thorough exploration of relevant attitudes, interviewing techniques, information provision skills, and training methods are laid out in this chapter. Effective communication is vital for first-rate psychosocial care.

Pam Firth has updated Frances Sheldon's chapter on social services following the death of this outstanding academic social worker. How do we respond to social isolation? How do we ration scarce resources such as day care? Self-help groups, carers' groups, and expanded programmes of family therapy are some of the creative ways we can use to respond to unmet social needs.

Care of the marginalized is described in a new, thought-provoking chapter by Philip Larkin from the National University of Ireland in Galway. The palliative care needs of those with chronic mental illness and intellectual disability necessitate close liaison with the specialist services supporting these patients. Social death from dementia presents some ghastly challenges to family carers. Perhaps the most disenfranchised of all patients are prisoners who may die in an environment characterized by mistrust and despair. This challenges practitioners to rise above the prison culture to provide compassionate care. Substance addicted persons are another group who are often alienated from their family-of-origin and who present complex clinical challenges in their medical treatment. Finally, refugees, those ill with AIDS, and patients from underserved minority races exemplify the cultural sensitivity needed to serve potentially disparate groups of people. Larkin's chapter illustrates beautifully how we strive to 'cloak' suffering as we care for the dying.

Psychosocial distress is taken up as Trevor Friedman discusses its prevalence, determinants, and interventions. Service organization to deliver psychosocial care is considered, including screening approaches to better recognize those with psychiatric disorder. The treatment of psychiatric disorders is then discussed by experts from my own Department at Memorial Sloan–Kettering Cancer Center: Steven Passik writes with colleagues Kirsh and Lloyd-Williams about Anxiety and Adjustment Disorders, while William Breitbart combines with Pessin, Alici Evcimen and Apostolatos to provide an extensive discussion of depression. How does one differentiate suicidality from acceptance of dying? What medications can best help these ailments? What psychotherapies offer benefits to the dying? Psychotherapeutic interventions are reviewed in detail by Fritz Stiefel and Mat Bernard from Lausanne. Important contributions here include the use of Experiential Psychotherapy from the humanistic tradition, art and music therapy, and the non-specific elements of all therapies, which promote healing. Therapy that values the worth and recognizes the meaning of a person's life, can affirm this as if a story of accomplishment and success has been told, and is able to offer this understanding back to the patient and their family achieves much. The potential to move the patient to a position of psychological acceptance of one's dying, with expressions of gratitude for the life lived, will be too lofty for some but achievable for others.

Holistic approaches to healing are reviewed by Ezard Ernst from the Universities of Exeter and Plymouth using an evidence-based perspective. The contribution of a specific treatment such as acupuncture is contrasted with a host of complementary therapies that can be used to ameliorate patients' symptoms. Mindful of safety issues, Ernst provides frank commentary on what does not work alongside what might help.

While combining biopsychosocial and spiritual approaches to care provision, this book is explicit about the importance of the spiritual dimension at all times. Thus, Mark Cobb encourages us to understand the very soul of the person and to integrate spiritual care into our clinical practice. Religious traditions are one pathway, but we also need to be able to respond to the atheist and promote a sense of transcendent connection with the enduring universe. Concepts of legacy, metaphor, symbolism, and mystery come to the fore as we try to replace doubt and despair with reverence and courage.

St Christopher's Hospice in London is well represented by Michael Payne, who provides sage guidance about staff stress, burnout, and compassion fatigue. Finally, Sheila Payne from the University of Lancaster combines with Mari Lloyd-Williams and Vida Kennedy in a chapter on bereavement care. Theoretical concepts of grief and bereavement create the background to a detailed review of bereavement services, including due emphasis on the continuity of psychosocial care from before to after the death.

A particularly noteworthy and pleasing feature of this second edition is the incorporation of literature from the twenty-first century. In the process a solid rationale and evidence base for clinical practice are substantiated. The result is a text which comprehensively reviews psychosocial issues in palliative care and provides an up-to-date and scholarly guide suitable for both established clinicians and students from every discipline.

Anatole Broyard, in his book *Intoxicated by my illness*, wants his doctor to have a little magic, an aura, to be both a talented physician and a metaphysician, somebody who can get to the soul through the body. This is not about quackery but giftedness, an ability to recognize the crisis, appreciate the horror, value the person and create for them a sense of healing. We value our humanity as healers. This book offers practical direction towards achieving this critical aptitude.

I am left with a sense that Dame Cicely Saunders would be proud of the maturation of hospice and its ability to respond to 'total pain', the suffering of our patients. Congratulations to Mari Lloyd-Williams for her leadership and inspiration in collating the work of these authors into a fine and cohesive book.

Professor David Kissane, MD, BS, MPM, FRACGP, FRANZCP, FAChPM
Alfred P. Sloan Chair, Attending Psychiatrist and Chairman
Department of Psychiatry & Behavioral Sciences
Memorial Sloan–Kettering Cancer Center, New York
Professor of Psychiatry, Weill Medical College of Cornell University

Preface

No reader to this book needs reminding that much has changed in palliative care over the last 20 years. I accidentally came across palliative medicine as a medical student 20 years ago and knew this was the area in which I wished to specialize. Although trained in one of the new and forward thinking medical schools with an exciting and dynamic curriculum, palliative care was not an integral part of medical student training but was included as an option for an 'agency placement' where we could spend an afternoon in what was then the very new LOROS Hospice at Leicester.

We now have a situation where the majority of those training for medicine, nursing, and professionals allied to medicine spend at least some time gaining experience and awareness of what palliative care can offer. Palliative medicine is a very well established speciality in its own right and there are thousands of professionals working solely in palliative care in the UK. Yet we still have a situation where only a fraction of patients who need palliative care receive it; where patients suffering from conditions other than cancer rarely access palliative care and even more rarely access hospice care and where families still express disappointment and sadness at the care their loved ones received in the last days and weeks of life. This lack of care is not limited to suboptimum symptom control but more frequently to poor psychosocial care—to the communication issues and lack of co-ordination of multiprofessional services, which can make so much difference to patients and their families.

I hope this second edition of *Psychosocial issues in palliative care* with all the previous chapters updated and many new chapters will allow all those caring for patients with advanced disease to gain greater confidence in their skills and to therefore give better care to all those who require it.

It is so sad that two contributors to the first edition are no longer with us. The late Frances Sheldon and Peter Maguire contributed so much to improving psychosocial palliative care both in the UK and internationally and it is as a tribute to them that we incorporate their contributions to the first edition within this second edition.

I am very grateful to so many people for their support, guidance, and reflections when editing this second edition. My grateful thanks to Ann and to Sarah D' Agostino and Saga Graham for their kind assistance with the wonderful patient artwork contained in this book. My research team at the Academic

Palliative and Supportive Care Studies group have contributed directly to the book and also shaped its format; the service users who are engaged in our research programme also gave such useful perspectives and insights on what should be contained in this book for lay carers; all the contributors so kindly agreed to write a book chapter on top of already very busy clinical and research commitments; and clinical colleagues and academic colleagues within the School of Population. Community and Behavioural Sciences at the University of Liverpool have as usual given wise counsel and advice on many aspects of this work.

The final thanks goes to my patients—some of whom shared in the vision of this book and who so generously gave me their thoughts on what did and would make a difference to their care and how that could be incorporated within this edition—it is a constant privilege to be able to contribute some small part to the care of patients in the final stages of their lives; patients who have faced difficult surgery and treatment and who would describe themselves as very ordinary people but who display extraordinary courage and bravery in the face of great adversity.

Professor Mari Lloyd-Williams
Professor/Director of Academic Palliative and Supportive Care Studies
Group, University of Liverpool and Consultant in Palliative Medicine

Contents

Colour Plates: My Life's Mandala

The wonderful colour plates in this book were painted by Ann in order to create a visual journey that she could leave behind as a legacy of her life for her children.

Whilst she was painting Ann said:

"It is not that I feel that I wished this illness on me, but in some way I feel that I have had a surge of creativity that I have never previously experienced. Before I was operated on for my brain tumor, I was very worried that I would never be the same again, that I would lose my ability to think. In order for me to know that I was still in this world, I began to create a visual journey in my mind. I put together new pictures everyday for my imaginary journal and I received a flow of the most wonderful creative images. I feel that I am on a new journey."

Of the paintings Ann said:

"The blue in the outside is very soothing and it reminds me of serenity and water. Water is very important to me. But I could not continue on without giving it a soul. The red is my soul. It is my life and it is vibrant. The blue is like a cool cocoon holding the spirit. After my illness my soul and spirit has become very important to me. I am trying to combine spirit with logic. I feel that there must be some logic to my spiritual search. I feel that the mandala is my life. Everything is interwoven like these rings, there is nothing that is separate and it all influences each other. The yellow is for hope and life"

Contributors

Andreas J. Apostolatos
Department of Psychiatry and
Behavioral Sciences,
Memorial Sloan-Kettering
Cancer Center,
New York, USA

Mathieu Bernard
Psychiatry Service,
University Hospital,
Lausanne, Switzerland

William Breitbart
Chief, Psychiatry Service,
Memorial Sloan-Kettering Cancer
Center; Professor of Psychiatry,
Weill Medical College of Cornell
University,
New York, USA

Mark Cobb
Clinical Director of Professional
Services,
Royal Hallamshire Hospital,
Sheffield, UK

Edzard Ernst
Professor of Complementary
Medicine,
Peninsula Medical School,
Exeter, UK

Yesne Alici Evcimen
Department of Psychiatry and
Behavioral Sciences,
Memorial Sloan-Kettering
Cancer Center,
New York, USA

Pam Firth
Head of Family Support and Deputy
Director of Hospice Services,
Isabel Hospice,
Welwyn Garden City, UK

Trevor Friedman
Consultant Psychiatrist,
Department of Liaison Psychiatry,
Leicestershire Partnership Trust,
Leicester, UK

Cathy Heaven
Communication Skills Tutor,
CRC Psychological Medicine Group,
Christie Hospital,
Manchester, UK

Vide Kennedy
Research Associate,
Academic Palliative and Supportive
Care Studies Group,
University of Liverpool

Ken Kirsh
Department of Psychiatry and
Behavioural Science,
Memorial Sloan Kettering Hospital
New York, USA

Philip J Larkin
Senior Lecturer in Nursing
(Palliative Care),
School of Nursing and Midwifery
Studies,
The National University of Ireland,
Galway, Ireland

Mari Lloyd-Williams
Professor/Director,
Academic Palliative and Supportive
Care Studies Group,
University of Liverpool

Rod MacLeod
Professor,
Hibiscus Coast Hospice,
Whangaparaoa; Department of
General Practice and Primary
Health Care,
University of Auckland,
New Zealand

Peter Maguire (the late)
Professor of Psychiatry,
CRC Psychological Medicine Group,
Christie Hospital,
Manchester, UK

Steve Passik
Director,
Oncology Symptom Control
Research,
Indianapolis, USA

Malcolm Payne
Director,
Psycho-social and Spiritual Care,
St Christopher's Hospice; Honorary
Professor,
Kingston University/St George's
University of London,
London, UK

Sheila Payne
Help the Hospices Chair in
Hospice Studies,
Lancaster University,
Lancaster, UK

Hayley Pessin
Research Associate,
Department of Psychiatry and
Behavioral Sciences,
Memorial Sloan-Kettering
Cancer Center,
New York, USA

Frances Sheldon (the late)
Macmillan Senior Lecturer in
Social Work,
University of Southampton, UK

Frederick Stiefel
Professor of Psychiatry,
Psychiatry Service,
University Hospital,
Lausanne, Switzerland

Dedication

This book is dedicated to D, M, and F and to D, G, E, T, A without whom this book would not have been written.

Chapter 1

Setting the context: What do we mean by psychosocial care in palliative care?

Rod MacLeod

What is palliative care?

Caring for people who are dying has been seen as a special form of care for centuries. In the first millennium the church was closely involved with such care and the original hospices were set up as resting places for travellers. Religious orders advanced the notion of care for people who were dying in the nineteenth century and St Joseph's Hospice was founded in London in 1905. The modern hospice movement was born out of a response to perceived inadequacies of medical care (Clark 2002). The pioneering work of hospices such as St Christopher's Hospice, which opened in Sydenham, London in 1967, demonstrated that the principles of hospice care could be applied in a variety of settings. Dame Cicely Saunders introduced the concept of whole person care in that institution and developed the model of 'total pain', which highlighted not only the physical aspects of a person's pain, but also psychological, social, and spiritual dimensions of their distress (Saunders and Sykes 1993). The term 'palliative care' was coined in Canada in 1974 by Balfour Mount, a pioneering surgeon who had worked in London with Saunders and wanted to take the concept back to Canada where there could have been confusion among the French-speaking population about the term hospice. Using the term palliation to reflect the non-curative nature of care was not new—it had been used in the seventeenth century. This terminology was subsequently adopted in many countries and a new medical specialty was proposed—that of palliative medicine. The discipline received recognition by the Royal College of Physicians in 1987 as a speciality within medicine in the UK. Since that time other countries have adopted that approach and palliative medicine and palliative care are practised around the world in over 100 countries. A universally agreed definition of palliative care was disseminated by the World Health Organization (WHO) in 1986, followed by a revision in 1990. A revised and updated definition of palliative care was accepted by the WHO in 2002 (Sepúlveda *et al.* 2002).

Palliative care is an approach that improves the quality of life of patients and their families facing the problems associated with life-threatening illness, through the prevention and relief of suffering by means of early identification and impeccable assessment and treatment of pain and other problems, physical, psychosocial, and spiritual.

Palliative care:

◆ provides relief from pain and other distressing symptoms;

◆ affirms life and regards dying as a normal process;

◆ intends neither to hasten or postpone death;

◆ integrates the psychological and spiritual aspects of patient care;

◆ offers a support system to help patients live as actively as possible until death;

◆ offers a support system to help the family cope during the patient's illness and in their own bereavement;

◆ uses a team approach to address the needs of patients and their families, including bereavement counselling, if indicated;

◆ will enhance quality of life, and may also positively influence the course of illness;

◆ is applicable early in the course of illness, in conjunction with other therapies that are intended to prolong life, such as chemotherapy or radiation therapy, and includes those investigations needed to better understand and manage distressing clinical complications.

Definitions are helpful in gaining consensus about the limits of a specialty but what does it mean in practice? Generally speaking people with advancing disease need to be supported and cared for by clinicians with excellent skills.

The National Institute for Clinical Excellence (NICE) has defined supportive care for people with cancer. With some modification the definition can be used for people with any life-threatening condition (NICE 2004).

> Supportive care helps the patient and their family to cope with their condition and treatment of it—from pre-diagnosis, through the process of diagnosis and treatment, to cure, continuing illness or death and into bereavement. It helps the patient to maximise the benefits of treatment and to live as well as possible with the effects of the disease. It is given equal priority alongside diagnosis and treatment.
>
> Supportive care should be fully integrated with diagnosis and treatment. It encompasses:
>
> ◆ Self help and support
>
> ◆ User involvement
>
> ◆ Information giving

- Psychological support
- Symptom control
- Social support
- Rehabilitation
- Complementary therapies
- Spiritual support
- End of life and bereavement care.

Palliative care is therefore part of supportive care. It embraces many elements of supportive care.

Who provides palliative care?

Palliative care is provided by two distinct categories of health and social care professionals:

- Generalist palliative care is provided by those working to providing day-to-day care to patients, families, and carers in their homes and in hospitals:
  - they should be able to assess the care needs of each patient and their families across the domains of physical, psychological, social, and spiritual needs
  - meet those needs within the limits of their knowledge, skills, and competence in palliative care and know when to seek advice from or refer to specialist palliative care services.
- Specialist palliative care is provided by professionals with additional training in the discipline and who only work in palliative care (consultants in palliative medicine and clinical nurse specialists in palliative care, for example).

Specialist palliative care services

These services are provided by specialist multidisciplinary teams and include:

- Assessment, advice, and care for patients and families in any or all care settings, including hospitals and care homes.
- Specialist in-patient facilities (in hospices or hospitals) for patients and families who benefit from the continuous support and care of those specialist teams.
- Intensive co-ordinated home support for patients with complex needs who wish to stay at home (this may involve the specialist palliative care service working with the patient's own doctor and community nurse to enable someone to stay in their own home.)

- Many teams also now provide extended specialist palliative nursing, medical, social, and emotional support and care in the patient's home, often known as 'hospice at home'.
- Day care facilities that offer a range of opportunities for assessment and review of patients' needs and enable the provision of physical, psychological, and social interventions within the context of social interaction, support, and friendship. Many also offer creative and complementary therapies.
- Advice and support to all the people involved in a patient's care.
- Bereavement support services that provide support for the people involved in a patient's care following the patient's death.
- Education and training (and for many, research) in palliative care.

The specialist teams should include palliative medicine and palliative care nurse specialists together with a range of expertise provided by physiotherapists, occupational therapists, art and music therapists, dieticians, pharmacists, social workers, and those able to give spiritual and psychological support.

Who should receive palliative care?

Anyone with a life limiting disease should be able to have access to palliative care services. Historically modern palliative care services were primarily involved with providing care for people with cancer and some neurological disorders such as motor neurone disease or other degenerative disorders of the nervous system.

Cancer develops when cells in any part of the body begin to grow out of control. Normally the cells in the body grow in an orderly manner until they are replaced—in cancer the growth becomes disordered and disorganized. Although there are many kinds of cancer, they all start because of this disordered growth of abnormal cells. Cancer cells develop because of damage to DNA, the building blocks of all cells. Although damage occurs to DNA throughout our lives it can normally be repaired but in cancer this does not happen. Damaged DNA may be inherited (so producing inherited cancers) or it can be damaged by any number of triggers in the environment such as radiation, sunlight, or smoking. Frequently cancer cells spread to other parts of the body. This process is called metastasis. Different cancers have different patterns of metastasis.

The other major group of people who should receive palliative care are those with failure of one of the major organs of the body such as the lungs, heart, kidneys, or liver. In these situations people often have a prolonged period of time to adjust to the understanding that the body is failing.

One problem though can be that medical science has become so adept at propping up failing bodies that the realization that death is approaching may not be so apparent. This can produce problems for families and carers as death approaches. It may also explain why it is that in England, for example, the majority of people with chronic conditions die in hospital—58% of those with heart failure, 78% of those with renal failure, and 61% of those with COPD—most people who die in hospital do so in the first week after admission.

The clinical course of people who are dying tends to follow one of three trajectories (Dy and Lynn 2007). The first is the maintenance of relatively good function until a predicted decline a few weeks or short months before death. The second is the course of chronic organ failure, which shows a slow decline with exacerbations that may end in sudden death. The third trajectory is one where there is poor functional status over a long time with a slow but relentless decline; frail elderly people with many co-morbidities fit into this group. It is important therefore that services are developed for people who are dying in any of these ways. There are a number of models available—for example, the Gold Standards Framework in the UK, which incorporates resources and end of life tools into primary care so hoping to enable people to have real choice about where they wish to die (Thomas 2003; King et al. 2005).

Of course the majority of people who are dying would prefer to do so at home being cared for by their primary healthcare professionals. Primary care shares common values with specialist palliative care—holistic, patient centred, and delivered in the context of their families—but too often it becomes difficult for a number of reasons for people to be cared for in their own homes (Murray et al. 2004). Developing primary palliative care is essential if people are to exercise their right to die in the bed of their choice.

David Field (1998) identified two important differences between patients with cancer and those with non-malignant conditions. First, differences in disease progression mean there is a continuing benefit from curative/restorative interventions and treatments for the latter category. Second, there was greater uncertainty about the fact and likely time of death with non-cancer patients. Field identifies the latter as appearing to be the key obstruction to extending specialist palliative care services to non-cancer patients. This is because they will not be seen as suitable candidates for palliative care until they have been defined as terminally ill. One of the reasons that this may occur is because of the difficulty many clinicians have in dealing with uncertainty in general. In medicine, and possibly in other disciplines as well, uncertainty stimulates and propels activity (Hall 2002)—doctors have a 'propensity to resolve uncertainty and ambiguity by action rather than inaction' (Katz 1984).

Increasing diagnostic uncertainty leads to a reluctance to withdraw from 'active' interventions so leaving patients and families in a similar situation of ambiguity and doubt about the future (Christakis and Asch 1993) There is evidence from the SUPPORT Study (1996) suggesting widespread difficulty in predicting the life expectancy of hospitalized non-cancer patients. This relates to a tendency for the continuation of what might be deemed futile treatment in the face of relentlessly advancing disease. Taken out of context (i.e. without considering the person as a whole) almost any disease may be deemed 'treat-able'—such are the advances in medical science and technology. This confidence in the advancement of medical science is relayed not only to the medical and nursing professions but to the lay public as well, with a consequent sense of expectation that is unfortunately not wholly realized. This situation is compounded with the advancing age of people being treated. Many elderly patients have multiple clinical diagnoses involving multisystem pathology and the diagnosis of dying is often made only by exclusion. Communication may be more difficult due to a combination of a higher incidence of confusion in elderly patients with non-malignant disease than in younger cancer patients and reduced social networks in the elderly may lead to reduced care and support from family and friends. The incidence, duration, intensity, and type of symptoms follow a different pattern in cancer compared with other illnesses. People with non-malignant disease also tend to be older. People aged 75 and over who do not die from cancer are more likely to have outlived their spouses, brothers, and sisters, and even their children. They are predominantly women and many live alone or in residential care and therefore present differing challenges for the provision of social support.

The scope of palliative care therefore extends beyond people with a diagnosis of cancer to include patients with other chronic life-threatening diseases.

It is estimated that almost 300 000 people who die from non-malignant disease in England and Wales each year may benefit from specialist palliative care (NHS 2005) but are excluded by reason of their diagnosis. This figure suggests that there would be a significant increase in caseload if specialist palliative care services were made fully available to non-cancer patients. While the focus of much in palliative care is on the relief of physical symptoms there are equal, if not greater, burdens to be relieved in non-physical management.

A retrospective review identified the pattern of non-cancer referrals to a specialist palliative care service (Kite *et al.* 1999). Twenty-nine per cent of the hospital ward referrals had a non-cancer diagnosis, which were referred predominantly for symptom control. Of 130 outpatient referrals 23% had a non-cancer diagnosis and again were also predominantly referred for the management of pain. Nine per cent of 196 home care referrals had a non-cancer diagnosis, which tended to be referred for 'multi-professional care' of end-stage disease. Only 4% of 421 hospice inpatient admissions in that study were for patients with a non-cancer diagnosis and were predominantly for respite care.

Perhaps one of the greatest challenges for palliative care services is the provision of care for people with dementia—an area which modern palliative care has so far largely avoided. The annual incidence of dementia in Americans doubles nearly every 5 years from 7 in 1000 (65–69 years of age) to 118 in 1000 (86–89 years of age) (Hanrahan *et al.* 2001). Roger (2006) outlines challenges for palliative care provision for people with dementia and provides a number of recommendations including supporting the development of palliative care programmes for people with dementia and the development of a better understanding of assessment tools and treatment procedures related to pain management. Assessment of the ethics of advanced care documentation and evaluative tools for decision making with this group of people are encouraged.

Current provision of specialist palliative care services

For example as at January 2006, in England, Wales and Northern Ireland there were:

- ◆ 193 specialist inpatient units providing 2774 beds, of which 20% were NHS beds.
- ◆ 295 home care services—at present this figure will include both primarily advisory services delivered by hospice or NHS-based community palliative care teams and other more sustained care provided in the patient's home.
- ◆ In addition there were 314 hospital-based services, 234 day care services, and 314 bereavement support services.

http://www.ncpc.org.uk/palliative_care.html

Palliative Care Australia, in 2003, released an outline of the population-based resources necessary to provide palliative care services in that country (Palliative Care Australia 2002). It was evidence based and underwent a thorough consultation process Similarly, in the United States there are a number of initiatives that promote models for providing end of life care. Promoting Excellence in End-of-Life Care was a national programme of the Robert Wood Johnson Foundation dedicated to long-term changes in healthcare institutions to substantially improve care for dying people and their families. They produced a number of major programmes that can be utilized in many settings and all have been extensively researched and evaluated. Resources include clinical, evaluation, education, and organizational tools.

Another major contributor to understanding and practice in this area is the Centre to Advance Palliative Care (CAPC).

For example they published a report *A National Framework and Preferred Practices for Palliative and Hospice Care Quality*, which endorses a framework for palliative and hospice care that is intended to be the first step in developing a comprehensive quality measurement and reporting system for palliative care and hospice services (National Quality Forum 2006). The report also endorses a set of preferred practices designed to improve palliative and hospice care in the USA. Further examples of models of care can be found in a publication from the charitable organization Help the Hospices and the International Observatory on End of Life Care entitled Models of hospice and palliative care in resource poor countries (Wright 2003).

Psychosocial care

The National Council for Hospice and Specialist Palliative Care Services (now the National Council for Palliative Care—NCPC) has defined psychosocial care as 'concerned with the psychological and emotional well being of the patient and their family/carers, including issues of self-esteem, insight into an adaptation to the illness and its consequences, communication, social functioning and relationships' (National Council for Hospice and Specialist Palliative Care Services 1997).

Psychosocial care addresses the psychological experiences of loss and facing death for the patient and their impact on those close to them. It involves the spiritual beliefs, culture, and values of those concerned and the social factors, which influence the experience. Psychosocial care includes the practical aspects of care such as financial, housing and aids to daily living, and overlaps with spiritual care. Spiritual care is less easy to define and is often subjective, arbitrary, and personal. It is generally assumed to include an individual's beliefs, values, sense of meaning and purpose, identity, and for some people religion. It may also encompass the emotional benefits of informal support from relatives, friends, religious groups, and more formal pastoral care. For many, existential questions about the human condition can be ignored during many phases of life but are brought into acuity at the end of life (Williams 2006).

Psychosocial care also includes the professional carers who are inevitably affected by their experiences and who thus require support. Thus psychosocial care encompasses:

- ◆ Psychological approaches, which are concerned with enabling patients and those close to them to express thoughts feelings and concerns relating to illness.

◆ Psychological interventions to improve the psychological and emotional well being of the patient and their family/carers

In the past there has been a greater emphasis on psychological needs than social needs—the National Council for Hospice and Specialist Palliative Care Services (2002) have emphasized the importance of social care to patients: 'The social fabric of their lives is central to how they make sense of their illness experiences, the meanings they draw upon to understand these and the range of resources they can call upon to help them manage them.' In practice, the social aspects of palliative care are often limited to a focus upon the patient's family, ignoring community influences.

Palliative care in different settings

Palliative care is applicable in most settings. However, in the UK, as in many other countries, almost a quarter of occupied hospital bed days are taken up by patients who are in the last year of life and in many countries a majority of people die in hospital. Of those referred to palliative care services in England, Northern Ireland, and Wales in 2006 though the figures are somewhat different. Of 75 000 deaths recorded 36% were in hospital, 27% at home, and 31% in a palliative care unit (Eve 2006). In that survey it is estimated from home care data that about 101 000 new patients are cared for each year of whom 94% have cancer. This is approximately 69% of the number of patients dying of cancer. Seymour (2001) has commented on the social isolation of dying patients in hospital and of the failure of medical technology to coexist appropriately with dignified dying. Mola (1997) confirmed what many thought, that hospital is often perceived to be a place of insecurity, discomfort, intrusion, and demands for compliance. This can be contrasted with the home setting where generally there is a sense of social and physical security and where people who are dying may have a greater sense of control. It is after all, their place. A constant interruption to the running of their lives by visiting health and social care professionals threatens privacy. Professionals must ensure that the choices of the patient and family are honoured in a way that they want—not in a way that suits professional needs. In recent times it is apparent that the wishes of the users of palliative care services can be at variance with the policies of the providers (Clark *et al.* 1997). However, by listening to patients and those close to them, the nature of care that is appropriate to each individual becomes clear.

Psychosocial assessment

Patients and families face a range of issues that are not only related to illness and approaching death. The healthcare professionals need to assess individual strengths and coping styles, experience and stress and attend to previous losses.

The initial assessment of a patient is carried out by a member of the specialist palliative care team and will include a detailed medical/nursing assessment of the patient's and family/carers' needs. The time invested in this initial assessment is essential in creating a framework for the provision of future care; a partnership between patient and professionals. The initial assessment may indicate the need for more formal psychological or social assessment. This will include the need to maintain autonomy, which includes respect for dignity and the opportunity to exercise choice.

An empirically derived psychosocial assessment tool for use in advanced cancer has been described (Powazki and Walsh 1999) whereby physical, cognitive, social, and emotional dimensions were the framework for the assessment of both patient and caregiver functioning. The study of 150 patients found not surprisingly that specific high-risk psychosocial issues may impact on the discharge planning and overall care of the patient but that a comprehensive assessment such as the one described can guide interventions to maximize psychosocial interventions.

In order to identify caregivers at risk of poor psychosocial functioning, self-reported anxiety and competence rating is suggested as an aid to care provision (Hudson *et al.* 2006). A small group of caregivers (35) was studied. Using a screening tool, the researchers identified the possibility of low-level psychosocial functioning as a potential determinant for family caregivers at risk of psychosocial distress.

There are, however, a multitude of assessment tools and techniques that will illuminate elements of psychosocial well-being and identify psychological and social needs of patients and caregivers. They include:

- *After Death Bereaved Family Interview*: a survey used to measure quality of care at the end of life from the unique perspective of family members.

- *Beck Depression Inventory (BDI)*: a 21-item multiple choice test used for assessing the presence and degree of depression in adolescents and adults.

- *Caregiver Strain Index*: a tool that measures strain related to care provision. Used to assess individuals who have assumed the role of caregiver for an older adult.

- *Geriatric Depression Scale in two forms—long (30 item) or short (15 item)*: a screening tool for symptoms of depression in the elderly.

- *Herth Hope Index*: a 12-item interview containing three dimensions: temporality and future, positive readiness and expectance, and interconnectedness; tested in community and hospital patients and family members.

- *Mini Mental State Questionnaire:* a screening tool for assessing cognitive impairment.
- *Needs at the End-of-life Screening Tool (NEST):* NEST is a comprehensive assessment and outcome measures instrument.
- *Palliative Care Outcome Scale (POS):* a 10-item scale (plus an open question) that was specifically developed and validated for palliative care and covers physical symptoms, patient and family or caregiver anxiety/fears and well being.

(A comprehensive list of such tools may be obtained from a number of sources including http://www.npcrc.org/resources/resources.)

The psychosocial aspects of care of the dying person whatever their diagnosis includes the need for:

- *understanding:* of symptoms and the nature of disease and of the process of dying
- *acceptance:* regardless of mood, sociability and appearance
- *self-esteem:* involvement in decision-making
- *safety:* a feeling of security
- *belonging:* a wish to feel needed and not to feel a burden
- *love:* expressions of affection, human contact (touch)
- *spirituality:* an explanation of meaning and purpose, both religious and non-religious
- *hope:* for an improvement in any aspect of their life or of their living.

In the provision of psychosocial care for people at the end of life each of these needs must be identified and addressed.

Social context

Social elements of care are often influenced by the disease that is ending a life. Dying from a non-malignant disease, in many ways, creates a different social structure or standing than dying from cancer. The language that we use is quite different—for example, people who die from cancer are often referred to as 'brave' in their 'battle' with cancer. They often talk of 'beating' the disease or 'fighting' it. Non-malignant disease does not seem to have that same social cache. Death from end-organ failure is often silent and slow—in many ways relentless in its nature. Without heroic medical interventions to replace organs or use artificial means to support ailing bodies many of these people would die earlier and perhaps more suddenly. In identifying social or psychological care for these people it is important to recognize this significant difference in perception of disease that is possible to have originated both from the individual and from society.

For many people with cancer there are well-recognized social networks or programmes that may provide both psychological and social support. Social supports for people with non-malignant diseases should emerge from people in similar situations, family and friends, and from the wider community. Many of the current support systems for people with non-malignant disease are focused on raising awareness and funding for curative interventions rather than supporting people in the last stages of their disease. The professions, while openly supporting cancer networks and programmes have been slower to acknowledge the need for similar systems for people with incurable non-malignant disease.

Emotional context

Some feelings and emotions are almost universally experienced near the end of life.

- Fear of being left alone or having to leave loved ones; of breaking down or losing control—of the situation they are currently in, getting worse.
- A sense of helplessness in which physical and psychological crises show up human powerlessness. Alongside this is the knowledge of physical and emotional strength gradually deteriorating—loss of physical ability bringing with it attendant psychological and social helplessness.
- Feelings of sadness for what is not to be and for the loss to come.
- A sense of longing for all that has gone before and all that is not going to be, in the future.
- Feelings of guilt for being better off than others or regret for things that have been done or not done.
- A sense of shame for having been exposed as helpless, emotional and of needing others or for not having reacted, as one would have wished.
- Anger at what has happened, at whatever caused it or allowed it to happen, that the treatment hasn't worked, at the injustice and senselessness of it all and the shame and indignity and at the lack of proper understanding by others.

These feelings and emotions may also be influenced by memories of feelings or loss or of love for other people in their lives who have been injured or died, perhaps let down by doctors, by the system or society or by the family.

Psychological context

The fundamental clinical skill of medicine is acquiring the history of the illness from the patient and providing the patient with the opportunity to identify their concerns is mandatory. Specific questions need to be asked to elucidate psychological distress; in particular they should include questions concerning fatigue, hallucinations, and suicide risk (Macleod 2007). Examples of psychological interventions include (Chochinov and Breitbart 2000):

- psychosocial support and psychotherapy
- behavioural-cognitive therapies
- educational therapies.

Initially, it is helpful to look for indicators of pathological levels of psychological disturbance such as clinical depression or other mood disturbance or personality disorder. These lend themselves well to specific psychological interventions. Variables suggesting that the patient or family is at serious risk of psychological disorder or distress may be identified (for example, social isolation or a history of psychiatric hospitalizations). All members of the healthcare team may observe and subjectively report distress that they feel is psychological in nature (fear or anger) or psychologically mediated (pain or breathlessness) but may not meet the criteria of a discrete psychological disorder. The team should also look for the potential for preventative interventions that may forestall, minimize, or bolster resources for predictable areas or times of vulnerability and hardship (similar patterns of ill-health, pre-bereavement work, or anniversary calls to the bereaved).

Specific psycho-educational interventions that may enhance coping skills, psychological insights, and quality of life should be employed, regardless of the presence or absence of clinical levels of psychological distress. (For an extensive review of psychiatric syndromes and interventions see Macleod 2007.)

People with neuromuscular degenerative disorders, such as motor neuron disease, multiple sclerosis, muscular dystrophies, and less frequently seen disorders such as Creutzfeldt–Jacob disease may have particular psychological needs associated with their care. Such disorders bring with them potentially challenging communication issues. For example, some patients may not be able to communicate verbally but retain effective cognitive functioning (Oneschuk 2001). It is important to help families to differentiate between behavioural disturbances associated with cognitive impairment from other communication difficulties. Cognitive impairment, depressive symptoms, emotional incontinence, or lability all need expert assessment and careful explanation and management. All or any of these may significantly impact on coping ability, psychological adjustment, and communication both of the patient and family (Macleod 2001).

Cultural context

In palliative care, the cornerstone of practice is the holistic approach to care that is exemplified by the management of 'total' pain. This classically includes physical, psychological, social, and spiritual pain. Cultural pain or distress can be expressed through any of these dimensions (Oliviere 1999). Often closely allied to culture are spiritual and religious beliefs that have a bearing on how people approach and understand their disease. In many societies people define themselves by their religious, cultural, or tribal grouping, even when their faith or immersion in religion or culture is limited. There are wide variations between people of differing faiths, ethnic backgrounds, and national origins and their approach to the end of life. Although documented evidence is thin there is anecdotal evidence to suggest that there is a difference in approach to dealing with malignant and non-malignant disease. In order to understand these differences it is important to understand the culture from the perspective of the patient and family. Cultural safety was a term originally identified by a New Zealand nursing scholar, Irihapeti Ramsden, which became incorporated into guidelines for nurses and midwives in training in that country. The concept of cultural safety suggests that 'the effective nursing of a person/family from another culture recognizes the impact of the nurse's culture on his or her practice. Unsafe clinical practice is any action which diminishes, demeans or disempowers the cultural identity and wellbeing of an individual.' (Nursing Council 1996). Cultural safety is now a concept that is identified and embraced in all healthcare practices throughout New Zealand and many other parts of the world. In the management of non-malignant disease it is helpful to identify any particular taboos or discrimination that people may experience as a result of their diagnosis (for example, AIDS or neuromuscular disorders).

In caring from people of a different culture to our own it is imperative that we understand the expectations of that culture in order that we act appropriately (Kashiwagi 1995; Ho 2006; Schwass 2006). For example, the notion of individual autonomy is essentially a Western one—many people live together and make decisions together in extended families. People in China, Japan, and the Pacific Islands as well as many Maori in New Zealand, for example, consider the family as the fundamental unit of society and will expect the family to make medical decisions. Without the accurate and honest provision of information in the right form, at the right time, there can be little hope of an understanding being reached about the situation the patient and family are facing and the goals of care that are being formulated. Without asking, we cannot know what individuals need to make a difference to the end of their life. That asking must include an acknowledgement of difference—difference in culture, in religious beliefs, in understanding of the nature of disease, in expectations in a particular situation, and in perceptions for hope at the end of life.

Sexual context

Sexuality is an element of being that is often easily sidelined or overlooked when caring for people at the end of life, particularly if those people are elderly. It is too often assumed that because people approaching death are weak and tired that their sexual needs are minimized but this fails to recognize the many ways in which human beings can express their sexuality aside from sexual intercourse. Staff often view people's sexual interests as 'behavioural problems' rather than natural occurrences or expressions of needs for loving contact (Steinke 1997; McPherson *et al.* 2001). Many people approaching the end of life with a non-malignant disease have had a relentless decrease in their physical being for some time. Much of their time may have been spent in repeated hospital admissions and the physical isolation that encourages. Many treatments, as well as the diseases themselves, can affect sexual performance and of course sexual activity may not be at the forefront of people's minds as they approach death. Acknowledging that all people are sexual beings is a starting point in helping people address their sexual needs and wishes—it is in no way different to acknowledging that they are physical or emotional beings as well. Taking a sexual health history may be one way of ensuring this aspect of each individual's being is not overlooked. This is one aspect of their functional health that can contribute to their sense of self-worth or self-esteem. Changes in physical appearance, size, skin colour and texture as well as increasing fatigue often decrease an individual's sense of self-worth or attractiveness. Identifying psychological elements of their functional health may help to reverse this decrease. Providing information and advice on ways of expressing sexuality other than through sexual intercourse may help to restore an individual's sense of worth in this aspect of themselves.

Ethical context

In all of our care for people near the end of life one of our goals is to help people to do what they want in the way that they want. In many ways that is what has become known as autonomy. 'Autonomy has emerged as a modern criterion of moral worth providing the grounds to distinguish between being merely *alive* and being *meaningfully* alive' (Woods 2002). People's choices at the end of life are often different to those they may make earlier in their life. Patients' authority to choose what interventions they have and even to refuse interventions is seen as one way of protecting dignity and autonomy (Dy and Lynn 2007). Being in charge is better than having control taken away (Carter *et al.* 2004). That idea of being in charge though will be different for different ethnic groups. Professional carers need to ensure that they understand the nature of communication and decision making that is the norm for each person and family they encounter. Assessment of family dynamics from a different culture may help ensure that their ethical constructs are not over-ridden (Ho 2006).

The ethics of the provision of palliative care are really no different to those required for any form of healthcare; however, in providing care for the most vulnerable there are particular issues to address. Palliative care must be based on a philosophy that acknowledges the inherent worth and dignity of each person and in order to understand that worth and dignity every facet of their being should be explored—not just the physical (MacLeod 1997). This philosophy must be based on an ethical framework—this is most commonly represented by the 'famous four'—autonomy, beneficence, non-maleficence, and justice. These principles encourage a sharing of decision making between carer and cared for but also create the right environment for promoting patient well-being. In addition to this framework virtue-based ethics may give some indicators for the way in which we could practise our professions. Virtues are often thought to be 'old-fashioned' but they are particularly relevant to end-of-life care.

Integrity and trust are perhaps the cornerstones of the caring relationship. Development of these can be gained by attending to the psychosocial as well as the physical wants and needs of individuals and families. Trust is essential in any human relationship but in one where one party is so vulnerable then perhaps it is even more important. In all of our dealings with patients and their families we must be truthful and honest. However, unskilled attempts to inform patients have created a practice best described as the 'assault of truth'. If information or advice of any sort is given in an unsympathetic way it may serve to induce helplessness, hopelessness, and despair in the patient and family and 'the door to any creative future is slammed shut and the patient has nowhere to look except death' (Latimer 1991). People who are dying have lost so many elements of their being that it is essential that they can maintain trust in their professional attendants.

Compassion, a further virtue required in all our dealings with patients and their families could be described as suffering together *with* another or participation *in* suffering. Suffering is clearly not only related to the physical elements of our being and in order to understand suffering in its broadest sense we must address social, psychological, and spiritual elements as well.

Phronesis is a virtue rarely mentioned in modern practice but it is essentially prudence. Nowadays this can be regarded as timidity, undue self-interest, or unwillingness to take risks, but it might also be considered to be discretion or common sense. In history, phronesis was thought to be practical wisdom—the link between the intellectual and moral life. Phronesis urges us to look for 'the right way of acting' (MacLeod 2003).

In modern healthcare practice, working from an effective evidence base, where randomized controlled trials are sought for as many interventions as possible to guide us, it is often forgotten that practical wisdom, phronesis, can guide us where there is no concrete evidence to do so.

The virtue of justice, fairness, requires that people are not put down or labelled in any way. Such labels can determine how people are cared for in the future and they may often have arisen from isolated encounters. So often, labels can imply intolerance—this in turn can lead to an expectation that there is a particular 'right' way to live or a right way to die.

Integrity defines the nature of the individual and it also integrates all the virtues. A person with integrity is someone who can judge the relative importance in each situation of principles, rules, guidelines, and other virtues in reaching a decision. It implies honesty and righteousness. The integrity of a person is shown in the right ordering of the parts in relation to the whole, the balance and harmony between the various dimensions of human existence necessary for the healthy functioning of the whole organism (Pellegrino and Thomasma 1993). It is a balanced relationship between the physical, psychosocial, and intellectual elements of their lives. This could be a definition of what palliative care should be about.

The doctor/patient relationship relies on integrity and trust. Neither party must impose their values on the other. Overriding another person's values is an assault on their humanity and their person (MacLeod 1997).

Using these principles and virtues enables carers to address some of the challenging moral or ethical issues near the end of life. Aspects such as people asking for or insisting on futile treatments, balancing ordinary and extraordinary treatment, the doctrine of double effect and the relationship between killing and letting die have attracted much discussion and comment over the last three decades and the debate has been considerably better informed by research, investigation, and dialogue between those in the palliative care community and their colleagues in the field of medical bioethics. (For a brief summary see, for example, Brock (1993) or Ten Have and Clark (2002).)

The developments in the provision and understanding of palliative care have enabled a more informed discussion of these topics but resolution for many in our broader society is still a long way off. However, by attending to people as whole people within the context of their family whoever that may be, we stand a much better chance of meeting their needs—not just their physical needs but their psychological, social, and spiritual needs as well.

References

Brock D (1998). Medical decisions at end of life. In: Kuhse H, Singer P (ed.), *A companion to bioethics*. Oxford: Blackwell Publishers.

Carter H, MacLeod RD, Brander P, McPherson K (2004). Living with a terminal illness. *J Adv Nurs* 45(6):611–20.

Chochinov HM, Breitbart W (ed.) (2000). *Handbook of psychiatry in palliative medicine*. London: Oxford University Press.

Christakis N, Asch D (1993). Biases in how physicians choose to withdraw life support. *Lancet* 342:642–6.

Clark D (2002). Between hope and acceptance: the medicalisation of dying. *BMJ* 324:905–7.

Clark D, Hockley J, Ahmedzai S (1997). *New themes in palliative care*. Buckingham: Open University Press.

Dy S, Lynn J (2007). Getting services right for those sick enough to die. *BMJ* 334:511–13.

Eve A (2006). NCPC National Survey of patient activity data for specialist palliative care services MDS Full report 2005–2006. http://www.statistics.gov.uk/downloads/theme_health/Dh1_37_2004/DH1_no_37.pdf (accessed March 2007)

Field D (1998). Special not different: general practitioners' accounts of their care of dying people. *Soc Sci Med* 46:1111–20.

Hall KH (2002). Reviewing intuitive decision-making and uncertainty: the implications for medical education. *Med Educ* 36:216–24.

Hanrahan P, Luchins D, Murphy K (2001). Palliative care for patients with dementia. In: Addington-Hall J, Higginson I (ed.). *Palliative care for non-cancer patients*. New York: Oxford University Press, pp. 114–24.

Ho A (2006). Family and informed consent in multicultural setting. *Am J Bioethics* 6:26–8.

Hudson PL, Hayman-White K, Aranda S, Kristjanson LJ (2006). Predicting family caregiver psychosocial functioning in palliative care. *J Palliat Care* 22(3): 133–40.

Kashiwagi T (1995). Psychosocial and spiritual issues in terminal care. *Psychiatry Clin Neurosci* 49(Suppl. 1):S123–127.

Katz J (1984). *The silent world of doctor and patient*. New York: Free Press, pp. 195–7.

King N, Thomas K, Martin N, Bell D, Farrell S (2007). 'Now nobody falls through the net': practitioners' perspectives on the Gold Standards Framework for community palliative care. *Palliat Med* 19: 619–27.

Kite S, Jones K, Tookman A (1999). Specialist palliative care and patients with non-cancer diagnoses: the experience of a service. *Palliat Med* 13:477–84.

Latimer E (1991). Caring for seriously ill and dying patients: the philosophy and ethics. *Can Med Assoc J* 144(7):859–64.

MacLeod RD (1997). All patients need doctors who care as well as cure. *NZ Fam Physician* 24(6):7–9.

MacLeod RD (2003). Wisdom and the practice of palliative care. *J Palliat Care* 19(2):123–6.

Macleod S (2001). Multiple sclerosis and palliative medicine. *Prog Palliat Care* 9:196–8.

Macleod S (2007). *The psychiatry of palliative medicine—the dying mind*. Abingdon, Oxon: Radcliffe Publishing.

McPherson KM, Brander P, McNaughton H, Taylor W (2001). Living with arthritis—what is important? *Dis Rehab* 23:706–21.

Mola GD (1997). Palliative home care. In: Clark D, Hockley J, Ahmedzai S (ed.). *New themes in palliative care*. Buckingham: Open University Press

Murray S, Boyd K, Sheikh A, Thomas K, Higginson I (2004). Developing primary palliative care *BMJ* 329: 1056–7.

National Council for Hospice and Specialist Palliative Care Services (1997). *Feeling better: psychosocial care in specialist palliative care*. Occasional Paper 13. London: NCHSPC.

National Council for Hospice and Specialist Palliative Care Services (2002). *Definitions of supportive and palliative care*. A Consultation Paper. London: NCHPCS.

NHS Confederation (2005). Improving end-of-life care. *Leading Edge* 12:1–8. http://www.dyingwell.org.uk/docs/NHSConfederationBriefing.pdf (accessed March 2007)

National Institute for Clinical Excellence (2004). *Supportive and palliative care services for adults with cancer* http://www.guidance.nice.org.uk/csgsp/guidance (accessed March 2007).

National Quality Forum (2006). *A national framework and preferred practices for palliative and hospice care quality* http://www.qualityforum.org/publications/reports/palliative.asp (accessed March 2007).

Nursing Council (1996). *Guidelines for cultural safety in nursing and midwifery education*. Wellington: Nursing Council of New Zealand.

Oliviere D (1999). Culture and ethnicity *Eur J Pall Care* 6:53–6.

Oneschuk D (2001). Progressive multifocal leuko-encephalopathy and sporadic Creutzfeldt-Jacob disease: a review and palliative management in a hospice setting. *Prog Pall Care* 9:202–5.

Palliative Care Australia (2002). *Palliative care service provision in Australia: a planning guide*. Canberra: PCA available at http://www.pallcare.org.au/publications/planning-guide02.pdf (accessed Mar 2007).

Pellegrino, ED, Thomasma DC (1993). *The virtues in medical practice*. Oxford: Oxford University Press.

Powazki RD, Walsh D (1999). Acute care palliative medicine: psychosocial assessment of patients and primary caregivers. *Palliat Med* 13:367–74.

Roger KS (2006). A literature review of palliative care, end of life, and dementia *Palliat Supportive Care* 4:295–303.

Saunders C, Sykes N (ed.) (1993). *The management of terminal malignant disease*. London: Edward Arnold, Hodder & Stoughton.

Schwass M (2006). *Last words: approaches to death in New Zealand's cultures and faiths*. Wellington: Bridget Williams Books and FDANZ.

Sepúlveda C, Marlin A, Yoshida T, Ullrich A (2002). Palliative care: The World Health Organization's Global Perspective. *J Pain Symptom Manage* 24(2):91–6.

Seymour JE (2001). *Critical moments—death and dying in intensive care*. Buckingham: Open University Press.

Steinke EE (1997). Sexuality in aging: implications for nursing facility staff. *J Contin Educ Nurs* 28:59–63.

Ten Have H, Clark D (ed.). (2002). *The ethics of palliative care*. Buckingham: Open University Press.

The SUPPORT Principal Investigators (1996). A controlled trial to improve care for seriously ill hospitalized patients: the Study to Understand Prognoses and Preferences for Outcomes and Risks of Treatments (SUPPORT) *JAMA* 274:1591–8.

Thomas K (2003). *Caring for the dying at home. Companions on a journey.* Oxford: Radcliffe Medical Press.

Williams A-L (2006). Perspectives on spirituality at the end of life: a meta-summary *Palliat Supportive Care* 4:407–17.

Woods S (2002). Respect for autonomy and palliative care. In: Ten Have H, Clark D (ed.). *The ethics of palliative care.* Buckingham, Open University Press, p. 145.

Wright M (2003). Models of hospice and palliative care in resource poor countries. London; Help the Hospices.

Chapter 2

Communication issues

Cathy Heaven and Peter Maguire

This chapter reviews the problems health professionals involved in cancer and palliative care report in communicating with patients, families and colleagues. A three-step guide to improving practice is presented.

1. To understand how communication goes wrong and consider why this happens.

2. To identify the key skills necessary for effective interviewing.

3. To look at how good communication skills can be acquired and consider the difficulties of transferring training into clinical practice.

The need to improve communication skills within palliative care

Communication underpins every aspect of the care we offer to our patients their families, and is the key to effective team work. It is estimated that on average in a 40-year professional career the average doctor will conduct between 160 000 and 200 000 consultations (Lipkin *et al.* 1995), making communication the most used clinical skill any palliative care professional possesses.

Recent changes in UK and other government policies have meant that providing compassionate care, which assesses need, provides accurate information and gives people the choices in treatment and care, is a requirement (NICE 2004). These requirements are based on research showing not only the need to improve skills but also the value of those improvements to physical and emotional well-being of patients families and staff. They are also a response to analysis of hospital complaints, which, certainly in the UK, show that 90% of complaints dealt with by official bodies concern poor communication (Royal College of Physicians, London 1997) and that communication and insufficient information is the second most common cause for complain (Healthcare Commission 2007), despite that fact that it is known that 30–40% of patients who have begun litigation will not proceed if they receive an apology (Vincent 1994).

Assessment of need

Poor communication is linked to poor assessment of patients concerns (Heaven and Maguire 1996; Farrell *et al.* 2005) and this in turn is known to be associate with the development of anxiety and depression, in both newly diagnosed and palliative care patients (Parle *et al.* 1996; Heaven and Maguire 1998) and in relatives or carers of cancer patients (Pitceathly and Maguire 2000). A relationship has also been established between the types of concerns commonly found in palliative care, such pain (Derogatis *et al.* 1983), fatigue (Worden and Weisman 1977), breathlessness (Bredin *et al.* 1999), and psychiatric morbidity.

Given that one in three cancer patients suffer from an episode of anxiety or depression regardless of stage (Barraclough 1994; Ibbotson *et al.* 1994; Fulton 1998), and between 30 and 33% of relatives also suffer an episode of such morbidity (Kissane *et al.* 1994; Pitceathly and Maguire 2000), it is vital that healthcare professionals are able to identify concerns and recognize the associated distress. However, in practice, many concerns are not elicited, and psychological morbidity is missed (Heaven and Maguire 1997; Sharpe *et al.* 2004; Farrell *et al.* 2005). This failure to elicit problems is not restricted to the psychological domain, but also applies to physical concerns, for example, pain and fatigue (Glajchen *et al.* 1995; Heaven and Maguire 1997). Consequently, many patients are not given the appropriate help or support to resolve or come to terms with their difficulties.

Information giving

It has been found that patients cope better with their predicament if they perceive they are given adequate information (Butow *et al.* 1996; Schofield 2003). Yet, only a small proportion receive the information they require (Hinds *et al.* 1995). Some patients are given too much or too little, and this increases the risk of anxiety and depression (Fallowfield *et al.* 1990). The challenge for the health professional is to quickly establish what information individual patients need. However, many healthcare professionals do not have the strategies to do this (Butow *et al.* 1996; Ford *et al.* 1996). So, they tend to use routinized ways of giving the information, which take no account of individual needs or preferences (Maguire 1998).

Decision making

Non-involvement or overinvolvement in decision-making can lead to dissatisfaction and non-compliance (Dowsett *et al.* 2000) and affect patient outcomes adversely (Coulter 1999). There is some debate as to whether all seriously ill cancer patients want involvement in decision making (Cox 2002). Rothenbacher *et al.* (1997) established that the majority of patients with advanced cancer want a collaborative or active role in decisions, but a substantial minority (28%) desire a passive role. Thus, healthcare professionals need to identify those who wish to take part in decisions and respect those who wish the clinician to take decisions for them. Clinicians do not know how to assess patients' wish for involvement (Rothenbacher *et al.* 1997), and fear patients will blame themselves or lose confidence in the doctor, if treatment does not work (Richards *et al.* 1995). Doctors take refuge in a paternalistic approach, in which less disclosure and less patient participation are favoured (Fallowfield *et al.* 1990; de Valch *et al.* 2001) but this increases both anxiety and depression (Ashcroft *et al.* 1985; Morris and Royle 1987).

Interprofessional communication

Many health professionals report frustration in communicating with colleagues (Maguire and Faulkner 1988; Fallowfield *et al.* 1998; Madge and Khair 2000), but little research has been conducted in this area. A study of 48 nurses showed that much of the written interprofessional reporting was task orientated, focused on medical treatments, and failed to cover psychological and social aspects of care (Dowding 2001). The study also showed that during shift reports nurses recorded less than half the information given or discussed, and recalled less than 27%. There was a clear bias in recall towards medical information, treatment, and history. Professionals appear to only report and record a small amount of the information they have elicited from the patient (Heaven and Maguire 1997). The rules that govern which information is valued and passed on between healthcare professionals and which is not are complex and need further investigation, but it is clear that each person's professional training and background will mean that they attend to and value different cues, and that these will influence how they report a patient's situation to colleagues within the team (Crow *et al.* 1995).

These communication difficulties create problems for patients and relatives, and also affect healthcare professionals. Lack of confidence in their ability to communicate with patients and relatives contributes to high levels of burnout in cancer professionals (Delvaux *et al.* 1988; Ramirez *et al.* 1996; Taylor *et al.* 2005). Within palliative care and oncology nursing, communication problems have been identified as contributory factors to stress, burnout, illness, and staff turnover (Payne 2001; Wiseman 2002).

Improving communication

The key to improving communication is to understand how and why it breaks down.

Step 1: understanding how and why communication breaks down

How communication breaks down

Healthcare professionals often 'distance' from what the patients is saying. While this is often a conscious process (Booth *et al.* 1996) it may also happen unconsciously (Maguire 1999). From analysis of many consultation behaviours that have the function of distancing have been identified (Maguire *et al.* 1996a,b; Zimmerman *et al.* 2003; Eide *et al.* 2004; Heaven *et al.* 2006).

Selective attention A behaviour reported in both nurse and doctors (Crow *et al.* 1995; Bornstein and Emler 2001), which happens when the interviewer controls the content of the conversation, by picking up only certain areas, commonly those which are factual or which contain no feeling. In doing this, the interviewer limits the agenda to those topics they feel comfortable discussing or helping with. For example,

> *Patient:* I was in pain, weak and tired, and was absolutely terrified that the treatment wasn't working'
>
> *Interviewer:* 'Tell me about your pain. How bad was it?'

Switching This is the term used when the interviewer changes the focus of what is being said, so controlling the content, emotional depth, or focus of the conversation. Switching can happen in several ways.

1. *Switching the time focus.* This is when the interviewer changes the 'time-frame' of the interview, so preventing the patient from talking further about the concern they have offered. For example, responding to talk about initial fears, by encouraging a person to focus on current thoughts. In doing this the interviewer inhibits patients from expressing their emotions about past events, by focusing them on different events.

2. *Switching the topic.* This is when the interviewer, often unconsciously, changes the topic or content of the conversation completely.

3. *Switching the person focus.* This happens when the interviewer changes the focus of the interview from the interviewee, or person being spoken to, to a third party, either present at the interview or not. So inhibiting the interviewee from talking about how he or she feels.

Offering advice or reassurance One of the most common responses to expression of emotion is for the health profession to give reassurance or offer advice. However, Maguire *et al.* (1996a,b) in their investigation of facilitative and inhibitory interviewing behaviours found that giving advice prematurely, before patients concerns have been fully explored, significantly decreased patient disclosure. This early finding has been confirmed using a more robust system of sequence analysis (Zimmerman *et al.* 2003), which show that disclosure falls after advice or reassurance has been given. These findings create a difficulty for many healthcare professionals who struggle to resist the pressure to problem solve when a concern is heard and find allowing space for ventilation of feelings hard, when they feel that something can be done to help.

Patient: 'I was really very upset when she first mentioned the word hospice'

Interviewer: 'Well, it's only natural that you should feel that way at first, all patients do'

In the example above moving immediately into advice has the function of inhibiting the patient from saying more about their distress, and means that the health professional's advice or reassurance may not actually address the patients' real concern.

Passing the buck This is a particular form of advice giving in which the interviewer, in direct response to the patient's cue or concerns, advises the patient to talk to a third party. While this may be appropriate at the end of an interview, using it immediately a patient mentions a problem indicates that the interviewer does not want to hear the patients concerns.

Patient: 'I was so upset, I just didn't know what he meant'

Interviewer: 'Clearly you need to talk to the surgeon about that, to get things clear'

Using jargon Using medical jargon in communication can create an obstacle between the patient or relative and the healthcare professional. It is interesting to note that the use of medical terminology is not confined solely to the health professional. As information is now widely available from the internet there is increasing evidence that patients and relatives are using medical terms, which may or may not be fully understood. Health professionals need to be alert not only about their own use of language, but also to medical terms used by the patient, which may seem appropriate, but which may be a source of misunderstanding as the word may simply be being repeated without having been understood.

Why communication breaks down

Communication is a complex process that is dependent not just on skills, but also on a number of other factors that relate to both the professional and to the recipient of the communication, i.e. the patient, relative, or colleague. The healthcare professional's ability to use their skills, or the patient's willingness to come clean about concerns is dependent on many factors, including attitudes, beliefs, and fears. For communication to be effective these influences must be understood (Bandura 1977).

A number of very specific studies have been conducted in this area, and have focused on asking both staff (Booth *et al.* 1996; Heaven *et al.* 2006) and patients (Heaven and Maguire 1997) about specific distancing behaviours and disclosure of concerns and worries. These studies build on a large literature, which has reported communication problems and the potential reasons for these difficulties. Interestingly, in these specific studies for the majority of cases both nurses and patients were conscious of their non-disclosure and distancing behaviours, and gave clear explanations as to why they had withheld information of changed the focus or switched topic at the identified points (Booth *et al.* 1996; Heaven and Maguire 1997; Wiseman 2002; Heaven *et al.* 2006).

Professionals' lack of skills

One of the reasons given by the nurses in Booth *et al.*'s study was their perception that they lacked skills. Studies of communication in medicine and nursing have shown repeatedly that doctors and nurses lack the skills necessary to elicit and explore patients' concerns, identify and respond to patients' information needs and decision making preferences (Maguire *et al.* 1996a,b; Heaven and Maguire 1996; Wilkinson *et al.* 1998; Razavi *et al.* 2000; Fallowfield 2002).

Healthcare professionals experience other difficulties when interviewing, including: integrating factual, physical, emotional, social and spiritual modes of enquiry, and avoiding a purely bio-medical approach to the interview (Maguire *et al.* 1996; Ford *et al.* 1996; Butow *et al.* 2002); assessing less familiar aspects (for example, body image or anxious preoccupation), and knowing how to close an

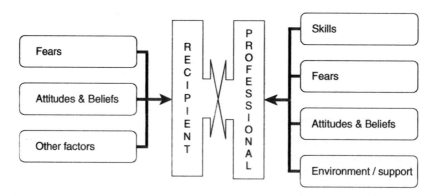

Figure 2.1 Factors affecting health care professionals' communication

interview that has been emotional (Parle *et al.* 1997). Coping with key tasks, for example, giving bad news about a poor prognosis, negotiating with a relative who wishes to withhold the truth from a patient, or supporting a dying patient (Maguire and Faulkner 1988; Fallowfield *et al.* 1998; Razavi *et al.* 2000; Schofield *et al.* 2003; Butow *et al.* 2006) are also areas that clinicians find difficult. Other communication tasks highlighted in the literature include: handling difficult questions (Hitch and Murgatroyd 1983; Maguire and Faulkner 1988), dealing with anger (Duldt 1982), and handling denial, collusion, and withdrawn and silent patients (Delveaux *et al.* 1988).

Professionals' fears

The literature points to a large number of fears that affect health professionals' use of communication skills. These include fear of upsetting the patient, fear of unleashing strong emotions such as anger or uncontrollable distress (Heaven and Maguire 1997). Many health professionals are aware of the depth and strength of patients and relatives emotions, and so fear encouraging the expression of them; for example, asking how a man feels when he has just been told he is dying could easily provoke extreme distress, or even anger. If the professional giving the bad news is fearful of handling such emotions, then the likelihood of giving the patient the chance to ventilate his or her feelings is remote.

Another fear is that of opening up a 'can of worms', and in doing so giving patients false expectations about the professionals' ability to alleviate concerns. Health professionals may fear that they could get out of their depth, or be unable to cope with the list of worries. They may fear that they might respond in a way that would make the situation worse for the patient worse or even damage the patient (Maguire 1985; Booth *et al.* 1996; Heaven *et al.* 2006).

Fear of taking up too much time is reported as a deterrent to exploring feelings by many nurses and doctors, who they envisage that once patients are encouraged to talk about emotions they will be difficult to stop, or they may somehow lose control (Maguire 1985; Fielding and Llewelyn 1987; Sellick 1991). Even in palliative care, where time is often less of an issue, the fear of getting stuck with a patient, or of not being able to complete our allocated workload, can be a powerful deterrent to exploring the concerns expressed (Booth *et al.* 1996).

In a study of in-depth interviews with general practitioners, Rosser and Maguire (1982) noted that the fear of having to face one's own sense of failure in not being able to help also influences health professionals' willingness to talk openly with their patients (Rosser and Maguire 1982). This is echoed by Baider and Porath (1981) in discussing nurses' difficulties in facing patients who are having difficult death experiences. One's own death anxieties have been identified as a factor mediating communication with patients by a number of authors (Field and Kitson 1986; Wilkinson 1991), and have therefore been part of a number of training schemes aimed at altering communication behaviours (Razavi et al.1993).

It is easy to see how such strong fears about what might happen inhibit and change the course of an interview. If these issues are not explored and addressed, they will inevitably result in professionals exhibiting 'blocking' behaviours to protect both the patient and themselves from what they perceive might be negative consequences (Parle et al. 1997; Razavi et al. 2000; Heaven et al. 2006).

Professionals' attitudes and beliefs

A broad number of attitudes have been associated with distancing. Beliefs about emotional problems being an inevitable consequence of a palliative situation encourages professionals to either ignore concerns, or normalize them, i.e. accept everyone feels like that (Peterson 1988; Booth et al. 1996). This, coupled with the belief that nothing can be done about certain types of concerns, for example, anxiety while waiting for results, can mean some worries get overlooked or minimized (Fallowfield et al. 2001; Sharpe et al. 2004). There is evidence that nurses and doctors believe there is no point in talking about things that cannot be changed. Opening up irresolvable issues will upset the patient unnecessarily (Booth et al. 1996). In a palliative situation this might be shown by reluctance to discuss issues such as 'what might happen when the cancer becomes worse'. While the professional does this to protect the patient, the patient who is experiencing such fears, realizes the health professional is reluctant to talk about them and so remains isolated with their concerns.

The belief that people from different cultures experience different problems or interpret things differently can be a powerful deterrent to open communication. This may explain why cultural differences were put at the top of the list of patient characteristics which oncologists found most difficult to handle (Fallowfield et al. 1998). An awareness of cultural differences will enhance professional communication and has been the focus of a recent training and resource handbook (Kai 2005). Evidence suggests that patients in different cultures experience similar worries and problems (Cheturvedi et al. 1996), experience the same range of emotional difficulties (Kai-hoi Sze et al. 2000), and that constructs such as quality of life are stable across several cultural boundaries (Lo et al. 2001). However, they are known to access services less and appear to receive less information about their cancer (Chattoo et al. 2002; Fazil and Kai 2004).

Beliefs that if patients have concerns they will volunteer them spontaneously can also hinder communication (Maguire 1985; Hardman et al. 1989), as can the notion that healthcare professionals should not intrude on patients' private feelings by asking directly about their fears and concerns (Booth *et al.* 1996).

The professional's environment and support

The final factor known to affect health professionals' use of their communication is the environment in which they work and how supportive it is. Direct links have been made between support and communication behaviour; demonstrating that lack of support for both senior and junior cancer professionals is likely to lead to blocking of patient cues, and that blocking is more evident when there is team conflict (Wilkinson 1991; Booth *et al.* 1996; Heaven *et al.* 2006).

Authors for many decades have discussed the role of stress and support in determining communication behaviour (Delvaux *et al.* 1988; Ramirez *et al.* 1996; Payne 2001; Taylor *et al.* 2005). In 1982 McElroy wrote that: 'Today the professional nurse realises the importance of giving emotional support and compassionate care to each patient and family. As a result of this involvement, the nurse is more vulnerable, and this adds to the stress already present in her job. The nurse who does not receive emotional support is not able to give emotional support.' There is continuing evidence to show that this statement is still true today (Payne 2001; Heaven *et al.* 2006).

Other influences created by the ward environment include a feeling of there being lack of time. However, the evidence, from early and more recent work, of the relationship of workload to communication behaviour shows that workload impacts on nurses' feelings of stress, but that reducing workload is not associated with increased communication with the patients (Huckaby and Neal 1979).

Patient behaviours

Relatively few studies have looked at the role of patients in breakdown of communication. A comparison of a patient-generated list of concerns with a list generated from ratings of the audio-taped interviews with nursing carers, revealed that the patients withheld up to 60% of the concerns they were experiencing. Patients experiencing most distress, as assessed by the Hospital Anxiety and Depression Scale, withheld most concerns (Heaven and Maguire 1997). Further analysis demonstrated that patients only revealed certain types of concerns to their nursing carers, the physical concerns, and withheld other types, e.g. emotional concerns and those relating to impact on life. This was despite the fact that the nurses considered themselves to be providing holistic care, and had undertaken basic skills training. Withholding of key information was also found in a more recent study of clinical nurse specialists assessments of patients (Heaven *et al.* 2006) and in a study of patient disclosure of pain to both nurses and doctors (Glajchen *et al.* 1995), showing little has changed since these early studies. However, Anderson *et al.* (2001) reported that patients disclosed over 90% of troublesome concerns, although some differences were found between disclosure of physical, psychological, and social areas.

Patients' fears

Patients fears, which reduce the likelihood of them being open about their concerns, include fear of the stigma of cancer, especially the elderly for whom cancer equates to death (Maguire 1985), those whose lifestyles could have contributed to the illness, e.g. smokers (Heaven and Maguire 1997), or those who come from a culture where cancer is less openly accepted (Parker and Hopwood 2000). Patients also fear that being troubled by concerns may make them less liked or less popular among staff, they fear allowing staff to see that they are not coping, or talking about difficulties with side-effects may make them seem ungrateful, or may lead to treatment being stopped.

An interesting finding from the Heaven and Maguire (1997) study was that patients worry about burdening the staff caring from them. It is well documented that patients withhold concerns from relatives in order to protection them (Pistrang and Barker 1992) but this protection is less often discussed in relation to professional carers. Insights into this phenomena were gained in the study (Heaven and Maguire 1997), when a patient who told two nurses completely different concerns on the same day, reported that she did this because: 'The first nurse was so sweet and nice, I did not want to hurt her by telling her all about that. Nurse 'X' on the other hand seemed stronger, less fragile, I felt I could tell her all my troubles.' (Hospice Patient, Heaven and Maguire 1997).

This response raises important issues for palliative care. The line between being a personal and professional friend should always be kept clear, least the patient starts to protect the professional and closes off to themselves a line of support.

Patients' attitudes and beliefs

Patients hold inaccurate beliefs or assumptions which get in the way of open communication. For example many patients believe that certain problems are an inevitable part of having cancer and thus they suppose that health professionals would automatically recognize the presence of such difficulties and would offer help is it was available. They assume, that the lack of help being offered must mean that the problem cannot be alleviated, and as they do not want to embarrass nurses and doctors, by asking for the impossible, they with-hold the concern (Rosser and Maguire 1982; Maguire 1985; Heaven and Maguire 1997).

Patients also believe that there is not enough time to go into all their worries. They, therefore, prioritize worries on the basis of what they think the professional will need or want to hear about, quite wrongly believing that certain types of professionals are only interested in certain types of prob-lems or concerns (Glajchen *et al.* 1995; Heaven and Maguire 1997). A palliative care doctor may thus be told about physical symptoms, treat-ments, etc., while a nurse may be told about deficits in self-care and the family situation, etc.

Other patient factors

Other factors that inhibit open communication include a lack of privacy from people overhearing what is being said, especially in a ward environment, or a lack of space away from key individuals in front of whom that patient or rela-tive may not wish to discuss certain fears, e.g. spouses, children, etc. Many health professionals do not consider the impact of the presence of a family member on an interview. Indeed in palliative care, professionals positively encourage the carer to be present when interviewing the patient (Heaven *et al.* 2006); however, this may lead to many concerns being withheld, as patients actively seek to protect their relatives (Pistrang and Barker 1992).

For many patients finding the right words is another difficulty that inhibits their ability to disclose concerns (Maguire 1985). Some individuals have a broad and extensive vocabulary for describing emotions, but some will have never talked about their emotions. They may simply not have the words to describe how they feel or what they are experiencing. This is particularly rele-vant for certain groups, for example, those who are conducting the interview in a language that is not their first or native tongue (Firth 2001; Chattoo *et al.* 2002); those who are mentally impaired due to illness (Morita *et al.* 2001) or learning difficulties, and those who are very young. The danger for health professionals is that they may jump to the wrong conclusion, by filling in too many gaps or not providing sufficient time and space.

Summary

The literature reveals a great number of reasons why communication difficul-ties occur. To date no study has compared the relative impact of the different influences identified, and therefore there is no way of knowing which repre-sents the greatest influence on behaviour. Indeed it is probable that the influ-ence is different for each individual. There are many valid reasons why healthcare professionals may be ill at ease in talking openly and frankly to patients, and why patients or relatives may withhold so much information about their fears and concerns.

Step 2: developing effective interviewing

What are effective interviewing behaviours?

The evidence for what constitutes an effective interview behaviour has been developed over a number of years. This review will draw on literature that has researched the effectiveness of medical student, GP, nursing, psychotherapy, and psychiatry interviews. Effective interviewing is about not only using facilitative micro-skills but also adopting a style that is patient centred and enables optimal disclosure.

Effective interviewing micro-skills

In the late 1970s and early 1980s studies were conducted with GPs that showed that a number of key skills were associated with better interview outcomes (Marks *et al.* 1979; Goldberg *et al.* 1980). Key skills were:

- using more eye contact at the outset of an interview
- clarifying more about the presenting complaint
- responding to verbal cues about possible distress
- asking directly about feelings
- asking about the home situation
- handling interruptions well
- making supportive comments
- using directive questions about specific problems and using open questions more generally
- coping with talkativeness
- responding to verbal and non-verbal cues
- showing empathy.

The studies also showed that reading notes as the patient talks was inhibitory and suggested that changes in question style seem appropriate when seeking specific information about a specific issue, or when establishing what the issues and events had been. Taking this evidence into the field of cancer and palliative care Maguire and colleagues (1980) showed that that nurses trained to ask open questions about feelings and respond to cues empathetically were more effective in establishing patients' emotional concerns and concerns about side-effects.

In 1996 a study was published that looked at the validity of certain interviewing behaviours in relation to cancer patient disclosure (Maguire *et al.* 1996a,b).

It involved assessment interviews conducted by 206 healthcare professionals, from different professionals disciplines. Result showed that disclosure of key information, emotions, and concerns was significantly enhanced by certain key skills and significantly inhibited by others. These key skills are shown and defined in Figure 2.2. Interestingly a ratio of 1 inhibitory to 1 facilitative behaviours was noted by the authors prior to training, regardless of interviewer's age, experience, or professional grouping.

Recent developments in both interviewer rating systems and also in conversation analysis tools have enabled researchers to look in more detail at the impact of individual behaviours within interviews. Evidence has been published, which confirms these early findings, showing that open questions are more likely to elicit cues than closed (Zimmerman *et al.* 2003), that giving information during an interview reduces the likelihood of further disclosure (Langowitz *et al.* 2006), and that pauses, or short silences are the most likely things to immediately precede patient disclosure (Eide *et al.* 2004). There is also new evidence generated from the field of linguistics that suggests that certain words have a positive or negative polarity or inference; i.e. they generate expectations and influence how somebody might respond. Testing out this hypothesis, Heritage *et al.* (2006) found that asking patients visiting a GPs whether they had 'something else' they would like to discuss was more than

Facilitative behaviours	
• open directive questions	- Questions which give a broad focus but are open. eg. "How have you been since I last saw you?"
• questions with a psychological focus	- Eliciting information about emotions, worries, concerns and fears
• clarification of psychological aspects	- any behaviour which seeks to understand more about any emotional aspect
• empathy	- a brief statement showing understanding of the patients experience
• summarising discussed	- A recapitulation of two or more items previously
• educated guesses. which the	- An educated guess is a tentative behaviour in interviewer makes share a guess or hypothesis about the situation, based upon feelings or 'gut reactions' with the patient, and then allows the patient to respond to confirm or refute it.
Inhibitory behaviours	
• leading questions	- Is one which suggests or presupposes the answer
• Physically focused questions	- Questions which limit the topic to the physical experience of the patient
• clarifying the physical aspects	- any behaviour which seeks to understand more about the physical experience of the patient
• giving of any advice	- any information given to the patient before or after exploration of the concerns (Maguire, Faulkner, Booth Elliot, Hillier 1996).

Figure 2.2

twice a likely to elicit new concerns than asking whether there was 'anything else' a person would like to discuss.

The most recent work done in this area has looked at the context in which skills are used, and has shown that it is not just what skills are used, but the context in which they are used which is important (Fletcher *et al.* 2006, pers. comm.). For example, open questions can be used to block if they chance the subject or switch the conversation, but they can also be used very effectively to explore key disclosure (Heaven *et al.* 2006). This is discussed more in the next section.

Effective interviewing style Using effective micro-skills is not sufficient in creating an effective interview. An efficient interviewer needs to adopt a style that will facilitate optimal disclosure and leave the patient feeling both listened to and understood.

The early studies (Marks *et al.* 1979; Goldberg *et al.* 1980) supported a probing, enquiring style of interviewing in which the doctor was encouraged to ask questions. However, there is much support for a less probing interviewer dominated approach within the field of psycho-oncology (Mead and Bower 2000). Testing out the benefits of a more passive approach to medical interviewing a Dutch group (Bensing and Sluijs 1985), evaluated the training of general practitioners to be more empathic, take more time and give the lead to the patient more. Interestingly, the outcome showed that this more passive approach led to patients giving a more confused and less sequenced history of events and that overall they said significantly less about their key problems. These results are backed up by an American study (Putnam *et al.* 1988), which confirmed that teaching medical residents a more passive interview style showed no improvement in clinical outcomes.

While we can conclude from this that a structured probing style is required, there is a great deal of evidence to show that taking a patient-centred rather that a disease-centred or medically focused approach to interviewing has benefits. The patient-centred approach has been shown to be both effective and acceptable to patients and their families (Bensing 2000; Mead and Bower 2000), and has been associated with increased satisfaction, reduced anxiety, more accurate recall of information, compliance with treatment, better management, and recovery (Laine and Davidoff 1996; Bensing 2000; Mead and Bower 2000).

One way of combining proactive interviewing skills and a patient-centred approach is to be 'cue focused' (Heaven *et al.* 2006). A cue is 'A verbal or non verbal hint which suggests an underlying unpleasant emotion and would need clarification from the health provider' (Butow *et al.* 2002). A European group set up to look at measuring good interviewing practice have identified seven categories of cue (Del Piccolo *et al.* 2006):

- Verbal cues
  - word of phrases suggesting vague undefined emotions (e.g. 'it felt odd')
  - verbal hints to hidden concerns (e.g. 'I cope with it')
  - words or phrases that describe psychological correlates or unpleasant emotional states (e.g. sleep disturbance, agitation, panic, irritability).
  - unusual or affect loaded emphasis or repeated mentions of issues of potential importance (e.g. 'hell of a day', 'left like I'd been hit by a car', use of profanity as emphasis)
  - communication of life-threatening events (e.g. 'doctor said I had cancer', 'I know I am dying')
- Non verbal cues
  - non-verbal expressions of emotion (e.g. crying)
  - non-verbal hints of emotion (e.g. signing, frowning, silence, looking away, looking uncomfortable).

The number of cues per interview has been shown to vary, Some studies show it to be as little as 1–2 per 15-minute interview while others consider it to be approximately 10–11 (Heaven *et al.* 2006). These differences can be accounted for in terms of definition. What is clear it that both emotional distress and the interviewers responsiveness to cues will increase the level of cue emission (Davenport *et al.* 1987; Del Piccolo *et al.* 2000; Fletcher *et al.* 2006, pers. comm.). The importance of picking up cues has been shown by a number of authors; most recently the importance of the first cue has been highlighted (Fletcher *et al.* 2006, pers. comm.). The group showed, using interviewed conducted by clinical nurse specialists in cancer care, that if the first cue in an interview is missed there is a 20% drop in the number of cues given by the patient over the course of the interview, irrespective of whether the second cue was picked up or missed. Linking effective interviewing skills to cues has been the focus of some of the most recent work in this area. Fletcher *et al.* (2006, pers. comm.) have shown that when open questions are used in an interview they have only a 50:50 chance of leading to disclosure; however, if they are linked to a cue they are 4.5 times more likely to facilitate more information.

Despite the fact that there is a great deal of evidence to support cue-based interviewing (Butow *et al.* 2002; Fletcher *et al.* 2006, pers. comm.) studies of interviewer behaviour continue to report difficulties in following patient cues (Ford *et al.* 1996; Levinson *et al.* 2000; Butow *et al.* 2002; Heaven *et al.* 2006).

A common concern is that allowing the patient or relative to dictate the course of an interview will increase its length; however, the evidence is to the contrary. Working with GPs, Levenson *et al.* (2000) showed that cue-based consultations were on average 15% shorter than those in which cues were missed, while Butow *et al.* (2002) showed that in oncology consultations, addressing cues reduced consultation times by 10–12%.

Summary To be effective an interviewer needs to be proactive and use open and directive questions to elicit cues about patient experiences (for example, 'how is chemotherapy going') and then acknowledge and clarify those cues to obtain further disclosure about their impact on the patient both physically and emotionally. The use of empathy and educated questions is likely to encourage patients to disclose associated feelings. Repeated summarizing of what the interviewer has heard lets patients know that they have been understood correctly or allows them to correct the interviewer. The establishment and maintenance of good eye contact is key. The integration of enquiry about physical symptoms, the psychological impact, social impact, and effect of spirituality is particularly important.

What are effective information giving skills?

So far effective interviewing has only been considered in terms of assessment. The process of giving information, specifically bad news is now considered. The importance of the bad news interview on patient adjustment has been shown (Butow *et al.* 1996); however, very little research has been conducted that identifies how aspects of the process affect patients outcomes.

Mager and Andrykowski (2002) established long-term distress was related to the 'caring skills', i.e. the empathy and responsiveness, and not the doctor's technical competence. Fallowfield *et al.* (1990) showed that adjustment was related to meeting patients' information needs appropriately. Too much or too little information can be detrimental to a patient's mental health (Fallowfield *et al.* 1990), indicating that the amount of information given should be tailored to need, that the pace of delivery should be dictated by the recipient (Maguire 1998). There is also evidence that using audio-recordings can assist patients in taking on board complex information (Hogbin *et al.* 1992), but that they may be detrimental if the news received is of a poor prognosis. (McHugh *et al.* 1995). Cultural background has not been found to affect a patient's desire to know about their diagnosis (Fielding and Hunt 1996; Seo *et al.* 2000), although relatives clearly have a greater influence in some cultures than in others (Mosoiu *et al.* 2000; Di Mola and Crisci 2001).

In 1995, Girghis and Sanson-Fisher created guidelines on breaking bad news that were drawn up on the basis of a comprehensive literature review, and recommendations of a panel of doctors and cancer patients. The guidelines covered: practical issues, privacy and adequate time; and strategy of approach, assess the patient's current understanding, provide information simply and honestly, being realistic concerning time frames and prognosis, avoiding euphemisms, encouraging patients to express feelings and being empathic. Miller and Maguire (2000, pers comm) drew similar conclusions from a systematic review of the literature; however, they found some evidence that using euphemisms to deliver bad news in a step-wise fashion was beneficial for patients who are totally unaware of diagnoses.

The longitudinal study conducted by Parle *et al.* (1996) suggested that a key element in bad news consultation was to acknowledge the distress the bad news had created and then invite the patient proactively to explain how they were feeling and the concerns that were contributing to that distress. The patient should then be invited to prioritize their concerns so each concern could be taken in order. Only then should further information be given based on what information patients wanted at that point.

This approach has been the subject of a randomized trial. The data suggest that this model not only increases the chances that patients will disclose their concerns, but also reduces their distress. Moreover, it helps the doctors feel better about the way they are breaking bad news and gives them validation that they are helping rather than upsetting patients (Green *et al.* 2007, pers comm).

Summary

While it is clear that the process of giving bad news is crucial to long-term adjustment little evidence exists as to what constitutes effective practice. It is clear that information must be tailored to individual needs no matter what culture the individual comes from, and that it should be given in 'bite-sized chunks' and delivered at a pace that is controlled by the patient. Empathy and understanding of the potential impact of the news on the patient appears is crucial.

Step 3: acquiring and transferring skills to the work-place and maintaining them over time

Acquiring effective interviewing skills

There are a large number of communication skills training studies published, some show admirable results; however few have been evaluated formally to assess their effectiveness in achieving desired outcomes. Those that can provide evidence of effectiveness are clearly most desirable. Within the UK, these types of course are now available to all senior healthcare professionals in cancer care, through the National Advanced Communication Skills Training Programme (Cancer Action Team 2007), although such courses are not as yet available to all within palliative care. This section, therefore, considers the key elements of effective communication skills training, so individual can assess the value of potential courses.

Early studies, conducted with medical students measured outcomes in terms of changes in interviewing behaviour, and ability to identify diagnoses and problems. These experimental studies showed the value in a didactic introduction to a model of interviewing behaviour, together with some kind of demonstration of that model working in practice (Rutter and Maguire 1976; Maguire et al. 1977). Subsequent evidence confirmed the value of feedback on individual performance as being essential, with video and audio feedback conferring equal benefit (Maguire et al. 1978). An alternative training approach developed in America, but shown to be effective in nurse and doctor training, is micro-counselling training (Daniels et al. 1988; Crute et al. 1989). This again uses the same core elements of training, but focuses on one microskill per session, rather than one strategy or task, as described in the studies already mentioned.

Studies of the problems of open and honest communication highlighted the important role of attitudes and beliefs (Wilkinson 1991; Booth et al. 1996). This led to training that focused on attitudes, but a comparison study showed that attitude training alone was not sufficient to change communication behaviour, and that training had to encompass a skills focus if skills were to be changed (Rickert 1982). The role of attitudes, however, must not be overlooked, as was shown by Razavi and colleagues (1988) and by a major evaluation of their workshop training programme by Maguire et al. (1996a,b). The 1996 UK-based evaluation showed that the training conferred many positive skill changes in communication skills, but did not confer changes in the key skills of empathy and educated guesses. Furthermore, it was found that while training which addresses skills alone leads to more significant and emotional disclosure from the patient, it also led to significantly more blocking on the part of the professional.

To overcome these difficulties changes were implemented so that workshops provided more time to practise skills and feedback on performance, and greater safety to address attitudes and beliefs and fears about possible consequences of the communication process (Parle et al. 1997). At the same time the structural issues of interviewing, for example, learning about how long to remain with one particular topic, when and how to move on, as well as how to integrate the factual, physical and emotional modes of interviewing was explored. The experimental evaluation showed that the optimal training method was one that addressed not only skills, but also interview structure, and professionals attitudes and feelings. This multidimensional focus in training has now been shown to be highly effective in different contexts (Wilkinson *et al.* 1998; Razavi *et al.* 2000; Fallowfield *et al.* 2002; Heaven *et al.* 2006).

Summary For communication skills training to be effective there appear to be key elements that need to be in place. These include: presentation of a clear, evidence-based model of communication; demonstration of that model; opportunity for trainees to practise skills in a safe environment; and explicit but constructive feedback on performance. Furthermore, to be effective training needs to take account not only of skills, but to challenge beliefs and overcome fears, and needs to teach integration of factual, physical, emotional, spiritual, and social domains.

Transfer of skills from training environment to the work-place

The final step to changing communication behaviour is to ensure the transfer of learning to the work-place and then maintain the improvement in skills over time. Those who have looked at the learning of skills in the training situation and then compared it with skills used with real patients have found discrepancies (Mumford *et al.* 1987; Pieters *et al.* 1994; Heaven *et al.* 2006). There appears to be a difference between competence (what a health professional can do in interviewing simulated patients, and what they actually do when faced with real patients or relatives). Parle *et al.* (1997) suggested that this difference could be accounted for by Bandura's learning theory. They highlighted the importance of considering self-efficacy, a persons confidence in their ability to perform a communication task successfully, and outcome expectancy, a personal belief that the outcome of using a specific skill or strategy would benefit both themselves and their patient.

Within the communication skills training literature 'drop off' in skills has been noted (Maguire *et al.* 1996a,b; Wilkinson *et al.*1998), as has the inability of trainees to apply skills in a clinically meaningful way (Putman *et al.* 1988; Razavi *et al.* 1993; Heaven and Maguire 1996). A much greater understanding of the problem of transfer can be gained from other applied psychology literature, where the phenomena has been researched in great depth (Gist *et al.* 1990). In a major literature review Baldwin and Ford (1988) point to a number of key factors in facilitating transfer. First, that before training there needs to be real commitment not only to learning but also behaviour change. Secondly, that the training has to be effective and, finally, that the environment into which the trainee is returning must be supportive. There is strong evidence to support the notion that for skills to be effectively transferred back into the work-place, both general support and more specifically facilitated integration of skills appears crucial (Gist *et al.* 1990; Bandura 1992).

These factors have been the focus of the authors' most recent work, in which the role of clinical supervision in affecting transfer of communication skills training from workshop to work-place was investigated. Sixty-one clinical nurse specialists 42 of whom were palliative care nurses, participated in a randomized controlled trial of workshop training alone versus workshop training plus a 4-week integration programme using clinical supervision (Heaven *et al.* 2006). Those nurses who had received supervision used significantly more facilitative communication skills with patients and relatives, responded to cues in a more facilitative fashion, and were more able to identify concerns of an emotional nature, than those who did not.

If the key to transfer is facilitating the integration of skills into practice then it is logical to assume that programmes of training that extend over a period of time, will be more effective. Wilkinson *et al.* (1998) published a study of nurses who had undergone a programme of communication skills training as part of a palliative care course. The results show significant improvements in the nurses' interviewing behaviours with real patients over the course of the training programme suggesting that this method of training may overcome the transfer problem. Wilkinson *et al.* (2001), however, compared workshop training with an integrated programme of training. They found both conferred equal learning and transfer, suggesting that the apparent transfer effect could be due to other factors. The use of intensive workshop training, following a similar format to that previously discussed, has been shown to have a clinically measurable effect, which was transferred back into the work-place by the senior doctors undergoing the training (Fallowfield *et al.* 2002). This training was highly intensive (one facilitator/four participants) and provided written feedback on performance for a randomized sample of participants. Written feedback was not found to confer greater learning or use of skills.

The conclusion of the studies is that transfer of skills to the work-place must not be assumed. To ensure integration of skills and facilitate maintenance over time support within the work-place and help during the integration process is key. Extended or highly intensive training may overcome some of these problems, as may work-place structures, such as clinical supervision (Heaven *et al.* 2006).

The key aim of any intervention aimed at facilitating transfer should be to provide a forum in which self-efficacy can be boosted, negative outcome expectancies challenged, and emotional and practical support provided

(Gist *et al.* 1990; Bandura 1992; Heaven *et al.* 2006). Other methods include informal peer supervision, in which two or three individuals meet together with the purpose of discussing specific difficulties. Alternatively individual reflection, a personal de-briefing of an event or encounter (Newell 1992) or alternatively de-briefing or critical event analysis can provide a forum in which the individual can challenge their assumptions, attribution, purpose, and outcomes; and gain confidence in their abilities and outcomes.

On a more informal level support for skills can be elicited during the course of a normal day through feedback from the patient, which it is noted may be positive or negative influence; 'chats' with colleagues about specific events and team meetings at which views can be validated, and ideas endorsed. There is evidence that many people leave courses with good intentions about using skills but often these are not put into practice. Goal setting may help avoid this, as may reviewing courses after a period of time to appraise how much trainees feel they have used the skills learned (Baile *et al.* 1997; Fallowfield *et al.* 1998). Another method of self-appraisal is audio recording of an interview, with the patients' full consent, and then to review it. It is important to remember that to boost self-efficacy positive reinforcement is very important; therefore, a balanced appraisal is critical. The final method available to maintain learning is to regularly reappraise learning needs and further training courses that offer the chance to re-look at skills or learn new skills (Razavi *et al.* 1993). Initiatives in Scandinavia have shown that initial training followed by shorter booster workshops have been very effective in changing practice, when evaluated subjectively (Aspegren *et al.* 1996).

The key to transfer appears to be recognizing that intentions and actions are not the same, and that without specific action and support, changes in competence are not necessarily translated into changes in performance.

References

Anderson H, Ward C, Eardley A, Gomm S, Connolly M, Coppinger T, Corgie D, Williams J, Makin W (2001). The concerns of patients' under palliative care and a heart failure clinic are not being met. *Palliat Med* 15:279–86.

Ashcroft JJ, Leinster SJ, Slade PD (1985). Breast cancer—patient choice of treatment: preliminary communication. *J R Soc Med* 78:43–6.

Aspegren K, Birgegard G, Ekeberg O, Hietanen P, Holm U, Jensen AB, Lindfors O (1996). Improving awareness of the psychosocial needs of the paient—a training course for experienced cancer doctors. *Acta Oncol* 35(2):246–8.

Baider L, Porath S (1981). Uncovering fear: group experience of nurses in a cancer ward. *Int J Nurs Stud* 18:47–52.

Baile W, Lenzi R, Kudelka A, Maguire P, Novack D, Goldstein M, Myers E, Bast R (1997). Improving physician-patient communication in cancer care: outcome of a workshop for oncologists. *J Cancer Educ* 12(3):166–73.

Baldwin TT, Ford JK (1988). Transfer of training: a review and directions for future research. *Personnel Psychol* 41:63–105.

Bandura A (1977). Self-efficacy: toward a unifying theory of behavioral change. *Psychol Rev* 84(2):191–215.

Bandura A (1992). Psychological aspects of prognostic judgements. In: Evans, Baskin, Yatsu (ed.). *Prognosis of neurological disorders*. pp. 13–28.

Baraclough J (1994). *Cancer and emotion*. Oxford: Radcliffe Medical Press.

Bensing JM (2000). Bridging the gap. The separate worlds of evidence-based medicine and patient-centrered medicine. *Patient Educ Couns* 39:17–25.

Bensing JM, Sluijs EM (1985). Evaluation of an interview training course for general practitioners. *Soc Sci Med* 20(7):737–44.

Booth K, Maguire P, Butterworth T, Hillier VF (1996). Perceived professional support and the use of blocking behaviours by hospice nurses. *J Adv Nurs* 24:522–7.

Bornstein B, Emler C (2001). Rationality in medical decision making: a review of the literature on doctors decision-making biases. *J Eval Clin Pract* 7(2):97–107.

Bredin M, Corner J, Krishnasamy M, Plant H, Bailey C, A'Hearn R (1999). Multicentre randomised controlled trial of nursing intervention for breathlessness in patients with lung cancer. *BMJ* 318:901–4.

Butow PN, Kazemi J, Beeney L, Griffiiiin A, Dunn S, Tattersall M (1996). When the diagnosis is cancer: patient communication experiences and preferences. *Cancer* 77(12):2630–2637.

Butow PN, Dowsett S, Hagerty R, Tattersall MH (2002). Communicating prognosis to patients with metastatic disease: What do they really want to know? *Suort Care Cancer* 10(2):161–168.

Cancer Action Team Advanced Communicaiton Skills Training Programme (2007). *Department of Health of United Kingdom* 2007.

Chattoo S, Ahmed W, Haworth M, Lennard R (2002). South Asian and White Patients with advanced Cancer: patients' and families experiences of the illness and perceived needs for care. Final report to Cancer Research UK. Centre for Primary Care, University of Leeds (unpublished).

Cheturvedi S, Shenoy A, Prasad K, Senthilnathan S, Premlatha B (1996). Concerns, coping and quality of life in head and neck cancer patients *Support Care Cancer* 4:186–90.

Coulter A (1999). Paternalism or partnership? Patients have grown-up and there's no going back. *BMJ* 319:719–20.

Cox K (2002). Informed consent and decision-making: patients' experiences of the process of recruitment to phase I and II anti-cancer drug trials. *Patient Educ Couns* 46:31–8.

Crow R, Chase J, Lamond D (1995). The cognitive component of nursing assessment: an analysis. *J Adv Nurs* 22(2):206–12.

Crute VC, Hargie ODW, Ellis RAF (1989). An evaluation of a communication skills course for health visitor students. *J Adv Nurs* 14:546–52.

Daniels TG, Denny A, Andrews D (1988). Using microcounseling to teach RN students skills of therapeutic communication. *J Nurs Educ* 27(6):246–52.

Davenport S, Goldberg D, Miller T (1987). How psychiatric disorders are missed during medical consultations *Lancet* 4:439–41.

Del Piccolo L, Saltini A, Zimmerman C, Dunn G (2000). Differences in verbal behaviours of patients with and without emotional distress during primary care consultations. *Psychol Med* 30:629–43.

Del Piccolo L, Goss C, Bergvik S (2006). The fourth meeting of the Verona Network on Sequence Analysis 'Consensus finding on the appropriateness of provider responses to patient cues and concerns'. *Patient Educ Couns* 61:473–5.

De Valch C, Bensing J, Bruynooghe R (2001). Medical student's attitudes towards breaking bad news: an emperical test of the world health organisation model. *Psycho-oncology* 10(5):398–409.

Delvaux N, Razavi D, Farvaques C (1988). Cancer care—a stress for health professionals. *Soc Sci Med* 27(2):159–66.

Derogatis LR, Morrow GR, Fetting J, Penman D, Piasetsky S, Schmale AM, Henrichs M, Carnicke CLM (1983). The prevalence of psychiatric disorders among cancer patients. *JAMA* 249(6):751–7.

Di Mola G, Crisci M (2001). Attitudes towards death and dying in a representative sample of the Italian population. *Palliat Med* 15:372–78.

Dowding D (2001). Examining the effects that manipulating information given in the change of shift report has on nurses' care planning ability. *J Adv Nurs* 33(6):836–46.

Dowsett SM, Saul JL, Butow PN, Dunn SM, Boyer MJ, Findlow R, Dunsmore J (2000). Communication style in the cancer consultation: preferences for a patient-centred approach. *Psycho-oncology* 9:147–56.

Duldt BW (1982). Helping nurses to cope with the anger-dismay syndrome. *Nurs Outlook*, March:168–74.

Eide E, Quera V *et al.* (2004). Physician-patient dialogue surrounding patients' expression of concerns: applying sequence analysis to RIAS. *Soc Sci Med* 59:145–55.

Fallowfield LJ, Hall A, Maguire P, Baum M (1990). Psychological outcomes of different treatment policies in women with early breast cancer outside a clinical trial. *BMJ* 301:575–80.

Fallowfield L, Lipkin M, Hall A (1998). Teaching senior oncologists communication skills: results from phase 1 of a comprehensive longitudinal program in the United Kingdom. *J Clin Oncol* 16(5):1961–8.

Fallowfield L, Ratcliffe D, Jenkins V, Saul J (2001). Psychiatric morbidity and its recognition by doctors in patients with cancer. *Br J Cancer* 84(8):1011–15.

Fallowfield L, Jenkins V, Farewell V, Saul J, Duffy A, Eves R (2002). Efficacy of a Cancer Research UK communication skills training model for oncologists: a randomised controlled trial. *Lancet* 359:650–6.

Farrell C, Heaven C, Beaver K, Maguire P (2005). Identifying the concerns of women undergoing chemotherapy. *Patient Educ Couns* 56:72–7.

Fazil Q, Kai J (2004). Quality and equity of care: learning from study of the CAPACITY advocacy service for people with cancer. University of Nottingham.

Field D, Kitson C (1986). Formal teaching about dealth and dying in UK nursing schools. *Nurse Educ Today* 6:270–6.

Fielding R, Hunt J (1996). Preferences for information and involvement in decisions during cancer care among a Hong Kong Chinese population. *Psycho-oncology* 5:321–9.

Fielding RG, Llewelyn SP (1987). Communication training in nursing may damage your health and enthusiasm: some warnings. *J Adv Nurs* 12:281–90.

Firth S (2001). *Wider horizons: care of the dying in a multicultural society.* The National Council for Hospice and Specialist Palliative Care Services, London.

Ford S, Fallowfield L, Lewis S (1996). Doctor-patient interactions in oncology. *Soc Sci Med* **42** (**11**):1511–19.

Fulton C (1998). The prevalence and detection of psychiatric morbidity in patients with metastatic breast cancer. *Eur J Cancer Care* 7:232–9.

Girghis A, Sanson-Fisher R (1995). Breaking bad news: consensus guidelines for medical practitioners. *J Clin Oncol* 13:2449—56.

Gist ME, Bavettw AG, Stevens CK (1990). Transfer training method: its influence on skill generalization, skill repetition, and skill performance level. *Personnel Psychol* 43:501–23.

Glajchen M, Blum D, Calder K (1995). Cancer pain management and the role of social work: barriers and interventions. *Health Social Work* 20(**3**):200–6.

Goldberg DP, Steele JJ, Smith C, Spivey L (1980). Training the family doctors to recognise psychiatric illness with increased accuracy. *Lancet* **September**:521–3.

Hardman A. Maguire P, Crowther D (1989). The recognition of psychiatric morbidity on a medical oncology ward. *J Psychosom Res* 33(**2**):235–9.

Healthcare Commission (2007). *Spotlight on complaints*. London: Commission for Healthcare Audit and Inspection.

Heaven CM, Maguire P (1996). Training hospice nurses to elicit patient concerns. *J Adv Nurs* 23:280–6.

Heaven CM, Maguire P (1997). Disclosure of concerns by hospice patients and their identification by nurses. *Palliat Med* 11:283–90.

Heaven CM, Maguire P (1998). The relationship between patients' concerns and psychological distress in hospice setting. *Psycho-Oncology* 7:502–7.

Heaven C, Clegg J, Maguire P (2006). Transfer of communication skills training from workshop to workplace: the impact of clinical supervision. *Patient Educ Couns* 60:313–25.

Heritage J *et al.* (2006). *Reducing patients' unmet concerns in primary care*. European Association for Communication in Healthcare. Conference Proceedings July 2006.

Hinds C, Streter A, Mood D (1995). Functions and preferred methods of receiving information related to radiotherapy. Perceptions of patients wth cancer. *Cancer Nurse* 18(**5**):374–84.

Hitch PJ, Murgatroyd JD (1983). Professional communications in cancer care: a Delphi survey of hospital nurses. *J Adv Nurs* 8:413–22.

Hobgin B, Jenkins VA, Parkin AJ (1992). Remembering 'bad news' consultations: an evaluation of tape-recorded consultations. *Psycho-oncology* 1:147–54.

Huckaby L, Neal M (1979). The nursing care plan problem. *J Nurs Admin* 9(**12**):36–42.

Ibbotson T, Maguire P, Selby P, Priestman T, Wallace L (1994). Screening for anxiety and depresson in cancer patients: the effects of disease and treatment. *Eur J Cancer* 30A:37–40.

Kai J (ed.) (2005). PROCEED. Professionals responding to ethnic diversity and cancer. A resource book. University of Notingham and Cancer Research UK.

Kai-Hoi Sze F, Wong E, Lo R, Woo J (2000). Do pain and disability differ in depressed cancer patients. *Palliat Med* 14:11–17.

Kissane D, Bloch S, Burns WI, McKenzie DP, Posterino M (1994). Psychological morbidity in the families of patients with cancer. *Psycho-Oncology* 3:47–56.

Laine C, Davidoff F (1996). Patient-centred medicine: a professional evolution. *JAMA* 275:152–6.

Levinson W, Gorawara-Bhat R, Lamb J *et al.* (2000). A study of patient clues and physicians responses in primary care and surgical settings. *JAMA* 284(**8**):1021–8.

Levinson W *et al.* (2005). Not all patients want to participate in decision making: a national study of public preferences. *J Gen Int Med* 20(6):531–5.

Lipkin M Jr, Putnam SM, Lazare A (1995). *The medical interview. Clinical care, education and research.* New York: Springer-Verlag.

Lo R, Woo J, Zhoc K, Li C, Yeo W, Johnson P, Mak Y, Lee J (2001). Cross-cultural validation of the McGill Quality of life questionnaire in Hong Kong Chinese. *Palliat Med* 15:387–97.

Madge M, Khair K (2000). Multidisciplinary teams in the United kingdom; problems and solutions. *J Paediatr Nurs* 15(20):131–4.

Mager W, Andryowski M (2002). Communication in the cancer 'bad news' consultation: patient perceptions and psychological adjustment. *Psycho-oncology* 11:11–46.

Maguire GP, Clarke D, Jolley B (1977). An experimental comparison of three courses in history-taking skills for medical students. *Med Educ* 11:175–82.

Maguire GP, Rutter DR (1976). History-taking for medical students. I—deficiencies in performance. *Lancet* **September** 11:556–8.

Maguire P (1985). Improving the detection of psychiatric problems in cancer patients. *Soc Sci Med* 20(**8**):819–23.

Maguire P (1998). Breaking bad news. *Eur J Surg Oncol* 24:188–91.

Maguire P (1999). Improving communication with cancer patients. *Eur J Cancer* 35(**10**):1415–22.

Maguire P, Faulkner A (1988). Improving the counselling skills of doctors and nurses in cancer care. *Br Med J* 297:847–9.

Maguire P, Roe P, Goldberg D, Jones S, Hyde C, O'Dowd T (1978). The value of feedback in teaching interviewing skills to medical students. *Psychol Med* 8:695–704.

Maguire P, Tait A, Brooke M, Thomas C, Sellwood R (1980). Effect of counselling on the psychiatric morbidity assiciated with mastectomy. *BMJ* 281:1454–6.

Maguire P, Faulkner A, Booth K, Elliot C, Hillier V (1996a). Helping cancer patients disclose their concerns. *Eur J Cancer* 32A:78–81.

Maguire P, Booth K. Elliot C, Jones B (1996b). Helping health professionals involved in cancer care acquire key interviewing skills—the impact of workshops. *Eur J Cancer* 32A(**9**):1486–9.

Marks JN, Goldberg DP, Hillier VF (1979). Determinants of the ability of general practitioners to detect psychiatric illness. *Psychol Med* 9:337–53.

McElroy AM (1982). Burnout—A review of the literature with application to cancer nursing. *Cancer Nurs* **June**:211–17.

McHugh P, Lewis S, Ford S. Newlands E, Rustin G, Coombes C, Snith D, O'Reilly S, Fallowfield L (1995). The efficacy of audiotapes in promoting psychological well-being in cancer patients: a randomised controlled trial. *Br J Cancer* 71(**2**):388–92.

Mead N, Bower P (2000). Patient-centredness: a conceptual framework and review of the empirical literature. *Soc Sci Med* 51:1087–110.

Morita T, Tsunoda J, Inoue S, Chihara S, Oka K (2001). Communication capacity scale and agitation dsitress scale to measure the severity of delirium in terminally ill cancer patients: a validation study. *Palliat Med* 15:197–206.

Morris J, Royle GT (1987). Choice of surgery for early breast cancer: pre and post operative levels of clinical anxiety and depression in patients and their husbands. *Br J Surg* 74:1017–19.

Mosoiu D, Andrews C, Perolls G (2000). Palliative care in Romania. *Palliat Med* 14:65–7.

Mumford E, Schlesinger H, Cuerdon T, Scully J (1987). Rating of video simulated patient interview and four other methods of evaluating a psychiatric clerkship. *Am J Psychiatry* 144(3):316–22.

Newell R (1992). Anxiety, accuracy and reflection: the limits of professional development. *J Adv Nurs* 17:1326–33.

NICE Guidelines (2004). National Institute for Clinical Excellence. Clinical Guidelines. London. http://www.nice.org.uk/pdf/

Parker R, Hopwood P (2000). Literature review—Quality of life (QL). in black and ethnic monority groups (BEMGs) with cancer. Report to the CRC.

Parle M, Jones B, Maguire P (1996). Maladaptive coping and affective disorders in cancer patients. *Psychol Med* 26:735–44.

Parle M, Maguire P, Heaven CM (1997). The development of a training model to improve health profesionals' skills, self-efficacy and outcome expectancies when communicating with cancer patients. *Soc Sci Med* 44(2):231–40.

Payne N (2001). Occupational stressors and coping as determinants of burnout in female hospice nurses. *J Adv Nurs* 33(3):396–405.

Peterson M (1988). The norms and values held by three groups of nurses concerning psychosocial nursing practice. *Int J Nurs Stud* 25(2):85–103.

Pieters HM, Touw-otten FWWM, de Melker RA (1994). Simulated patients in assessing consultations skills of trainees in general practice vocational training: a validity study. *Med Educ* 28:226–33.

Pistrang N, Barker C (1992). Disclosure of concerns in breast cancer. *Psycho-oncology* 1:183–92.

Pitceathly P, Maguire P (2000). Preventing affective disorders in partners of cancer patients; an intervention study. In: Baider L, Cooper CL, De-Nour AK (ed.). *Cancer and the family*, pp. 137–54, John Wiley, oxford.

Putnam SM, Stiles WB, Jacob MC, James SA (1988). Teaching the medical interview: an intervention study. *J Gen Intern Med* 3:38–47.

Ramirez AJ, Graham J, Richards MA, Cull A, Gregory WM (1996). Mental health of hospital consultants: the effects of stress and satifaction at work. *Lancet* 347:724–8.

Razavi D, Delvaux N, Farvaques C, Robaye E (1988). Immediate effectiveness of brief psychological training for health professionals dealing with terminally ill cancer patients: a controlled study. *Soc Sci Med* 27(4):369–75.

Razavi D, Delvaux N, Marchal S, Bredart A, Farvacques C, Paesmans M (1993). The effects of a 24-h psychological training program on attitudes,communication skills and occupational stress in oncology: a randomised study. *Eur J Cancer* 29A:1858–63.

Razavi D, Delvaux N, Marchal S, De Cock M, Farvaques C, Slachmuylder J-L (2000). Testing health care professionals' communication skills: the usefulness of highly emotional standardized role-playing sessions with simulators. *Psycho-Oncology* 9:293–302.

Richards M, Ramirez A, Degner L, Maher E, Neuberger J (1995). Offering choice to patients with cancers. A review based on a synposium held at the 10th annual conference of the British Psychosocial Oncology Group, December 1993. *Eur J Cancer* 31A:112–16.

Rickert ML (1982). Terminal illness, dying and death: training for caregivers. *Dissertation Abstr Int* 42(8):3443A.

Rosser J, Maguire P (1982). Dilemmas in general practice: the care of the cancer patient. *Soc Sci Med* 16:315–22.

Rothenbacher D, Lutz M, Porzsolt F (1997). Treatment decisions in palliative cancer care: patients' preferences for involvement and doctors' knowledge about it. *Eur J Cancer* 33(8):1184–9.

Royal College of Physicians London (1997). Improving communication between doctors and patients. A report of a working party. March 1997.

Rutter DR, Maguire GP (1976). History-taking for medical students. II—evaluation of a training programme. *Lancet* **September** 11:558–60.

Schofield T, Elwyn G, Edwards A, Visser A (2003). Shared decision making. *Patient Educ Couns* 50:229–30. No abstract available.

Sellick KJ (1991). Nurses' interpersonal behaviours and the development of helping skills. *Int J Nurs Stud* 28:3–11.

Seo M, Tamura K, Shijo H, Morioka E, Ikegame C, Hirasako K (2000). Telling the diagnosis to cancer patients in Japan: attitude and perception of patients, physicians and nurses. *Palliat Med* 14:105–10.

Sharpe M, Strong V, Allen K, Rush R, Postma K, Tulloh A, Maguire P, House A, Ramirez A, Cull A (2004). Major depression in outpatients attending a regional cancer centre: screening and unmet needs. *Br J Cancer* 90:314–20.

Taylor C, Graham J, Potts HW, Richards MA, Ramirez AJ (2005). Changes in mental health of hospital consultants since the mid 1990s. *Lancet* 366:742–4.

Vincent C, Young M, Phillips A (1994). Why do people sue doctors? A study of patients and relatives taking legal action. *Lancet* 343:1609–13.

Wiseman T (2002). *An ethnographic study of the use of empathy on an oncology ward.* Unpublished PhD thesis, Royal College of Nursing.

Wilkinson S (1991). Factors which influence how nurses communicate with cancer patients. *J Adv Nurs* 16:677–88.

Wilkinson S, Roberts A, Aldridge J (1998). Nurse-patient communication in palliative care; an evaluation of a communication skills programme. *Palliat Med* 12:13–22.

Wilkinson S, Leliopoulou C, Gambles M, Roberts A (2001). *The long and short of it: a comparison of outcomes of two approaches to teaching communication skills.* Paper presented at the 17th Annual scientific meeting of the British Psychosocial Oncology Society, London 2001.

Worden JW, Weisman AD (1977). The fallacy of post-mastectomy depression. *Am J Med Sci* 273(2):169–75.

Zimmerman C, Del Piccolo L, Mazzi MA (2003). Patient cues and medical interviewing in general practice: examples of the application of sequential analysis. *Epidemiol Epsichitria Soc* 12(2):115–24.

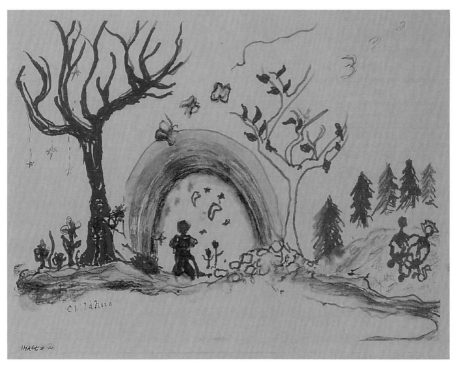

Plate 1

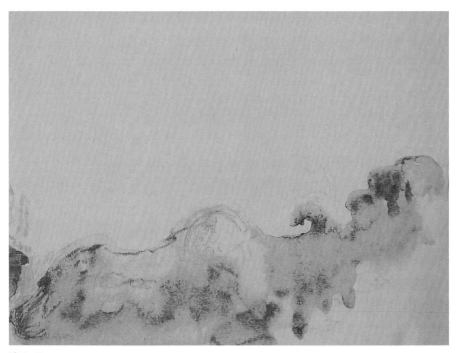

Plate 2

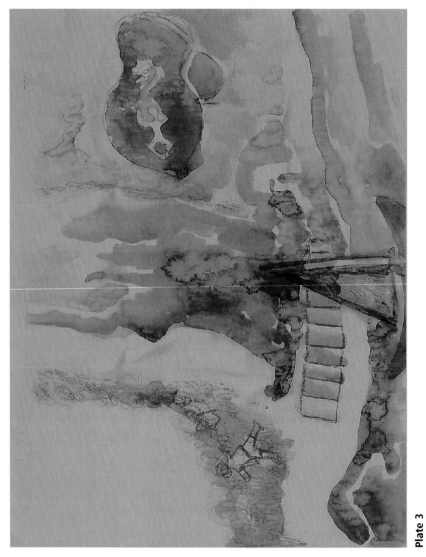

Plate 3

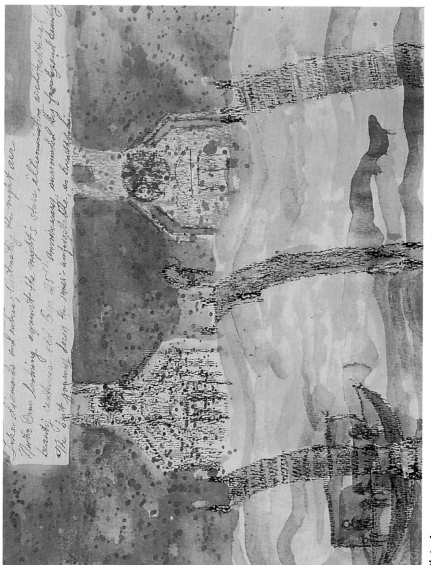

Plate 4

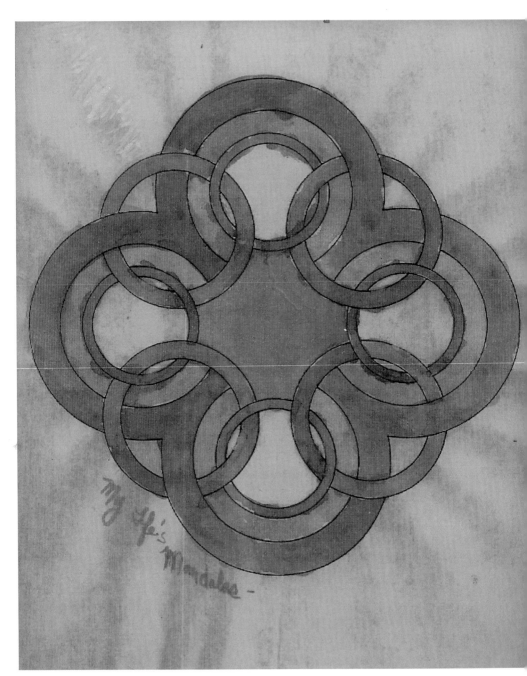

Plate 5

Chapter 3

Social impact of advanced metastatic cancer

Frances Sheldon, With an Introduction by Pam Firth

Introduction

I am honoured to be asked to update this chapter written by Frances Sheldon who died of cancer in 2005. Frances was a highly regarded academic, social worker, colleague, and friend who contributed much to our understanding of the psychosocial effects of cancer on patients and their families.

Palliative care is changing rapidly as new treatments bring advances to the medical and nursing care of patients. Pain and symptom control moves forward and good end of life care planning is the goal for all terminally ill patients. The drive to involve service users in the planning and delivery of services is giving more insights into what is needed. Initiatives by the UK government to encourage more carer support, recognizes the effects on the health of family carers of people with long-term conditions.

New laws are also going to impact on the care of the very sick and frail particularly the Mental Capacity Act 2005 whose main provisions become law in 2007. This update will try to capture the effects of the changes on the social lives of those suffering from advanced cancer.

Social workers have a particular expertise to offer psychosocial palliative care with their understanding of how social factors, social processes, and social change affect the lives of all of us. Beresford *et al.* (2006) have researched the value of the contributions of specialist palliative care social work by interviewing service users.

Social issues can lead to a multitude of distress in patients and families. This is particularly evident if we look at current research into the stress faced by patients with advanced cancer where it is clear that financial issues (Mcllfatrick 2007) and social isolation are exacerbated by smaller family units, family splits, social mobility, and a UK society that often values people in terms of their earning power.

The issue of social isolation becomes a major issue for patients who have been suffering from cancer for a long time. A number of recent studies of patients, suffering from metastatic cancer, highlight this issue. Patients and their spouses also experience a decrease in sexual, recreational and style and content of communication (Filek and Jennifer 2004). In a study by Navon and Morag (2003) looking at the way wives of men with advanced prostrate cancer dealt with their relationships, communication issues that included distancing and self-solacing cognitive tactics were common. Craib (1999) described the loneliness of cancer patients and their feeling that it is their duty to die quickly. Mulkay (1993) coined the phrase 'social death', which can be the effect/response of very sick people to the pain caused by the distancing they experience by their relatives and friends.

Recently there have been examples of family therapy models designed to help families adjust to the suffering of a close family member who has cancer such as the Family Focused Grief Therapy, an intervention used by Kissane and Bloch (2002).

In this chapter Frances Sheldon discusses the value of day care services but wisely points out the problem of discharge. How can patients with advanced disease be discharged and should they be? One solution is to target scarce resources more purposely by offering a set number of sessions and discharge patients for short periods when their disease is relatively stable. The creative use of day care for palliative care patients needs more research and development if we are to help provide good social support. In a recent patient satisfaction survey (2007) at Isabel Hospice Day Hospice when asked why they came to day care, emotional support was rated much higher than nursing care etc.

The use of self-help groups is one way forward. The author has been involved with the development of service user groups both for the bereaved and for patients. The groups with a well defined purpose enabled patients to feel that they were making an important contribution to the formation and shaping of services that would help others after they themselves had died. There is now a body of knowledge about the value and use of different types of group therapy for patients (Firth 2000). Research by Goodwin et al. (2001) and Classen et al. (2001) demonstrates that group therapy for women with metastatic breast cancer, aimed at psychosocial support, can reduce distress.

Harding (2005) discusses the development of carers support and again psycho-educational groups for carers have been found to offer valuable information and social support. The effects of caring for patients for a long time have been identified and the need for healthcare professionals to provide information both written and verbal is valued. A very good example of this is the leaflet, produced by the team who have developed the Liverpool Care Pathway, which describes the dying process.

One major effect of the changes in cancer treatment has been the experience of the children of patients with advanced disease. Many children live much of their childhood with a sick parent. They can often become young carers and as such can make use of services provide by social services for young carers. Information and support services have developed and organizations such as Winston's Wish, a service for bereaved children, have extended their work to children facing bereavement. They have collaborated with Macmillan Cancer Relief to produce an excellent book for young children called *The secret C* (Stokes 2000). Christ (2000) suggests her research demonstrates that it can be a worse experience for children when their parent is ill than afterwards. She describes the crippling fear and roller coaster affect that is talked about by many families we work with.

Conclusions

The experience of serious illness has a profound psychosocial affect on the patient and family. Services are expanding but they are often patchy with a heavy reliance on voluntary sector hospices to provide the specialist palliative care. When resources are scarce it can be services focused on psycho-social care, which are reduced and yet these needs are important if we listen to service users. The UK government recommendations contained in the NICE (2004) guidelines emphasize the need for social care. One weakness of these guidelines is the separation out of the elements of total care. In reality patients needs require professionals to be able to respond with care, which overlaps and acknowledges individuality.

The Mental Capacity Act (2005) is designed to rationalize the UK law for the most vulnerable members of our society, those that lack capacity. This act will impact on the care and treatment of these people as well as their financial arrangements. Teams of multiprofessionals will be asked to examine the mental capacity of some of their patients when decisions about care and treatment are made. We wait to see the impact of this law on services for patients with advanced cancer.

References

Beresford P, Adshead L, Croft S (2006). *Palliative care, social work and service users. Making life possible.* London: Jessica Kinsley.

Christ G (2000). *Healing children's grief, surviving a parent's death from cancer.* Oxford: Oxford University Press.

Classen C, Butler L, Koopman C, Miller E, DiMiceli S, Giese-Davis J, Fobair P, Carlson R, Kraemer H, Spiegel D (2001). Supportive-expressive group therapy and distress in patients with metastatic breast cancer: a randomised clinical intervention trial. *Arch Gen Psychiatry* 58(5):494–501.

Craib I (1999). Reflections on mourning in a modern world. *Int J Palliat Nurs* 5:87–9.

Filek V, Jennifer M (2004). Communication patterns and marital satisfaction of couples when wives are undergoing initial cycles of chemotherapy for metastatic breast cancer in *Dissertation Abstr Int B Sci Eng* 65(5-B):2623.

Firth PH (2000). Picking up the pieces: groupwork in palliative care. In: Manor O (ed.). *Ripples*. London: Whiting & Birch.

Goodwin P, Leszcz M, Ennis M Koopman J, Uircent L, Guither H Drysdete E, Hundleby M, Chochuor H, Navaro M, Speca M, Hunter J (2001). The effect of group psychosocial support on survival in metastatic breast cancer. *N Engl J Med* 345(24):1719–26.

Harding R (2005). Carers: current research and developments. In: Firth PH, Luff G, Oliviere D (ed.). *Loss change and bereavement in palliative care*. Buckingham: Open University Press. McGraw-Hill Education.

Kissane D, Bloch B (2002). *Family focussed grief therapy*. Buckingham: Open University Press.

Mcllfatrick S (2007). Assessing palliative care needs: views of patients, informal carers and healthcare professionals. *J Adv Nurs* 57:77–86.

Mulkay M (1993). Social death in Britain. In: Clark D (ed.). *The sociology of death*. Oxford: Blackwell.

Navon L, Morag A (2003). Advanced prostrate cancer patients' ways of coping with the hormonal therapy's effect on body, sexuality, and spousal ties. *Qual Health Res* 13(19):1378–92.

National Institute for Clinical Excellence (2004). *Guidance on cancer services: improving supportive and palliative care for adults with cancer*. London: NICE.

Stokes J (2000). *The secret C*. Gloucester: Winston's Wish.

Social impact of advanced metastatic cancer

Frances Sheldon

Introduction

From the moment that someone learns that there is no further curative treatment for their advancing metastatic cancer that person sees themselves differently and is perceived differently by those around them. How differently depends on the meaning attributed to the news and the coping styles of those individuals. One person may see this as a challenge to a fight that they are still determined to win, another as a death sentence, to which they can only respond with sadness and withdrawal. Those around the dying person may subscribe to that person's approach or see the situation quite differently. So understanding what may be involved as both the dying person and those connected with them struggle with a changing identity is crucial in working with those experiencing the social impact of advanced cancer. Of course not every dying person or every family member is specifically told of the situation, but the physical and possibly also mental deterioration experienced necessarily changes relationships and function in the short or long term. This developing awareness may occur early in the trajectory of the illness or after many years of relapse, treatment, and remission.

That there is social pain alongside physical, psychological, and spiritual pain has long been recognized in palliative care but it is probably the least-understood aspect of 'total pain' (Field 2000). This chapter aims to change that and to explore in more detail some of the components of social pain (Plate 2, pp. 98–99). We will first consider some of the broad issues relating to identity at this time, to dependence and independence, in the light of different contexts and different cultural backgrounds. Then we will look more specifically at the impact of advanced cancer on family relationships and the dying person's social situation and ways in which professional interventions and service provision may support those involved and ameliorate that impact.

Social contexts for death and bereavement

Our identity is developed in a social context over our lifespan, though, as Lawton (2000) indicates in her research study of the bodily realities of dying, this is also inextricably bound up with our inner sense of being. The social context in which death and bereavement take place is changing. Walter (1994) has charted three types of context for dying. The first is the traditional context where death occurs in a community setting with close involvement of family and friends and where religion often provides the framework that offers both meaning and ritual. The second is the modern context where the authority of medicine is paramount, the hospital is the predominant setting, and emotion and information are kept private and controlled, both by family members and by staff caring for the dying person. The third is a neo-modern approach where the dying person is much more self-determining. There is again more openness about what is happening, as in the traditional context. The dying person may even write about their emotions and experiences in a regular newspaper column, seek to control where death occurs, and plan the funeral.

As Walter (1994) points out, in a country like the UK all these three contexts may be operating. The traditional context may be found in some rural or migrant communities. The neo-modern approach is probably more often found among younger people (John Diamond and Ruth Picardie are well-known examples) than among older people who grew up through the middle of the twentieth century when medical and other types of authority were more highly respected. Families too develop their own individual cultures in response to the family history, the society in which they live, and the balancing of the contributions of the different members. So a particular family may wish to operate in neo-modern mode even when living in a traditional society.

In addition to the societal context and the familial culture, the cultural history and current cultural orientation of both the dying person and their family play a significant part in shaping the social impact of advancing cancer. As so many writers on cultural aspects of palliative care have observed, 'cultures are dynamic and not homogeneous' (Firth 2001). So knowing that someone emigrated from the west of Ireland as a young man forty years ago may provide useful background information but only a respectful and sensitive exploration of his present attitudes and beliefs will determine how influential those current in his childhood still are for him (Donnelly 1999). Firth (1997) reports that many hospitals in India send those that are dying back home because of the importance in Hindu culture of dying at home, well prepared and surrounded by a particular set of rituals. A younger generation of Hindus born in the UK may have very different expectations from their parents who were born in India and there may in any case be no qualified priest available to perform the rituals, so lay members of the community may need to substitute.

Culture links to the spiritual aspects of life, which are dealt with elsewhere in this book, and these too will influence the impact of advancing cancer on social relationships. In the Jewish faith it is important to maintain hope (Neuberger 1993). This may mean that openness about a terminal prognosis with the patient may not be acceptable to a Jewish family, with the consequences that may bring for resolution of unfinished business or acceptance of support from a Macmillan nurse. Culture similarly influences decision making in families and perceptions of dependence and independence. The anxiety about 'being a burden' and loss of autonomy, so evident in Western societies (Seale and Addington-Hall 1994), is less weighty in cultures where older people are more valued, where parents are still the decision makers in the family even when old, and where the family rather than the individual is significant.

Finally, gender is a factor to be considered in how the dying person and those involved with that person respond to advancing cancer. It has been most explored in bereavement where research by Stroebe (1998) indicates that on the whole men in Western societies are more problem focused and women more emotion focused in their reactions. Although it has not so far been specifically researched in relation to men or women caring for dying people, it does appear from the literature on caring in general that men carers (the minority) are more task oriented and adopt a more 'formal' approach than women carers, for whom a sense of duty and the expectation that it is part of a woman's identity are still significant (Neale 1991). Interestingly Lawton (2000) observes that for the seriously ill patients in the hospice she studied, gender differences in response to their illness were not marked. The bodily deterioration that these men and women had experienced had made them feel that they had lost much of what made them 'masculine' or 'feminine'. However professionals working with dying people and those involved with them need to be clear about all the particular influences from their social and cultural contexts if they are to offer appropriate care.

The nature of social pain

Employment and income

The losses experienced by people with advanced cancer in relation to their social world are concerned with their engagement with the world outside home and with the roles and relationships within the family. By the time the cancer is advanced many people of working age will have had to reduce or give up altogether their engagement in employment. For some this is the biggest loss and is resisted.

> Bill, aged 45, was a scaffolding erector. His marriage had broken up and he had become homeless as a result of this and his difficulty in earning because of his brain tumour which was producing frequent dizzy spells. He had a new girlfriend who was still married herself and living in the matrimonial home. Her husband was often away on business and had agreed that Bill could live in the cellar room of their house on a temporary basis. So much of his former identity had gone and he hated being dependent on the whim of his girlfriend's husband. So he tried at all costs to maintain his view of himself as a worker. When prospective clients called to book him he would tell them that he could not manage it this week but he would book them in next week. This considerably alarmed his girlfriend and the teams caring for him. They tried to confront him with the impossibility of clambering on roofs and up ladders but he brushed this aside. Over time it became clear that confrontation was not necessary because, although Bill remained in denial, he would always ring up and defer the client for yet another week when the booked date arrived. Thus he minimized the only aspect of his social pain that he felt he could control.

Financial hardship often goes hand in hand with serious illness. There may be additional expense for heat, food, and clothes at a time when income has stayed the same or reduced. For many this will be the first time in their lives they will have encountered the welfare benefits system or applied for charitable funds. Despite the efforts that have been made in the UK in recent years to simplify the language and layout of benefit application forms, they present a formidable challenge to a new user; for example, Jenny, caring for her bedridden husband and applying for 'attendance allowance' commented 'When they ask "Why do you want this help?" I don't know where to start.' But it is not just a practical issue. Stevenson (1973) has identified both the moral opprobrium that is often linked with poverty and the fact that being a claimant may also identify that person as someone who has 'failed' in some way. Particularly if you have always seen yourself as different from 'those layabouts on benefit who are given huge sums at the tax payer's expense', contemplating joining this group is extremely distressing. Similarly the symbolism of being a recipient of charity when you have always been a giver can prevent an application being made unless this issue is talked through first. It is interesting that this is an area often neglected by professionals (Sykes *et al.* 1992), perhaps because of fear of its sensitivity, though that does not stop detailed exploration of a patient's bowel habits! By acknowledging that this can be a problem, exploring what is most painful, not being too quick to reassure that somehow the ill person is different from other benefit or charity applicants (because in reality they are unlikely to be), but communicating that their worth and value are not changed, professionals can help claimants to tackle this step with less pain. Practical help in treading through the maze may well be needed alongside. Cancer and palliative care services can provide this, perhaps through a social worker, a volunteer who develops an expertise in this area, or through a link with the Citizens' Advice Bureau or local welfare benefits service.

Social engagement

As mobility and energies decline it becomes harder to participate in social events and maintain friendships that were built on sharing activities and interests. Social isolation is a frequent source of social pain for both the person with advanced cancer and any carers. Accessing local volunteer transport groups may help in maintaining old interests, if the loss of an ability to drive or use public transport is the problem. Even the provision of a disabled parking badge may make someone feel part of society again, through enabling common activities like shopping. Going on holiday is another valued social activity and charities like Macmillan Cancer Relief can provided support to make this possible. Hospice Information's booklet *Flying home—or on Holiday*, which gives advice about travel arrangements for very sick people, is a useful resource here, or for those who wish at a late stage to return to the country of their birth (Myers 2002).

For some, the change in the way they feel about themselves and their declining function create too big a gap between past social engagement and the present. For them a solution may be to participate in new social groups, such as cancer support groups, where they can both learn how others deal with a changed identity, compare their own situation, and continue to feel they can make a contribution. Some cancer support groups focus on simply providing a regular meeting where people with cancer can share experiences. Often professionals linked to a cancer centre or a palliative care service will facilitate these. Elsewhere the emphasis may be on self-help, through a well-developed voluntary organization that provides a range of services from information to advocacy, even training for patients to enable them to advocate for themselves if they wish. Here the focus is on empowering patients who have felt overwhelmed by their disease and are seeking to regain some control. The organization Cancerlink provides a directory of voluntary self-help and support groups. Active self-help groups can sometimes be perceived as challenging by professionals. The questioning they can promote can feel like criticism of a service that is struggling to cope with limited resources. Here there is a real need to be clear about the possibility of anger about the disease being projected onto the cancer service. A regular meeting between service providers and the voluntary organization, which provides a channel to deal with issues as they come up, can be helpful. Meetings set up only at times of crisis have to operate in a heated atmosphere, which makes dispassionate discussion very difficult.

A day-care service is another way of providing a new social group where members have in common the experience of advancing illness, however different their other social circumstances. Two observational studies of day care both comment on the way day care provided an 'alternative reality' (Lawton 2000) or a new 'normality' (Richardson 2001) for those attending. Lawton's participants seldom discussed the future, for it is this loss of future that particularly sets them apart from friends and acquaintances in their past. For Richardson's participants 'normality' seemed to consist of a structured opportunity to get out of the house, the potential for making new relationships and learning new skills, and a determination to divert from the illness that dominated life elsewhere. In day-care settings the deterioration of a fellow attendee can be challenging because of the reminder of the power of the illness. Staff in some settings may conceal or gloss over this despite the commitment to openness in palliative care philosophy. It can help if how such an event may be handled is discussed by the staff group when setting up the day-care service and monitored regularly to see whether the system devised meets the needs of attendees and staff.

While palliative day-care services expanded rapidly in the UK from 1980 to 2000 and were claimed to improve quality of life and increase time spent at home, models of care have been varied, not necessarily relating to an assessment of need and not rigorously evaluated. Higginson *et al.* (2000) are carrying out an evaluation of palliative day care and as part of this have examined what day-care services in a sample area of the UK are offering. They have found no clear distinction between medical and social approaches to care but different layers of activity provided in varying ways. Physical, social, and emotional support were a common base layer but then different services might offer a selection, including medical support, symptom control, creative activities, or therapy services. In the week the researchers surveyed the services, 25 per cent of patients had attended for over a year. This does raise the question of the objectives of the service and of the continued monitoring of need. Richardson (2001) pointed out from her study how difficult discharge might be for patients having become attached to a new social group.

Family culture and roles

In Western countries, thanks to improved living conditions and improved healthcare, most deaths now occur in old age, when people are less engaged in formal public roles, and even, because of declining functions, in private and familial roles. So their deaths may make less impact than a younger person's on their community and family. But we cannot necessarily assume this, because what is important is the actual role that person plays in the family and what the meaning for individuals in the family is of the advancing death.

> Ann Jones, aged 81, was now clearly very frail but still insisted that the family gather at her house once a month for Sunday lunch, though her daughters and daughters-in-law now prepared the meal. Her older, unmarried daughter, Jeanette, valued this tradition, still lived at home, and desperately wanted to maintain things 'as they always had been' for as long as possible. Her middle son, Paul, had always felt under-valued but paralysed by his imperious mother and the rest of the family and his wife longed for her mother-in-law's death, hoping at last for freedom from his damaging family.

Using a systems perspective we recognize that a change in one part of the system will reverberate through the whole system to different degrees. So some assessment of how roles are distributed in the family of the person with advanced cancer will help us in working appropriately with the social and emotional pain that changing roles may bring. Is the person with advanced cancer the one that acts as the link between family members? Mothers or oldest daughters often play this role in the majority white culture in the UK, as in Ann Jones' family. Are they the conciliator or the one who breaks tension by making people laugh? Vess *et al.* (1983–4), considering bereaved families, distinguished between person-oriented and position-oriented families, and their analysis has relevance for families before the death. They suggest that positionoriented families, where roles are ascribed on the basis of age and gender, rather than interest or ability, will adapt less well to crisis and new demands. Person-oriented families, where communication is open and roles are negotiated on the basis of achievement and not on culturally prescribed norms, are likely to deal more easily with the declining health of one member of the family system. It would be wrong to imply that there may not be considerable emotional pain in person-oriented families despite their adaptability. However there may be less social pain than in a position-oriented family, where resentment at the changes and at inability to sustain valued ways of operating may make the family feel they are failing to maintain what they see as a social norm.

Carers

Carers too have a changed identity. They may be struggling to sustain other commitments to a job or to other needy family members, or life may be 'on hold' as they put the needs of the dying person first. They may feel ambivalent about calling on professional help (Hull 1990).

> Mary was a lively, active woman in her sixties but small and overweight. She had cared lovingly for her husband who had lost the use of his legs but he was now too heavy for her to manage. She agreed to have two paid carers each evening to put him to bed and felt relieved that there would no longer be an undignified and exhausting struggle in the evening. On the first evening they came she showed them into the bedroom and then retreated to the kitchen and wept bitterly. She perceived that their coming marked a point at which the privacy of her home would be increasingly invaded and hammered home her husband's continuing deterioration.

Since the passing of the Carers (Recognition and Services) Act in 1995, carers in the UK who are providing 'regular and substantial care' have been entitled to a formal assessment of their ability to care and any support needed. But as Smith (2001) found in her research, it is the more long-standing carers who embrace the title of 'carer' and who grasp what is expected of them by professionals in terms of responsibility in that role. Newer carers might be much less clear and more diffident about asking for support for themselves as well as the ill person. Those who do make demands for themselves can be challenging to professionals.

> Jane and Richard had been married for two years when he developed cancer of the pancreas aged 27. They were young professionals and ambitious. Both were paragliding enthusiasts. As he became more ill and dependent he became quieter and more contemplative. After a few weeks of full-time caring, Jane announced that she wanted to go back to work. Richard's mother was available to look after him and in a short time he returned to his family home with Jane's agreement, to be cared for there by his mother until he died. Jane's behaviour was very difficult for many of the married women professionals involved in the care and for some of her friends and family. While they did not necessarily expect Jane to be a full-time carer, to be so ready, so cheerfully, to relinquish her 'wifely duty' totally did not accord with their expectations of a woman's roles. There was quite an expectation that she would pay the price by having a painful and guilty bereavement but Jane lived quite comfortably with her decision.

Sexuality

One area where the social impact of advanced cancer is still undervalued by professionals is the changes it brings in the life of the sick person and their sexual partner. The effect of surgery and drugs on sexual function is well established. For example, Stanford et al. (2000) showed that 24 months after surgery for prostate cancer, maintaining an erection was still a moderate to big problem for 42% of the men involved. What is also well established is that patients expect that professionals will bring this topic up if appropriate and professionals expect that patients will bring this topic up if they have a problem. So the issue frequently falls into the gap. A barrier for professionals is of course the sensitivity of this issue, a wish not to be intrusive or to seem to be making assumptions about this person's sexual life. Here there may be a value in breaking one of the standard rules of counselling—only ask one question at a time. Monroe (1993) suggests that a question like 'Has your illness changed your family relationships, your life as a couple, your ability to get close to each other physically?' signals that you are open to discussion about these issues. Then the dying person or their partner can choose to focus on the general family relationships aspect of the question or can use it as an opportunity to discuss any difficulties, whether practical or emotional.

> Mabel, aged 59, had bone metastases from her breast cancer. She and her husband were anxious about putting undue strain on her fragile bones but wanted to continue their active sexual life. They were able to do so after simple advice about appropriate positions.

Helpful resources in this area of care are the local psychosexual clinic or SPOD, the London–based, national Association to Aid the Sexual and Personal Relationships of People with a Disability. This organization produces a number of leaflets and has a helpline for anyone, professionals and carers included, seeking advice.

Dependants

One of the most painful issues that those with advanced metastatic cancer may have to confront is the change the illness and their death will bring to those dependent upon them. The emotional distress for healthy, independent adults who love them may be hard enough to contemplate, how much more difficult to consider the losses for a vulnerable dependant. That person may be a child, or an adult with learning disabilities, or a frail, confused partner for whom the dying person has been the main carer. In all these situations there is a need for some preparation before the death and this of course may be particularly painful for a dying person who has been wishing to deny this possibility or at the least avoid discussing it. If after the death there will still be someone living in the same house who will continue to be able to care for the vulnerable person, for example the other parent, then it may be possible to offer the dying person some protection. What is then most important is that the vulnerable person is prepared for the change by the person who will continue the care. Where this element of continuity is not possible, preparation and planning for the transition are vital. All too often people with learning disabilities, for example, have been moved quite suddenly into a residential setting following the expected death of their carer with no recognition of their distress (Oswin 1991). The existence now of a National Network for the Palliative Care of People with Learning Disabilities and the growing number of research and practice projects in this field demonstrate that this group's needs are at last beginning to be addressed. It is important not to make assumptions about what they do or do not understand. Overprotection can be counterproductive. This was nicely demonstrated by a contributor to the national meeting of the network in November 2001 who had cared for her sister with learning disabilities. 'When our mother died I told her the angels had come to take her away. She was crying uncontrollably and when I asked her why she said "I want Mummy to have a proper coffin like everyone else".' Certainly children from the Liverpool Bereavement Project who drew up a leaflet for other bereaved children were clear. 'It's best to be involved in and given choices about how you say good bye' (Barnard *et al.* 1999).

There are a number of principles that are helpful to guide practice in supporting children facing the death of a parent, some of which apply equally well to other vulnerable groups.

1. **Find out what the child knows or believes about the situation.** Children pick up much more than adults think from overheard conversations, from atmospheres, and from what their friends have heard from their parents. They may not always interpret what they hear or perceive accurately—all the more reason for checking out that they are not inappropriately distressed, perhaps blaming themselves for causing the illness.

2. **Help parents to talk to their children.** They know their child best, and can take advantage of a good moment for a conversation. Sometimes they may need reassurance that this is good parenting, trying to give the child knowledge and a greater sense of control in an uncontrollable situation. Sometimes they are keen to talk but uncertain how to go about it. So checking out with them what they think the child knows, offering support as they work out how to open up a discussion, and hearing how that went, are all valuable roles professionals can play. Clearly pacing and age-appropriate language must be considered. It is not necessary to tell children their mother is dying when her bone metastases have only just been picked up and it is likely that she will live for some time yet. It is important that they know that Mum and Dad are upset and distracted because the doctors have found some more signs of a serious illness.

3. **Help parents to consider what resources there might be within their family or community that could also be helpful to their children while they themselves have so much to cope with.** Schools can be very supportive but may also welcome some advice from palliative care professionals if they have not encountered this situation before. One important ethical principle here—consult children before talking to the school. Otherwise it may be more difficult if they are suddenly faced with the fact that their personal private grief is known by all.

4. **Use play.** There are many storybooks and workbooks now for children that can help them both to develop their understanding and express their feelings through art or games. *Finding a way through when someone close has died* (Mood and Whittaker 2001), produced by a group of young people, focuses most on the period after a death but has a list of books and resources, many of which are also useful beforehand.

Who has parental responsibility?

In the twenty-first century families are becoming ever more complex in their relationships. A couple may have come together, each bringing children from a previous relationship and then had children of their own. Marriage is becoming less common and it is now more usual for children to be born out of wedlock than in it. None of this may cause any problem unless the couple decides to separate or the partnership is threatened by advancing serious illness. Then who has parental responsibility and who does not may well become an issue. At the time of writing, the effective act is the Children Act (1989), though the Human Rights Act may in the end affect this. The Children Act (1989) changed rights to responsibilities. The mother always has parental responsibility. The father only has it if he was married to the mother when the child is born. He does not automatically acquire it even if he marries her subsequently. The non-married father can acquire parental responsibility in two ways. He and the mother can draw up a parental responsibility agreement made in the form prescribed by the Lord Chancellor and registered in the High Court or he can apply to the High Court to make a parental responsibility order in his favour. If the mother does not wish the father to have it, any other person with whom the child is living, for example grandparents, can apply for a residence order under the Children Act (1989) and through this acquire parental responsibility while the child continues to live with that person. Alternatively the mother can agree to a deed of guardianship before her death nominating whoever she feels suitable and can then bequeath her parental responsibility to that guardian. If a father is in dispute with a mother over this issue, he can take her to court and the court can make a parental responsibility or a residence order permitting the child to live with the father. With any family where parental responsibility is not straightforward these issues need to be considered, and for complex, reconstituted families early advice from a solicitor is vital.

> Yvonne and Peter had two children from their relationship, Paul, aged 5 and Vicky, aged 3. Yvonne also had a child by a previous relationship, Martin, aged 10, who saw his father intermittently and whose relationship with Peter was difficult. He often stayed with Yvonne's mother, who did not have a great deal of time for Peter. When it

became clear Yvonne would die in the next few weeks from her cancer of the pancreas, Peter asked her to marry him. She refused. Her mother, an active 55-year-old, who had become increasingly distraught at the likely loss of her only child and fearful that she would lose all contact with her grandchildren once Yvonne died, was offering to look after all the children. Yvonne was worried that Peter would find another partner after her death who would not look after her children properly. In those circumstances she preferred her mother to care for them and talked of making a will in her favour. As she sank into a coma, battle raged between Peter and his family and Yvonne's mother and her family. The children's behaviour—Vicky wetting the bed again, Martin playing up at school, and Paul having nightmares—demonstrated the insecurity that they all felt. A much earlier discussion, which could have acknowledged some of the adults' fears and given time to work out a compromise, could have made this death much less horrific and divisive.

If parents are reluctant to tackle this issue because it feels like giving up the fight to acknowledge that one parent is dying, the strategy of 'what if' or 'hoping for the best and planning for the worst' can be helpful here. Confirming that while it may be important to continue to hope, and even struggle, for the best outcome, the professional can alongside this suggest that as good parents they may also want to prepare for the worst outcome so that the children are protected whatever the eventuality.

Who am I? What did I contribute?

In an earlier section we looked at the challenges to identity that the losses of advancing cancer bring. For many these may be explored within a spiritual framework but there is also a social aspect to the challenge. This is a time when reviewing the past to put the present in context can be very affirming to the dying person. This may be done in several ways. For some people informal talk with family and friends may well give the opportunity to go over past triumphs and tragedies and to receive confirmation from them that their contribution has been valued. For others a more formal life review may be helpful in settling anxiety and uncertainty. Formal life review processes have been developed in many parts of the world following the seminal article by Butler (1963). Lichter (1993) trained volunteers in a New Zealand hospice to assist patients to complete oral or written accounts of their lives. Lester (1997) has built on the work of Haight *et al.*(1995) with older people in the USA to develop a structured questionnaire covering childhood, adult life, and the present for work with people with advancing illness. An improvement in life satisfaction and reduction in stress have been found following such a review. Reminiscence sessions in day care, encouraging members to bring materials focusing round a historical period like the Second World War or round a common interest such as fashions through the participants' lifetimes, can also provide an affirmation of the importance of an experience with others who have shared it.

What am I leaving behind?

Associated with life review can be a wish to leave a legacy or be involved in planing for the future of loved ones. Many patients value participating in creative activities in day care because it enables them to produce a painting or poem that provides concrete evidence of a contribution. A parent with young children who is dying may wish to leave a letter, an audio- or videotape for the children to keep and refer to as they grow up. The child welfare organization Barnardo's have produced a framework both for a 'memory book' and a 'memory box' to help parents and those working with them on this. It is important when embarking on such a project for the professional to be aware of some of the pitfalls. The dying parent will not be able to control how the memorial is kept or what use is made of it. Nor will it be helpful for the children to be too prescriptive about the future. To say 'I hope you keep a strong Christian faith' or 'I know the family business will be safe in your hands' may create a burden of guilt for the child in the future. Material which concentrates on demonstrating the value of the child for that parent and reminders of times they shared is likely to be greatly treasured.

Making a will is another way of ensuring that your wishes continue to carry weight after your death. As with sorting out parental responsibility, tackling this may feel like giving up or bringing death uncomfortably close. So the strategy recommended in that situation may be helpful here—focusing on planning for the worst while hoping for the best, so that the issue can then be set on one side. Legal advice should be sought in all cases, to avoid additional unnecessary distress for the bereaved, because the laws of inheritance are complex. An interesting project funding the appointment and training of funeral advisers in two hospices reinforced how problematic it can be to plan for an unwelcome future. It was clear that people were often misinformed and unaware of their rights, but referrals came slowly, though they came from both dying and bereaved people. The project did generate considerable interest and mixed feelings among staff (Heatley 2001).

Support services

Most people spend 90 per cent of the last year of their life at home and indeed wish to die at home. Grande *et al.* (1998) have reviewed the factors that make death at home more likely. These are

- the existence of a fit and well-supported family carer, particularly a woman partner
- being a man
- being in a higher socio-economic group

- being younger rather than older

- good symptom control.

Hinton (1994) in his longtitudinal study found that provision of social work support and improved day care increased the percentage of home deaths.

Grande *et al.* (1998) conclude that the number of home deaths is more likely to be increased by improving access to the services available for those in lower socio-economic groups and by enabling men to take on the carer role. Interestingly they found the one study that showed women and older people more likely to die at home came from Italy, so the cultural and family context may in fact be more significant than age or gender. The supportive and palliative care guidance from the National Institute of Clinical Excellence is likely to recommend that a range of social support services should be available in the cancer network, many of which have already been alluded to in this chapter. These range from the availability of respite care and personal and domestic support at home, 24 hours a day, to laundry and meals services, adapted housing, and training for carers in moving and handling. Hopefully it will identify the importance of support to maintain adolescent and young cancer patients and carers in education and suggest that each in-patient setting should have at least one member of staff who has had training in working with children who have a parent with cancer.

For some people with advanced cancer there may come a point when they can no longer manage at home even with support and they are faced with the particular social pain of having to consider moving into a residential home or nursing home. This is a further challenge to identity and can bring a real sense of bereavement as someone gives up the home in which perhaps children were born and grew up, in which every corner carries memories. Different countries have different arrangements for financing institutional care and the current debates in the UK provide a good example of some of the practical and symbolic issues at stake. Over the last fifteen year of the twentieth century there was huge shift, never democratically decided, in the provision of long-stay beds from the National Health Service to the social care providers, the local authorities, and voluntary and private homes. Because healthcare is free at the point of access and social care is means-tested, a generation that expected to receive free services 'from the cradle to the grave' suddenly found they had to pay, even if they required substantial care. This raised issues about reciprocal obligation in families and of equity and justice. Parents might expect and hope for care from their adult children as they become more disabled and wish to pass on a financial legacy to those they love; children may expect to receive some financial benefit from their parents' estate. Should family members be expected to support each other practically,emotionally, and financially? Is it just that a successful businessman should receive the profits from the sale of his mother's house and expect that the tax payers, some of whom may be much poorer than him, should cover the cost of her nursing home fees? Professionals working with someone with advanced cancer who is facing giving up their home may well find themselves caught up in these debates and in the anger and disagreement which they bring. These are intensified by the different approaches now being taken by the four countries within the UK.

Conclusion

A holistic approach to the care of people with advanced metastatic cancer must take into account the issues raised in this chapter to provide comprehensive care. Each team needs access to a specialist in these areas, who is most likely to be a social worker.

However each team member has to have some appreciation of the power of social pain and what may help to reduce its impact. Working in this area requires good negotiation skills, a breadth of understanding, stamina, and sensitivity but the benefits for patients and those close to them of providing good social care are high.

References

Barnard P, Morland I, Nagy J (1999). *Children, bereavement and trauma: nurturing resilience*. London: Jessica Kingsley.

Butler RN (1963). The life review: an interpretation of reminiscence in the aged. *Psychiatry* 26:65–73.

Donnelly S (1999). Folklore associated with dying in the west of Ireland. *Palliative Med* 13:57–62.

Field D (2000). What do we mean by 'psychosocial'? London: National Council for Hospice and Specialist Palliative Care Services. Briefing Paper No.4.

Firth S (1997). *Death, dying and bereavement in a British Hindu community*. Leuven: Peeters.

Firth S (2001). *Wider horizons: care of the dying in a multicultural society*. London: National Council for Hospice and Specialist Palliative Care Services.

Grande G, Addington-Hall J, Todd C (1998). Place of death and access to home care: are certain patient groups at a disadvantage? *Social Science Med* 47:565–79.

Haight B, Coleman P, Lord K (1995). The linchpins of successful life review: structure, evaluation and individuality. In: Haight B, Webster J (ed.). *The art and science of reminiscing: theory, research, methods and application*. Washington DC: Taylor and Francis, pp. 179–92.

Heatley R (2001). *Funeral advisors: is there a need? A pilot study*. Bristol: National Funerals College.

Higginson I, Hearn J, Myers K, Naysmith A (2000). Palliative day care: what do services do? *Palliative Med* 14:277–86.

Hinton J (1994). Which patients with terminal cancer are admitted from home care? *Palliative Med* 8:183–96.

Hull M (1990). Sources of stress for hospice-based care-giving families. In: Kirschling JM (ed.). *Family-based palliative care*.New York: Howarth, pp. 29–54.

Lawton J (2000). The dying process: patients' experiences of palliative care. London: Routledge.

Lester J (1997). Life review with the terminally ill. Proceedings of the Fourth Congress of the European Association for Palliative Care; 6–9 December 1995; Barcelona. Milan: European Association for Palliative Care.

Lichter I (1993). Biography as therapy. *Palliative Med* 7:133–7.

Mood P, Whittaker L (2001). *Finding a way through when someone close has died. A workbook by young people for young people.* London: Jessica Kingsley.

Monroe B (1993). Psychosocial dimension of palliation. In: Saunders C, Sykes N (ed.). *The management of terminal malignant disease*.London: Edward Arnold, pp. 174–201.

Myers K (2002). *Flying home—or on holiday.* Hospice Information: London. http://www.hospiceinformation.info.

National Institute of Clinical Excellence (in preparation). *Supportive and palliative care guidance: the manual.*

Neale B (1991). Informal palliative care. a review of research on needs, standards and service evaluation. Sheffield: Trent Palliative Care Centre. Occasional Paper No. 3.

Neuberger J (1993). Cultural issues in palliative care. In: Doyle D, Hanks G, Macdonald N. (ed.). *Oxford textbook of palliative medicine.* Oxford: Oxford University Press, pp. 507–513.

Oswin M (1991). *Am I allowed to cry? A study of bereavement among people who have learning difficulties.* London: Souvenir Press.

Richardson H (2001). A study of palliative day care using multiple case studies [presentation]. Palliative Care Research Forum, Royal College of Physicians; 7 June 2001; London.

Seale C, Addington-Hall J (1994). Euthanasia; why people want to die earlier. *Soc Sci Med* 39:647–54.

Smith P (2001). Who is a carer? Experiences of family caregivers in palliative care. In: Payne S, Ellis-Hill C (ed.). *Chronic and terminal illness: new perspectives on caring and carers.* Oxford: Oxford University Press, pp. 83–99.

Stanford J, Feng Z, Hamilton AS, Gilliland FD, Stephenson RA, Eley JW (2000). Urinary and sexual function after radical prostatectomy for clinically localised cancer. The prostate cancer outcomes study. *J Am Med Assoc* 283:354–60.

Stevenson O (1973). *Claimant or client?* London: Allen and Unwin.

Stroebe M (1998). New directions in bereavement research: exploration of gender differences. *Palliative Med* 12:5–12.

Sykes N, Pearson S, Chell S (1992). Quality of care: the carer's perspective. *Palliative Med* 6:227–36.

Vess J, Morland J, Schwebel A (1983–4). Understanding family role reallocation following a death. *Omega* 16:115–28.

Walter T (1994) *The revival of death.* London: Routledge.

Chapter 4

Family-centred care: psychosocial care for the marginalized

Philip J Larkin

Introduction

Arguably at some point in everyone's life, they feel excluded for a variety of reasons. Usually, these experiences are transient and people resume their place within their social community. However, for some, exclusion and marginalization represent the totality of their experience. Koffman and Camps (2004) define this as 'no way in.' (p. 354). There is a broad literature defining the attributes of social exclusion and the need to reduce inequity has been seen as a founding principle of healthcare provision, not least in end of life care (Higginson 1993; Grande *et al.* 1998; Addington-Hall 2000; O'Neill and Marconi 2001;) Social exclusion encompasses a plethora of problems, including unemployment, low income, poor housing, high crime, bad health, and family breakdown. Some of these hold true for people in receipt of palliative care services. An overriding theme is poverty; either in monetary terms or the poverty of spirit, which can be experienced through prejudice and ignorance. Tickle (2007), in his discussion of a UK community health service for patients described as 'those shunned by others' (p. 69) highlights how clients live in conflict situations with authority for many reasons, often addiction or mental health problems. Where communication breaks down and services seem unable or unwilling to respond, the need for statutory services to examine mutual values and motivations is as imperative as any attempt to alter potentially destructive behaviours.

Given the breadth of exclusion, this chapter will explore specific care groups where the growing body of evidence indicates that palliative care has been highlighted as a significant issue.

- people with mental health problems
- people living with an intellectual disability (ID)
- the palliative care needs of older people with dementia
- the palliative care needs of those in prison

- ◆ the issues of chemical dependency in end-of-life care
- ◆ the complexity of end-of-life care for ethnic minority communities.

Through a series of case studies from an Irish context, the psychosocial dilemmas faced by this varied group of patients are described. The studies reflect a rural community in the west of Ireland but offer insight into more global issues experienced across the health and social care spectrum in many countries. Key issues will be highlighted at the end of each section. To begin, there are two questions to be considered. What is family care and what do we mean by 'the marginalized'?

What is meant by family-centred care?

Family-centred care derives from paediatrics or child health focus. This is not to say that family-centred care is relevant only to parental–child relationships. Indeed, a current definition suggests that: 'Family-centred care is an approach to the planning, delivery, and evaluation of healthcare that is governed by mutually beneficial partnerships between healthcare providers, patients and families. Family-centred care applies to patients of all ages and it may be practiced in any healthcare setting' (Institute for Family Centred Care 2005, website).

This definition has resonance with the World Health Organization (2002) definition of palliative care, which espouses an approach to end-of-life care that is eclectic, equitable, and relevant to a broad population. One of the most important skills in this approach is the ability to listen compassionately to the illness stories families share (Svavarsdottir 2006). How families respond to clinician's interventions in their lives, particularly in the case of chronic illness has been a focus of research in recent years (Bohn *et al.* 2003; Limacher and Wright 2003; Duhamel and Talbot 2004). These studies have demonstrated that addressing global family need involves listening and questioning skills, a belief in personhood, the ability to explore the illness experience in a way that does not alienate but rather normalizes the experience. Chesla (2005) identifies that collaboration with families during the chronic illness experience is best achieved by the willingness of the clinician to enter the lifeworld of the family and to be open to the narrative of families daily lives in order to understand their needs better. Therapeutic relationships with families are not based on lengthy conversation. Rather, affirmation and acknowledgement of the situation offers a more positive outcome (Wright and Leahey 2005).

These descriptions hold true for palliative care as the relationship underpins the philosophical early writings of its founder Cecily Saunders. Questions raised include the meaning of ideal family to palliative care patients and how it differs from our own world view. What if family is not seen in the context of a wholesome nurturing framework, but rather as a destructive element in their lives that has contributed to their experience of exclusion? Clearly, there is evidence that family breakdown ranks high among the reasons cited for homelessness, particularly in women (Rowe and Wolch 1990; Geissler *et al.* 1995; Pollio 1997; Kang *et al.* 2000; Anderson 2001; Lee *et al.* 2003; Anderson and Ravens 2004; Muir-Chochrane *et al.* 2006).Given that family-centred care seeks a reciprocal relationship between the professional and the cared-for, it is incumbent on palliative care practitioners to articulate how they mean to provide care that is seen as socially equitable. In the delivery of palliative care, and particularly for those who consider themselves to be marginalized, a 'one size fits all' mentality is clearly inappropriate.

What do we mean by the marginalized?

Morrell (2001) argues that the term 'marginalized' describes the unconscious social processes that underpin people's sense of isolation and powerlessness to challenge the system that has dictated their exclusion. Palliative care practitioners need to ask if their clinical discipline currently sustains a society that unconsciously divides its citizens. Until recently, the exclusion of palliative care for cancer patients may be one example Therese Vanier, described the parallel between the vision of L'Arche (faith communities for the intellectually disabled) and Cecily Saunders hospice movement as: 'somebody listening very carefully to some very fragile and vulnerable people'.

The fear that palliative care has in some way diluted its original aims (Praill 2000; Egan and Labyak 2001; McNamara 2001; Skilbeck and Payne 2005; Seymour 2005; Van Kleffens *et al.* 2004;) can be set against this simple description of what it means to be a palliative care practitioner and how we view the key determinants of a good quality service. In each case study presented here, the frailty and vulnerability of the individual presents the starting point of good palliative care.

The needs of people with mental health problems

Martin was a 45-year-old single man who lived with his elderly mother on their farm. Martin had a long-standing history of bi-polar disorder and was supported by local mental health services, although his mother had acted as his main carer for many years.

Following his diagnosis and treatment for rectal cancer, he was referred to the home care team who were able to provide guidance on his symptom management. Martin became increasingly withdrawn and reluctant to engage with the team, which his mother interpreted as part of his mental health disorder. His mother and the local mental health team wished him to be transferred to the hospice but the hospice were concerned about their ability to deal with his mental health issues.

The global prevalence of mental disorders in adults may reach 48% by 2020 (World Health Organization 2000). Mental health problems may be exacerbated by physiological imbalance associated with metabolic disturbances, unrelieved symptoms, infection or the progression of disease (Tuma and DeAngelis 2000; Garssen 2004; Thewes *et al.* 2004). Mental health patients may be unable to engage with palliative care practitioners due to a range of challenging and demanding behaviours that the latter are ill-equipped to deal with (McCormack and Sharp 2006). Depression is as a common symptom noted in end of life patients (Lloyd-Williams and Payne 2003; Meyer *et al.* 2003; Lawrie *et al.* 2004; Lloyd-Williams *et al.* 2004; Robinson and Crawford 2005). Wide variance in the rates of depression in palliative care patients are reported, attributable to the complexity of utilizing depression measurement instruments within an already frail and vulnerable population (Steifel *et al.* 2001; Hoptof *et al.* 2002). There is also evidence of a correlation between physical symptoms and the presence of depression (Lloyd-Williams *et al.* 2004) and a focus on physical rather than psychological symptoms in clinical assessments (Lloyd-Williams and Payne 2003).

Palliative care and mental health practitioners share common skills to engage therapeutically with patients or clients (Cutcliffe *et al.* 2001a,b). Addington-Hall (2000) argues for a partnership approach between mental health and palliative care services to enhance mutual skills and knowledge to ensure that those with severe mental health problems receive equitable care. Partnership has worked to alleviate clinicians mutual concerns and consolidated strong relationships between practitioners from disparate disciplines (McCormack and Sharp 2006). In the case presented here, palliative care concerns expressed about Martin's bi-polar disorder were ill-founded and based upon a limited knowledge of the treatment and maintenance of the disease. Equally, mental health practitioners were unfamiliar with the treatment that Martin had received for his cancer, how to deal with its side-effects and compounded his mothers fears regarding the use of opiates. Martin's reluctance to engage with palliative care services was based on his belief that to do so would hasten his death. Evidently, the need for cross-communication and joint care planning were paramount, involving both Martin and his mother as far as possible. By offering a weekly palliative day care place to Martin and inviting his community psychiatric nurse to visit him at the hospice on that day created the structure where Martin could feel safe and secure and have both his palliative and mental health needs monitored. Once inpatient care was necessary, Martin had built up a significant relationship with staff to reduce his tension about the move. The mental health services were also able to provide an outreach support service to his mother through Martin's final illness and into bereavement, as they had built a strong relationship with her during the time span of Martin's mental healthcare.

Key issues in caring for people with mental health problems at end-of-life

- ◆ There is a need to encourage liaison between the palliative care and mental health services beyond episodes of care to enhance mutual understanding of diverse perspectives.
- ◆ Close liaison with the local mental health practitioner who holds strong family knowledge is essential to securing trust with both family and mental health team.
- ◆ Be clear about role expectations, e.g. who will deliver bereavement support to the family.

The needs of people with intellectual disability

Catherine was a 48-year-old woman with Down syndrome in long- term residential care. She has lived in the same group home since the age of 19 and was employed in a workshop attached to the local day centre for young adults with ID. Catherine has received treatment for breast cancer, which has been largely unsuccessful and she is now developing clinical symptoms suggestive of extension of her disease and the need for palliative care. Catherine's parents are dead and she has one sister, Siobhan, who visits her occasionally. Catherine has a bright personality but evident speech and comprehension difficulties. She has strong attachments to her carers and this dependency has become increasingly problematic for the staff at her home. She is supported by the home care team and plans are being discussed for her care in the terminal phase of her life.

In the UK, approximately 25 people per 1000 have an ID with between three and four of those having severe or profound disability (Department of Health 2001; Tuffrey-Wijne 2003). Given the complex spectrum of ID, a flexible global definition (Luckasson *et al.* 1992) concludes that ID is characterized by altered intellectual function before the age of 18 with concurrent limitations in at least two of the following areas (among others): communication and social skills, academic skills, utilizing community resources, and self-care. Increased life expectancy due to better medical treatment has led to an increasing incidence of progressive illness in this client group, including cardiovascular disease, Alzheimer's disease, and cancer (Jancar 1993) Up to 16% of recorded deaths of persons with ID are from cancer and mortality from cancer in Down syndrome is particularly documented (Cooke 1997; Hollins *et al.* 1998; Mertens *et al.* 1998; Patja *et al.* 2001; Tuffrey-Wijne 2003).

It is suggested that people with an ID are among the most marginalized in society (Tuffrey-Wijne 2003) and their dying has been described as a 'hidden transition' within the ID community (Todd and Read 2006). End-of-life care of patients with ID is an area of increasing research interest. A series of papers presented at the ISSAID-Europe Conference in Maastricht (presented as a series of short reports in the *Journal of Applied Research in Intellectual Disabilities* in 2006) demonstrates a range of studies that explore the palliative care needs in ID, including tools to identify distress in people with communication difficulties (Tuffrey-Wijne *et al.* 2006), service delivery and planning (Tuffrey-Wijne *et al.* 2006a), the specific issues of bereavement (Blackman 2006) and the importance of user involvement (Tuffrey-Wijne *et al.* 2006). However, there still remains limited empirical evidence about the specific palliative care needs of people with ID. There are reports where ID has rendered someone ineligible for cancer treatment or symptoms are misinterpreted as attributable to their ID (Tuffrey-Wijne 1997, 2003; Miki *et al.* 1999). People with ID needs are not always offered the same range of treatment options as others, nor involved in the decision-making about their care, leading to distress and fragmentation of care (Kastner *et al.* 1993; Beange *et al.* 1995; Keywood *et al.* 1999; Keenan and McIntosh 2000; Northfield and Turnbull 2001). This is compounded by palliative care practitioners concerns that they lack appropriate skills on the management of ID patients (Tuffrey-Wijne 1998). Studies have also reported that healthcare professionals make assumptions about the capability of people with ID to give informed consent (Department of Health 2001; Tuffrey-Wijne 2002). Mild cases of ID may not be fully recognized by professionals (Howells 1997; Cumella and Martin 2000).

There is clear reference to the needs of this disadvantaged group in terms of access, information and supportive care (Department of Health 2000, 2001; National Institute for Clinical Excellence 2004). A key ethical premise of working with people with ID is the belief that the life of all persons holds equal value (Tuffrey-Wijne 2003). The case history opens the debate on what we mean by family. Blackman (2005) considers that people with learning disability are more likely to experience profound insecurity due to disrupted patterns of attachment in childhood, often through prolonged hospitalization. This is exacerbated when, for example, transfer to a residential setting is required if the parents die or are unable to cope. In Catherine's case, her family ties had been redirected to the care staff and away from her sibling, Siobhan, which required the palliative care team to redefine the goals and objectives 'family' meetings. The group home believed that Siobhan should make the decisions about her sister's care but she felt that the care staff were more sensitive and better placed to define Catherine's needs. In ID care settings, the bond between carer and resident can be very strong, which can have negative consequences when the need to involve a wider team of carers is warranted. Jacquemin (2005) describes this as balancing between active presence and respectful distance. In all cases, assessing the palliative needs of the person with ID must include an understanding of emotional investment on the part of the person, family, and carer. The biological family may choose to withdraw and this should be respected. Carers may be overprotective and even though people may seek information, they lack education and training to impart this. Given the emphasis on open communication around end-of-life care for patients and families, people with ID should receive information, albeit in a framework that is understandable to them (Tuffrey-Wijne et al. 2006). This is particularly important for bereavement. Research demonstrates that people with ID are likely to be excluded from the knowledge that someone close to them is going to die (Raji and Holmes 2001; Dowling et al. 2003; Todd 2004; Blackman 2005). For the other residents of Catherine's group home, it was important to prepare them for Catherine's final illness and death. In caring for Catherine in her own environment, the choice of the client's preferred location is essential. Catherine chose to stay in her group home and her carers undertook a short 1-week palliative care course in the earlier days of her illness to equip themselves with additional knowledge and skills. Supported by the local GP and home care team, Catherine died peacefully in the presence of her sister and close friends from the group home.

Key issues in intellectual disability

- People with ID are likely to be excluded from knowledge about their disease and prognosis but have the right to be fully informed within the scope of their understanding.
- ID covers a broad spectrum and end of life care needs to be tailored to the individual's ability to understand and participate in their care.
- The concept of family may need to be revised in terms of biological family versus 'meaningful family' to the person with ID.
- Grief support should be extended to the carers of the person with ID given the strength of long-term relationship developed in most cases.

The needs of older people with dementia

John is an 83-year-old widower who has been living in a residential nursing home for the past 3 years. Over the last year, John has become increasingly frail with marked deficits in terms of his neurocognitive and functional status. Initially confused, he became incoherent in speech, uncommunicative, and disorientated. He lost his appetite, became incontinent and eventually bed bound, which left him at risk of chest infection and decubitus ulcers. The GP and local community nurse were extremely supportive but felt that they lacked knowledge in terms of John's pain and symptom management. A referral to the local hospice was made and an agreement for home care support confirmed. John was not listed for inpatient care in the hospice.

It is a misnomer to assume that the needs of an older populations are similar to younger adults (Teunissen *et al.* 2006; Duggleby and Raudonis 2006). Older people are likely to suffer discrimination in terms of underassessment and treatment of symptoms and inappropriate judgements that symptoms are related to the ageing process and not exacerbation of disease (Seale and Cartwright 1994; Davies and Higginson 2004). One area of increasing clinical interest is care in dementia at end-of-life—approximately 100 000 people per annum will die from dementia (Bayer 2006). Few will receive specialist palliative care services even though their needs may not be markedly different from patients with malignant disease (Luddington *et al.* 2001). The principles of palliative care are clearly resonant with the needs of patients with end-stage dementia, from whom the progressive loss of cognitive and motor function results in increased dependency (Lloyd-Williams and Payne 2002; Abbey 2003; Chang *et al.* 2005). Although strategic developments emphasize the shift away from an overt cancer agenda (Commonwealth Department of Health and Ageing 2004; World Health Organization 2002) the case of dementia highlights the ongoing debate about whom palliative care is really intended? Services for people with dementia remain fragmented and scant (Brodaty *et al.* 2003; Shega *et al.* 2003; Bayer 2006). Lack of a clear trajectory towards death and the implicit burden on already stretched palliative care resources, in addition to a perceived knowledge deficit in determining the care needs of a dementia patient (as opposed to a cancer patient, for example) are often cited as reasons for the failure to include this group in a palliative care brief (Ahronheim *et al.* 2000; Schuster 2000; Connolly 2001; Kirchhoff 2002). However, the burden experienced by the family and carer of a person with dementia is known to have a significant impact on their health, social well-being, and financial status (Ory *et al.* 1999; Albinsson and Strang 2003). There are concerted efforts to highlight the palliative care needs of this group of patients. The concept of *end-stage dementia* (ESD) implies that palliative care has something concrete to offer in terms of symptom management and care (Chang *et al.* 2005; McQuillan 2006; Formiga *et al.* 2007). Studies demonstrate the clinical and social importance of understanding the unique perspective that dementia brings to the palliative care agenda (Evans 2002; Froggatt 2006; Mitchell *et al.* 2007). Key among these is being able to interpret needs appropriately when normal cues used by professionals to gauge the effectiveness of their intervention are absent due to cognitive frailty. ESD also raises two issues for the delivery of palliative care. The first is the prevalence of dementia patients in nursing and residential homes, outside the scope of the inpatient palliative care services and as such, unlikely to seek or receive admission. Second is a lack of education and training in appropriate end-of-life care skills for carers in non-specialist settings. Both aged care and acute care nursing staff lack basic knowledge around pain management and dealing with death and dying for older people (Moss *et al.* 2002). Educational interventions can significantly improve carer's ability to provide cohesive and comprehensive care planning and families ability to cope in complex care situations (Evans 2002; Froggatt and Hoult 2002; Albinsson and Strang 2003). Jack's case cited above is a clear example of how education can lead to a positive outcome for dementia patients. The rationale behind referral to the hospice had been motivated by a need to seek transfer, rather than any innate desire to increase knowledge in order to provide better care. However, the intervention of the home care team and the establishment of a short teaching programme on 1 day per week in addition to Home care support visits meant that staff were increasingly empowered to attend to Jack's management in a proactive way. Liaison between the nursing home and the home care team meant that telephone support was often sufficient to enable staff to confirm their decisions about Jack's needs and the appropriate action to take. Even when complex changes were proposed, such as the introduction of percutaneous gastrostomy, the nursing home was keen to retain his care within the home, rather than transfer to hospital. Jack died in the nursing home, supported by the home care team, GP, and community nursing service.

Key issues in dementia care

◆ Older people are likely to experience marginal care because of their age.
◆ Dementia is an important issue at end-of-life but patients are often denied access to the benefits of a palliative care service.
◆ The burden of family caring for a person with dementia cannot be underestimated.
◆ Education is key to improving access and management of end-stage dementia.

The end-of-life needs of people in prison

Mark is a 58-year-old man, currently serving 25 years in prison for armed robbery and aggravated assault. His diagnosis of lung cancer and cerebral metastases was confirmed 1 year ago and despite two course of chemotherapy, his prognosis is extremely poor. He is currently in the prison infirmary following an exacerbation of breathlessness and back pain. The palliative care team were invited to offer consultation. Mark's wife has petitioned for compassionate leave for Mark to be allowed to return home for his final days.

There is remarkably little written about the palliative care needs of people in prison. Maddocks (2004) describes prisoners with advanced disease as a truly marginalized population. Estimates suggest that the UK has the second highest rate of prisoners per capita in Europe (Elkins and Olugundoye 2001). Rold (2002) considers that the care and treatment given to prisoners at end-of-life is a reflection of the moral standing of a society and the dying prisoner is entitled to humane care, irrespective of the reasons for their incarceration.

An opposing argument would suggest that the purpose of incarceration is to correct errant behaviour through segregation and punishment (Dubler 1998; Byock 2002). The prison population demonstrate higher risk factors in terms of health and well-being. There is an increased incidence of drug abuse and therefore HIV/AIDS (Carvell and Hart 1990; Jeanmonod *et al.* 1991; Turnbull *et al.* 1993). Up to 75% of inmates have a history of chronic alcohol dependency, may age faster in physiological terms than people in the non-prison population and be susceptible to health problems often associated with chronic disease (Bick 2002). The structure of prison life divides family cohesion and relationships can breakdown, leaving the prisoner isolated and without external social support.

Colleran and O'Síorán (2006) highlight the following as key issues of the complexity of palliative care provision in the prison system:

◆ Many prisons lack the infrastructure to care for dying inmates.

◆ The focus may be on extending life as far as possible as the death of an inmate can pose a threat to prison security (Dubler 1998).

◆ Compassionate release to allow the prisoner can be a lengthy bureaucratic procedure (Lum 2004).

◆ Prison security measures such as 'lock-down' and the use of physical restraints mitigate against the ideal of death with dignity.

◆ Palliative caring can be limited by restricted access to the prison hospitals and medication and the continuing presence of prison officers by the patient bedside on 'bedwatch' (Finlay 1998; Lum 2004; Maddocks 2004).

Physical restraint of prisoners at end-of-life is a topical issue. Byock (2002) identifies that more than 2500 US inmates are manacled at the time of death. Finlay (1998) reports on a prisoner's experience of end-of-life care, where restraint became the subject of media debate. Restraint depends on the nature of the crime and the risk to the population. In the UK, prisoners are categorized from A (high risk) to D (low risk). Continual liaison between the palliative care team and the prison service is needed to ensure that the dignity and appropriate treatment are afforded to the patient in the most appropriate manner. Both the palliative care team and prison service have a duty of care towards the prisoner, the latter having an additional duty of safe custody. This includes discretion in supervising the dying prisoner.

Yampolskya and Winston (2003) have determined both the components and outcomes of best practice in US prison hospice services. Most institutions offered spiritual and psychological counselling to dying prisoners, a relaxation of visitation rules for families and the use of trusted inmates to act as volunteers to be with the dying person. The degree of support to the family, particularly in the bereavement phase was variable. Given the nature of incarceration, and the separation and isolation experienced by both prisoner and family, this would appear to be an area in need of redress.

The management of prisoners at the end-of-life is a multifaceted concept that warrants careful consideration on how best to match the palliative team skills to patient need. Maul's (1991) description of the prison environment as one of distrust and despair, juxtaposes the essence of palliative care as a cohesive and supportive network for all at the end-of-life. Palliative care practitioners need to practise their craft out of the defined ethical frameworks that govern best practice, different to non-clinical professionals. Confidentiality and sharing of information may have a very different meaning for a palliative care physician and a prison governor. In Mark's case, a twofold approach was needed: one to direct clinical management in the prison setting and the other to support the family in their struggle to obtain a compassionate release for him. Given his crime, home release was unlikely and the hospice was suggested as an alternative place of care, following agreement with the hospice management team. However, in Ireland, formal policies for this do not exist and the extended delay in organizing release meant that Mark died in prison before the release could be sanctioned.

Key issues in caring for people in prison at end-of-life

- ◆ The needs of prisoners is multifaceted and complex.
- ◆ Family and prisoner work involves addressing issues of despair, loss, and isolation.
- ◆ Bureaucracy can impact on the reality of palliative care service delivery.
- ◆ Mutual dialogue between the clinical team and the prison service is essential.
- ◆ The clinician's duty of care may exceed the containment and segregation requirements of the prison services and should be explicit at the outset.

The needs of patients with chemical dependency

Mary is 35-year-old woman with an astrocytoma grade IV, which has left her with a left-sided hemiparesis. She has a long-standing history of heroin and alcohol addiction and has been supported by community addiction services and her local mental health team. She lives alone, but has some family support from her own siblings some of whom are themselves in rehabilitation programmes or known addicts. Transfer to the hospice is imminent. Mary has two children in the care of social services who only have had limited contact with their mother and are currently fostered.

Chemical dependency and substance abuse is defined as an uncontrollable situation that results in adverse legal, health, and social consequences (Diagnostic and Statistical Manual for Mental Disorders, DSM-IV). In this case, we focus on heroin and alcohol addiction in one cancer patient. Bruera *et al.* (1995) estimated that over 25% of patients admitted to a palliative care unit had alcohol addiction problems. Evident in addiction is an internal struggle between the 'high' of elation as effected and the isolation, loneliness, and depression of a life-seeking procurement of the drug, notwithstanding the trauma of withdrawal and rejection by family and society at large (Kirsch and Passik 2006).

Mary's case raises a number of issues. How can her children be reincorporated into her end-of-life care plan and is that possible? How do a palliative care team work with substance abuse at a family level and where do the boundaries overlap with other services? Even the language of palliative care may need to be adapted. Concepts such as physiological dependence and tolerance, which are clearly understood in palliative care terms may hold different meaning for patients and families living with addiction (Kirsch and Passik 2006). Reticence in admitting addicted patients for end-of-life care is due to misconceptions that trying to manage such patients is too complex and intractable (Passik and Theobald 2000).

Passik and Theobald (2000) illustrate through case exemplars the extent to which addiction can impact on palliative care interventions. They note the deleterious effects of the addiction on the family and carers, the suffering endured by the patient as they fluctuate between their continual need for the 'fix' and the increasing burden to family as symptoms proliferate. The complexities identified include:

- increased suffering for the patient
- increased stress for the family
- difficulties in assessment, particularly the extent of symptom burden
- poor compliance (patient) and fear about prescribing (practitioner).

In addiction, a cancer diagnosis can compound already negative emotions, such as loss of self-worth and hopelessness. A high level of co-morbidity with psychiatric disorders is noted, with up to 85% of addicts having a non-substance-related psychiatric diagnosis (Khantzian and Treece 1985). The continual need to source drugs weakens the already compromised cancer patient and exacerbates symptoms of addiction, such as insomnia and fatigue. This can be then confusing to the palliative care practitioner who may misinterpret symptoms as related to cancer and not the addiction, or vice versa.

The successful transition to palliative care treatment may be best achieved through the construction of some degree of control over a potentially uncontrollable situation (Passik and Portenoy 1998). Again, this may be dependent on the type and depth of addiction. Support of a multidisciplinary team, supplemented by specialist workers in addiction counselling or addiction work will help to create a cohesive plan of care that meets the patient and family need. The impact on the family is such that a clear understanding of the existent family dynamic is essential before care is proposed. The dynamic of the family and the relations between members, including dependency and co-dependencies need to be identified. The family may harbour resentment, guilt, anger, or fear, which inhibit their ability to receive help and be a part of the care plan offered. They may clearly not wish to be part of the care team but find it difficult to move away from the situation. Families may have fears over the use of certain medications and specific safeguards may be necessary to ensure that drugs are safely managed outside the hospice setting. Palliative care staff have an educational role with families to enable them to understand the differences between dependence and addiction. Further, practitioners need to respond to families at the physical and emotional point in which they find themselves, which warrants specific supports for the practitioner. Families who are 'burnt-out' from living with an addicted family member need to hear that it is possible from them to withdraw from the situation and still play some part in being present to their family member at end-of-life.

As practitioners, key philosophical issues are addressed. For example, how do the goals of addiction 'recovery' fit with a model of palliative care? Patients at end-of-life are not likely to find the personal resources to seek recovery from their addiction and the best that may be achieved is a reduction in use and a satisfactory degree of compliance with a treatment and care protocol. Patients and families need to believe that their suffering can be supported and that pain does not have to be a necessary part of living. The safe surroundings of a hospice or similar environment may be protective to the family and patient, or in contrast, viewed as restrictive, as access to the drug is limited. Naturally, the decision to admit a patient with an addiction problem is a point of negotiation for the inpatient and community teams. As trust is a key determinant of how far a programme of care in addiction is successful, there is a need to focus on goals of stability and reorientation, which may prevent disturbing an already fragile existence and equilibrium.

Mary's initial needs were clearly based around the need to provide a regimen of sound symptom management, which kept her pain-free in order for her to address the psychosocial needs in her life, such as child care after her death. The complexity of addiction in other members of her family meant that stringent protocols were put in place to enable access in a controlled fashion. Ground rules were laid, including the fact that any member who came to the hospice under the influence of drugs would not be admitted. Initial staff fears over theft of drugs were unfounded as the medication room was not accessible to the public. Mary was able to be part of discussions with social services over the future care of her children and although a planned visit from the children was not fulfilled, she died peacefully 6 weeks after admission.

Key issues in addiction

- A clear understanding of how team members values around addiction is important.
- Symptom management can be complicated but possible, given flexibility.
- Families may not be willing or able to act in that capacity for the patient any longer.
- Addiction is about suffering and a palliative care response must encompass the context of suffering endured by the patient with dependency.

The needs of ethnic minority communities

Jean-Paul is a 38-year-old asylum seeker recently arrived in the country. Originally from Sierre Leone, he has applied for refugee status and is awaiting the outcome of this decision. Jean-Paul was unwell on arrival and diagnosed with an invasive carcinoma of the large bowel. He is also HIV positive. Following surgery, it was evident that further treatment options were limited. Jean-Paul speaks only French and some Portuguese. His wife and daughter remain in Sierre Leone and he has had no contact with them for the last 3 months. He was living in a hostel for refugees and asylum seekers until an exacerbation of his disease precipitated a hospital admission and now decisions need to be made regarding his place of care for his end-of-life management.

Concepts such as race, ethnicity, and culture lack definition, are largely immeasurable, problematic, and contradictory (Coker 2001; Koffman and Higginson 2001; Koffman 2006). British data suggest that black and ethnic minority communities are less likely to avail of palliative care services than white people (Haroon-Iqbal *et al.* 1995; Smaje and Field 1997; Spruyt 1999; Karim *et al.* 2000; Koffman and Higginson 2001). This has been attributed, in part, to a lower incidence of cancer in the black and ethnic minority population and a younger socio-demographic profile (Balarajan and Raleigh 1993). More recently, an ethos of mistrust is reported to play a part in the health decision-making of black and ethnic minority groups (Cort 2004). How far palliative care is culturally acceptable, is debatable (Bonifant 2000). Racial prejudice has also been noted in healthcare encounters (Gerrish *et al.* 1996; Koffman and Higginson 2001). From the professional perspective, little is known about their experience of caring for ethnic minority groups. One study suggests that the inability to communicate because of language barriers was a significant problem (Richardson *et al.* 2006). Professional staff needed to avoid erroneous assumptions about beliefs or behaviours.

There are notable differences of definition between the terms refugee and asylum seeker, which may impact on their ability to access services. The 1951 Geneva Convention dictates the terms under which countries offer asylum to people and the definition offered here is based upon a UK interpretation of terms and may differ across other jurisdictions. Refugees are those who have indefinite leave to stay within the country and may seek permanent residence. Asylum seekers have made application to remain in the country and are waiting for an official decision to be made (Burnett and Peel 2001; Burnett and Fassil 2002). In the UK, there are an estimated 250 000 people who fit within the category of refugee or asylum seeker. This is a conservative estimate as the transient nature of refugee life makes assessments unpredictable and difficult to develop healthcare services that are accessible and sustainable, including palliative care (Bardsley and Storkey 2000; Koffman and Camps 2004).

The case described here is somewhat unique as there is limited exposure to a process of acculturation in Ireland, i.e. the blend into the existing society over time. Palliative care practitioners must adapt their care to patients who are still immersed in their home culture with little, if any, understanding of the society in which they are now living. Immigration has had a significant impact on the legislature, including legal challenges to citizenship and residency, which only serve to enhance the sense of displacement felt by those people living in the refugee/asylum seeker vacuum (Fanning and Mutwarasibo 2007).

Refugees and asylum seekers exhibit a range of health problems associated with social deprivation (Jones and Gill 1998). Clearly of concern is the

HIV/AIDS pandemic and presentation with AIDS-related illnesses, often in advanced stages. HIV patients are more likely to be socially disadvantaged and only present when symptomatic (Brogan and George 1999). In the case of Jean-Paul, the local hospice had limited knowledge and resources to care for a HIV patient, as patients were only treated in tertiary centres.

A recent study from the Netherlands has suggested that refugees felt general practitioners were prejudiced in assuming that their background was always a causative factor in their symptoms. This said, there is increasing evidence that the traumatic experiences faced by refugees and asylum seekers impacts on their mental health, particularly when faced with detention on arrival in the host country (Maffia 2006; Peate and Richens 2006; Australian Human Rights and Equal Opportunity Commission (HREOC) 2007).

Practitioner's lack knowledge and skills needed to effect successful adaptations to refugee care (Richardson *et al.* 2006). Working with interpreters, practical and philosophical differences in culture, racial bias, and the need for training are key concerns for palliative care practitioners (Richardson *et al.* 2006). The problems interpretation is well reported in the literature (Robinson 2002; Randhawa *et al.* 2003). Patients may not understand or misinterpret the seriousness of their illness. Literacy can be a problem and the use of family interpreters has been considered unsatisfactory (Cox *et al.* 2002), especially if a child is involved. Professional interpreters may also have limited supports to de-brief from the emotional effort of having to deal with people's distress. Important decisions may be made by senior family members and not the patient. Cultural differences may impact on how care is viewed and relate to personal biases and unconscious judgements, such as an implicit assumption that working with people from ethnic backgrounds is going to be difficult. Opportunities for education and training remain scarce (Gatrad *et al.* 2003) and that which is available often provides global information that fails to capture the key case-specific communication strategies.

There is a call for a compassionate approach that transcends stereotypes (Molassiotis 2004; Richardson 2004). Education around cultural diversity needs to embrace eclectic methods of experiential learning, which focus on learning about personal attitudes and beliefs, as well as those of the different culture. Culturally specific knowledge can open dialogue between the patient and professional. Misplaced assumptions that a general understanding is enough usually closes that dialogue (Kemp 2005). There are important questions raised for the palliative care practitioner. How far are/can the family be involved? Does everyone understand the process clearly? Is talk about death culturally acceptable? What is the meaning of death and dying and how can the body be best respected after death? The development of cultural competence embraces dimensions of knowledge, experience, and the willing-ness to explore further (Davidhizar and Giger 2004; Doorenboos and Schim 2004; Lyke and Colón 2004). In the case of Jean-Paul, the decision about this place of care was resolved by a sudden deterioration in his health, which meant that the hospice was the only option in terms of their expertise to care for him. Two French-speaking nurses from the local district hospital were identified and willing to provide interpretation where required, usually when key decisions needed to be made. The experience was sufficiently positive that one of these nurses later transferred to the hospice. Social workers sought advice on making links with the Sierre Leone community but were advised to be sure that Jean-Paul wished to meet others from this community as there were always risks involved. Jean-Paul did not want to meet members of his own community and although his wishes were respected, it raised certain anomalies in the story given for his asylum status. Jean-Paul died in the care of the hospice 3 weeks after admission but before his refugee status was finally decided.

Conclusions

In this chapter, a number of possible scenarios have been explored that exem-plify the complexities of providing palliative care to patients who either consider themselves, or are considered to be, marginalized. There are initia-tives to address ways in which to provide palliative care services for the disen-franchised, often based on accessing charitable funding (Gibson 2001). For palliative care practitioners, the need to become 'contextually educated' would be an important factor in how patients such as those described here are supported in their final illness. Contextual education implies that textbook materials are only useful as resources for knowledge and not definitive guides to practice. Each case will be significant and unique and should open the opportunities for multiagency working. This requires that palliative care is clearly able to demonstrate how it can contribute to this complex situation, so to prevent transition to palliative care being seen as a last resort for a hopeless case. Neither can it be assumed that palliative care can provide all the resources to cater for such a wide and disparate group of people and again, the bound-aries of practice need to be clearly defined at the outset so that all, including the patient and family, understand what care is available to them.

References

Abbey J (2003). Ageing, dementia and palliative care. In: O'Connor, M, Aranda, S (ed.). *Palliative care nursing, a guide to practice*. Ausmed Publications, Australia, pp. 329–40.

Addington-Hall J (2000). *Positive partnerships: palliative care for adults with severe mental health problems*. London: National Council for Hospices and Specialist Palliative Care Services.

Ahronheim J, Morrison R, Morris J, Baskin S, Meter D (2000). Palliative care in advanced dementia: a randomized controlled trial and descriptive analysis. *J Palliat Med* 3:265–73.

Albinsson L, Strang P (2003). Differences in supporting families of dementia patients and cancer patients: a palliative perspective. *Palliat Med* 17:359–67.

American Society of Clinical Oncology (1998). Cancer care during the last phase of life. *J Clin Oncol* 16:1986–96.

Anderson DG (2001). Families of origin of homeless and never-homeless women. *West J Nurs Res* 23:394–413.

Anderson DG, Rayens MK (2004). Factors influencing homelessness in women. *Public Health Nurs* 21:2–23.

Australian Human Rights and Equal Opportunity Commission [HREOC] (2007). Detention worsens mental health. *Aust Nurs J* 14(8):7.

Balarajan R, Raleigh V (1993). *Ethnicity and health: a guide for the NHS*. London: Department of Health.

Bardsley M, Storkey M (2000). Estimating the numbers of refugees in London. *J Public Health Med* 22(3):406–12.

Bayer A (2006). Death with dementia—the need for better care. *Age Ageing* 35:101–2.

Beange H, McElduff A, Baker W (1995). Medical disorders of adults with mental retardation:a population study. *Am J Ment Retard* 99:595–604.

Bick JA (2002). Managing pain and end-of-life care for inmate patients: the California Medical Facility experience. *J Correctional Health Care* 9:131–47.

Blackman N (2006). Supporting bereaved people with intellectual disabilities. *Eur J Palliat Care* 12(6):247–8.

Bohn U, Wright LM, Moules NJ (2003). A family systems nursing interview following a myocardial infarction. The power of commendations. *J Fam Nurs* 9(2):151–65.

Bonifant J (2000). Palliative care—a universal discipline? *Prog Palliat Care* 8:351–3.

Brodaty H, Draper B, Low L (2003). Behavioural and psychological symptoms of dementia:a seven tiered model of service delivery. *Med J Aust* 179 (Suppl. 6):526–8.

Brogan G, George R (1999). HIV/AIDS: symptoms and the impact of new treatments. *Palliat Med* 1(4):104–10.

Bruera E, Moyano J, Seifert L, *et al*. (1995). The frequency of alcoholism among patients with pain due to terminal cancer. *J Pain Symptom Manage* 10:599.

Burnett A, Fassil Y (2002). *Meeting the health needs of refugees and asylum seekers in the U.K: an information and resource pack for health workers*. London: Department of Health.

Burnett A, Peel M (2001). What brings asylum seekers to the United Kingdom? *BMJ* 322:485–8.

Byock I (2002). Dying well in corrections:why should we care? *J Correctional Health Care* 9:107–17.

Carvell AL, Hart GI (1990). Risk behaviours for HIV infection among drug users in prison. *BMJ* 300:1383–4.

Chang E, Hancock K, Harrison K, Daly J *et al*. (2005). Palliative care for end-stage dementia: a discussion of the implications for education of health care professionals. *Nurs Educ Today* 25:326–32.

Chesla CA (2005). Nursing science and chronic illness:Articulating suffering and possibility in family life. *J Fam Nurs* 11(4):371–87.

Coker EM (2004). 'Traveling pains':embodied metaphors of suffering among Southern Sudanese refuges in Cairo. *Culture Med Psychaitry* 28:15–39.

Colleran M, O'Síoráin L (2006). Providing palliative care for prisoners. *Eur J Palliat Care* 13(6):257–9.

Commonwealth Department of Health and Ageing (2004). *Guidelines for a palliative approach to residential aged care*. Canberra: Commonwealth Department of Health and Ageing.

Connolly M (2001). The disadvantaged dying: care of people with non-malignant conditions. In: Kinghorn S, Gamlin R (ed.). *Palliative nursing, bringing comfort and hope*. Edinburgh: Baillière Tindall.

Cooke L (1997). Cancer and learning disability. *J Intellect Disabil Res* 41(4):312–16.

Cort MA (2004). Cultural mistrust and use of hospice care: challenges and remedies. *J Palliat Med* 7:63–71.

Cox CL, Leahey G, Malik F (2002). Counting the cost of cultural diversity. Final report of the bilingual and interpretation research project. City University: Health Care Research Unit.

Cumella S, Martin D (2000). *Secondary healthcare for people with a learning disability*. London: Department of Health.

Cutcliffe JR, Black C, Hanson E, Goward P (2001a). The commonality and synchronicity of mental health nurses and palliative care nurses: closer than you think? *J Psychiatric Ment Health Nurs* 8:53–9.

Cutcliffe JR, Black C, Hanson E, Goward P (2001b). The commonality and synchronicity of mental health nurses and palliative care nurses: closer than you think? *J Psychiatric Ment Health Nurs* 8:61–6.

Davidizhar R, Giger JN (2004). A review of the literature on care of clients in pain who are culturally diverse. *Int Nurs Rev* 51:47–55.

Davies E, Higginson I (ed.) (2004). *Better palliative care for older people*. Geneva: World Health Organization.

Department of Health (2001). Seeking consent: working with people with learning disabilities. London: Department of Health.

Duggleby W, Raudonis BM (2006). Dispelling myths about palliative care and older adults. *Semin Oncol Nurs* 22:58–64.

Department of Health (2001). *Valuing people: a new strategy for learning disability for the 21st century*. A White Paper. London: Department of Health.

Doorenbos AZ, Schim SM. Cultural competence in hospice. *Am J Hospice Palliat Care* 21:28–32.

Dowling S, Hubert J, Hollins S (2003). Bereavement interventions for people with learning disabilities. *Bereavement Care* 9:8–15.

Duhamel F, Talbot LR (2004). A constructivist evaluation of family systems nursing interventions with families experiencing cardiovascular and cerebrovascular illness. *J Fam Nurs* 10:12–32.

Dubler NN (1998). The collusion of confinement and care: end-of-life care in prisons and jails. *J Law Med Ethics* 26:149–56.

Egan KA, Labyak MJ (2001). Hospice care:a model for quality end-of-life care. In: Ferrell BT, Coyle N (ed.), *Textbook of palliative nursing*. Oxford: Oxford University Press, pp. 7–26.

Elkins M, Olugundoye D (2001). *The prison population in 2000: a statistical review.* London: The Home Office.

Evans B (2002). Improving palliative care in the nursing home: from a dementia perspective. *J Hospice Palliat Nurs* 4:91–9.

Fanning B, Mutwarasibo F (2007). Nationals/non-nationals: immigration, citizenship and politics in the Republic of Ireland. *Ethnic Racial Stud* 30(3):439–60.

Finlay I (1998). Managing terminally ill prisoners: reflection and action. *Palliat Med* 12:457–61.

Formiga F, Olmedo C, López-Soto A, Navarro M *et al.* (2007). Dying in hospital of terminal heart failure or severe dementia: the circumstances associated with death and the opinions of caregivers. *Palliat Med* 21:35–40.

Froggatt K (2006). A survey of end of life care in care homes: issues of definition and practice. *Health Soc Care Community* 14:341–8.

Froggatt K, Hoult L (2002). Developing palliative care practice in nursing and residential care homes: the role of the clinical nurse specialist. *J Clin Nurs* 11:802–8.

Garssen B (2004). Psychological factors and cancer development: evidence after 30 years of research. *Clin Psychol Rev* 24:315–38.

Gatrad A, Brown E, Sheikh A (2003). Palliative care needs of minorities. Understanding their needs is key. *BMJ* 327:176–7.

Geissler L, Bormann CA, Kwiatkowski CF, Braucht GN, Reichardt CS (1995). Women, homelessness and substance abuse:moving beyond the stereotypes. *Psychol Women Q* 19:65–83.

Gerrish K, Husband C, Mackenzie J (1996). *Nursing for a multi-ethnic society.* Buckingham: Open University Press.

Gerritsen AAM, Bramsen I, Devillé W, van Willigen LHM, Hovens JE, van der Ploeg HM (2006). Use of health care services by Afghan, Iranian, and Somali refugees and asylum seekers living in the Netherlands. *Eur J Public Health* 16(4):394–9.

Gibson R (2001). Palliative care for the poor and disenfranchised: a view from the Robert Wood Johnson Foundation. *J R Soc Med* 94:486–9.

Grande GE, Addington-Hall JM, Todd CJ (1998). Place of death and access to home care services: are certain patient groups at a disadvantage? *Soc Sci Med* 47(5):565–79.

Haroon-Iqbal H, Field D, Parker H, Iqbal Z (1995). Palliative care for ethnic groups in Leicester. *Int J Pallat Nurs* 1:114–16.

Higginson I (1993). Palliative care: a review of past changes and future trends. *J Public Health Med* 15:3–8.

Hollins S, Attard MT, von Fraunhofer N, McGuigan S, Sedgwick P (1998). Mortality in people with learning disability: risks, causes, and death certification findings in London. *Dev Med Child Neurol* 40:50–6.

Hoptof M, Chidgey J, Addiongton-Hall J, Lan Ly K (2002). Depression in advanced disease: a systematic review. Part 1: prevalence and case finding. *Palliat Med* 16:81–97.

Howells G (1997). A general practice perspective. In: O'Hara J, Sperlinger A (ed.). *Adults with learning disabilities: a practical approach for health professionals.* Chichester: John Wiley and Sons, pp. 61–79.

Institute for Family Centered Care (2005). Family Centered Care, questions and answers. Institute for Family Centered Care, Bethesda. Maryland. Available at http://www.familycentered-care.org/pdf/fcc_qa.pdf

Jacquemin D (2006). Caring for people with learning difficulties. *Eur J Palliat Care* 12(6):249–50.

Jancar J (1990). Cancer and mental handicap:a further study. *Br J Psychiatry* 156:531–3.

Jancar J (1993). Consequences of a longer life for the mentally handicapped. *Am J Ment Retard* 98(2):285–2.

Jeanmonod R, Harding T, Staub C (1991). Treatment of opiate withdrawal on entry to prison, *Br J Addict* 86:457–63.

Jones D, Gill PS (1998). Refugees and primary care: tackling the inequalities. *BMJ* 317:1444–6.

Kang M, Alperstein G, Dow A, Van Beek I, Martin C, Bennett D (2000). Prevalence of tuberculosis infection among homeless young people in central and eastern Sydney. *J Paediatr Child Health* 36:382–4.

Karim K, Bailey M, Tunna K (2000). Nonwhite ethnicity and the provision of specialist palliative care services:factors affecting doctors' referral patterns. *Palliat Med* 14, 471–478.

Kastnerm T, Nathanson R, Friedman D (1993). Mortality among individuals with mental retardation living in the community. *Am J Ment Retard* 98:285–92.

Keenan P, McIntosh P (2000). Learning disabilities and palliative care. *Palliative Care Today* 9(3):11–13.

Kemp C (2005). Cultural issues in palliative care. *Semin Oncol Nurs* 21:44–52.

Keywood K, Forvargue S, Flynn M (1999). *Best practice? Health care decision making by, with and for adults with learning disabilities.* Manchester: National Development Team.

Khantzian EJ, Treece C (1985). DSM-III psychiatric diagnosis of narcotic addicts. *Arch Gen Psychiatry* 42:1067–72.

Kirchoff M (2002). Lack of knowledge and training affects quality of hospice care for persons with dementia. *Am J Hospice Palliat Care* 19:372.

Kirsch KL, Passik SD (2006). Palliative care of the terminally ill drug addict. *Cancer Invest* 24(4):425–31.

Koffman J (2006). The language of diversity:controversies relevant to palliative care research. *Eur J Palliat Care* 13:18–21.

Koffman J, Camps M (2004). No way in. Including the excluded at the end of life In: Payne S, Seymour J, Ingleton C (ed.). *Palliative care nursing principles and evidence for practice.* Bucks: Open University Press, pp. 364–84.

Koffman J, Higginson IJ (2001). Accounts of carers' satisfaction with health care at the end of life: a comparison of first generation black Caribbeans and white patients with advanced disease. *Palliat Med* 15(4):337–45.

Lawrie I, Lloyd-Williams M, Taylor F (2004). How do palliative medicine physicians assess and manage depression. *Palliat Med* 18:234–8.

Lee BA, Spratlen-Price T, Kanan JW (2003). Determinants of homelessness in metropolitan areas. *J Urban Affairs* 25:335–56.

Limacher L, Wright, LM (2003). Commendations:Listening to the silent side of a family intervention. *J Fam Nurs* 9(2):130–50.

Lloyd-Williams M, Payne S (2002). Can multidisciplinary guidelines improve the palliation of symptoms in the terminal phase of dementia? *Int J Palliat Nurs* 8:370–5.

Lloyd-Willams M, Payne S (2003). A qualitative study of palliative care nurses' perceptions on depression. *Palliat Med* 17:334–9.

Lloyd-Williams M, Dennis M, Taylor F (2004). A prospective study to compare three depression screening tools in patients who are terminally ill. *Gen Hosp Psychiatry* 26:384–9.

Luddington L, Cox S, Higginson I, Livesley B (2001). The need for palliative care for patients with non-cancer diseases: a review of the evidence. *Int J Palliat Nurs* 7:221–6.

Lum KL (2004). Palliative care behind bars: the New Zealand prison hospice experience. In: Rajagopal MR, Mazza D, Lipman AG (ed.). *Pain and palliative care in the developing world and marginalized populations: a global challenge.* New York: Haworth Press Inc.

Lundberg JC, Passik SD (1998). Alcoholism and cancer. In: Holland JC (ed.) *Psycho-oncology.* New York: Oxford University Press, pp. 587–94.

Lyke J, Colón M (2004). Practical recommendations for ethnically and racially sensitive hospice services. *Am J Hospice Palliat Care* 21:131–3.

Luckasson R, Coulter DL, Polloway EA, Reiss S *et al.* (1992). *Mental retardation: definition, classification and systems of supports.* Washington: American Association of Mental Retardation.

Maddocks I (2004). Commentary: prisoners with advanced disease—a truly marginalized population. *J Pain Palliat Care Pharmacother* 17(3/4):139–40.

Maffia C (2006). The mental health of asylum seeking men. *Ment Health Nurs* 26(3):16–17.

Maull F (1991). Dying in prison: sociocultural and psychosocial dynamics. *Hospice Journal* 7: 127–142.

McNamara B (2001). *Fragile lives: death denying and care.* Buckingham: Open University Press.

McCormack P, Sharp DMM (2006). Palliative care for people with mental health problems. *Eur J Palliat Care* 13:198–201.

McQuillan R (2006). An exploration of the end-of-life needs of dementia patients: palliative perspectives. *J Palliat Care* 22:215.

Mertens A, Wen W, Davies S, Steinbuch M *et al.* (1998). Congenital abnormalities in children with acute leukaemia: a report from the Children's Cancer Group. *J Pediatr* 133:617–23.

Meyer HAM, Sinnott C, Seed PT (2003). Depressive symptoms in advanced cancer. Part 2. Depression over time; the role of the palliative care professional. *Palliat Med* 17:604–7.

Miki M, Ohtake N, Hasumi M, Ohi M *et al.* (1999). Seminoma associated with bilateral cryptorchidism in Down's Syndrome: a case report. *Int J Urol* 6:377–80.

Mitchell SL, Teno JM, Intrato O, Feng ZL *et al.* (2007). Decisions to forego hospitalization in advanced dementia: a nationwide study. *J Am Geriatr Soc* 55:432–8.

Molassiotis A (2004). Supportive and palliative care for patients for ethnic minorities in Europe: do we suffer from institutional racism? (Editorial). *Eur J Oncol Nurs* 8:290–2.

Moss M, Braunschweig H, Rubenstein R (2002). Terminal care for nursing home residents with dementia (ethics). *Alzheimer's Care Q* 3:233–49.

Muir-Chochrane E, Fereday J, Junedini J, Drummond A, Darbyshire P (2006). Self-management of medication for mental health problems by homeless young people. *Int J Ment Health Nurs* 15:163–70.

National Institute for Clinical Excellence (2004). *Supportive and palliative care services for adults with cancer: understanding NICE Guidance—information for adults with cancer, their families and carers and the public.* London: National Institute for Clinical Excellence.

Northfield J, Turnbull J (2001). Experiences from cancer services. In: Hogg J, Northfield J, Turnbull J (ed.). *Cancer and people with learning disabilties: the evidence from published studies and experiences from cancer services*. Kidderminster: BILD Publications, pp. 39–56.

O'Neill J. (1994) Ethnic minorities—neglected by palliative care providers? *J Cancer Care* 3:215–20.

O'Neill J, Marconi K (2001). Access to palliative care in the USA: why emphasize vulnerable populations? *J R Soc Med* 94:452–4.

O'Neill J, Akhter M, Poliquin L (2002). Terminally ill offenders: an international dialogue. *J Correctional Health Care* 9:119–24.

O'Rawe AM, Tehan C (ed.). (1991). *AIDS and the hospice community*. New York: Haworth Press Inc.

Ory M, Hoffman R, Yee J, Tennsedt S, Schultz R (1999). Prevalence and impact of caregiving: a detailed comparison between dementia and nondementia caregivers. *Gerontologist* 39:177–85.

Passik SD, Portenoy RK (1998). Substance abuse disorders, In: Holland JC (ed.). *Psychooncology*. New York: Oxford University Press, pp. 576–86.

Passik SD, Theobald DE (2000). Managing addiction in advanced cancer patients: why bother? *J Pain Symptom Manage* 19(3):229–34.

Patja K, Eero P, Iivanainen M (2001). Cancer incidence among people with intellectual disability. *J Intellect Disabil Res* 45:300–7.

Peate I, Richens Y (2006). Bring a male refugee or asylum seeker. *Pract Nurs* 17(12):602–4.

Pollio DE (1997). The relationship between transience and current life situation in the homeless services-using population. *Soc Work* 42:541–551.

Praill D (2000). Editorial: Who are we here for? *Palliat Med* 14:91–2.

Randhawa G, Owens A, Fitches R, Khan Z (2003). Communication in the development of culturally competent palliative care services in the UK: a case study. *Int J Palliat Nurs* 9:24–31.

Raji O, Hollins S (2001). Exclusion for funerary rituals and mourning: implications for social and individual identity. In: Hubert J (ed.). *Madness, disability and social exclusion: the archeology and anthropology of difference*. London: BILD Publications.

Richardson A (2004). Creating a culture of compassion:developing supportive care for people with cancer. *Eur J Oncol Nurs* 8:293–305.

Richardson A, Thomas VN, Richardson A (2006). 'Reduced to nods and smiles': experiences of professionals caring for people with cancer from black and ethnic minority groups. *Eur J Oncol Nurs* 10:93–101.

Robinson JA, Crawford GB (2005). Identifying palliative care patients with symptoms of depression: an algorithm. *Palliat Med* 19:278–87.

Robinson M (2002). *Communication and health in a multi-ethnic society*. Bristol: Policy Press.

Rold WJ (2002). Introduction. *J Correctional Health Care* 9:103–5.

Rowe S, Wolch J (1990). Social networks in time and space:homeless women in skid row, Los Angeles. *An Assoc Am Geog* 80:184–204.

Saunders CM, Clark D (2002). *Cicely Saunders: founder of the hospice movement: selected letters 1959–1999*. Buckingham: Open University Press.

Schuster J (2000). Palliative care for advanced dementia. *Clin Geriatr Med* 17:377–91.

Seale C, Cartwright A (1994). *The year before death*. Brookfield, VT, Ashgate.

Seymour JE (2005). Using technology to help obtain the goals of palliative care. *Int J Palliat Nurs* 11:240–1.

Shega J, Levin A, Hougham G, Cox-Hayley D *et al.* (2003). Palliative excellence in Alzheimer care efforts (PEACE): a program description. *J Palliat Med* 6:315–20.

Skilbeck JK, Payne S (2005). End of life care:a discourse analysis of specialist palliative care nursing. *J Adv Nurs* 51:325–334.

Smaje C, Field D (1997). Absent minorities? Ethnicity and the use of palliative care services. In: Field D, Hockey J, Small N (ed.). *Death, gender and ethnicity*. London: Routledge.

Spruyt O (1999). Community-based palliative care for Bangladeshi patients in East London. Accounts of bereaved carers. *Palliat Med* 13:119–29.

Stiefel F, Die Trill M, Berney A, Nunez Olarte JM, Razavi D (2001). Depression in palliative care:a pragmatic report from the Expert Working Group of the European Association for Palliative Care. *Supportive Care Cancer* 9:477–88.

Stevens J, McFarlane J, Stirling K (2000). Ageing and dying. In: Kellehear A (ed.). *Death and dying in Australia*. Melbourne: Oxford University Press, pp. 173–89.

Svarvarsdottir EK (2007). Listening to the Family's Voice. Nordic Nurses'Movement Toward Family Centred Care. *J Fam Nurs* 12(4):346–67.

Teunissen SC, de Haes HC, Voest EE, de Graeff A (2006). Does age matter in palliative care? *Crit Rev Oncol/Haematol* 60:152–6.

Thewes B, Butow P, Girgis A, Pedlebury S (2004). The psychosocial needs of breast cancer survivors. A qualitative study of the shared and unique needs of younger versus older survivors. *Psycho-oncology* 13:177–89.

Tickle S (2007). Why we treat patients shunned by others. *Pulse Careers* 69–70.

Titia Feldman C, Bensing JM, de Ruijter A (2007). Worries are the mother of many diseases: general practitioners and refugees in the Netherlands on stress, being ill and prejudice. *Patient Educ Couns* 65:369–80.

Todd S (2004). Death counts:the challenge of death and dying in learning disability service. *Learning Disabil Pract* 7(10):12–15.

Todd S, Read S (2006). Inclusion, exclusion and separation: a short history of death and disability. *J Appl Res Intellect Disabil* 19:252.

Tuffrey-Wijne I (1997). Palliative care and learning disabilities. *Nurs Times* 93(31):50–1.

Tuffrey-Wijne I (1998). Care of the terminally Ill. *Learning Disabil Pract* 1:8–11.

Tuffrey-Wijne I (2002) The palliative care needs of people with learning disabilities: a case study. *Int J Palliat Nurs* 8:222–32.

Tuffrey-Wijne I (2003). The palliative care needs of people with intellectual disabilities: a literature review. *Palliat Med* 17:55–62.

Tuffrey-Wijne I, Bernal J, Jones A, Butler G, Hollins S (2006). People with intellectual disabilities and their need for cancer information. *Eur J Oncol Nurs* 10:106–16.

Turnbull PJ, Dolan KA, Stimson GV (1993). HIV testing and the care and treatment of HIV positive people in English prisons. *AIDS Care* 5:199–206.

Tuma R, DeAngelis LM (2000). Altered mental status in patients with cancer. *Arch Neurol* 57:1727–31.

Van Kleffens T, Van Baarsen B, Hoekman K, Van Leeuwen E (2004). Clarifying the term 'palliative' in clinical oncology. *Eur J Cancer Care (Engl)* 13:263–71.

World Health Organization (2000). WHO International Consortium in Psychiatric Epidemiology. Crossnational comparisons of the relevances and correlates of mental disorders. *Bull WHO* 78:413–25.

World Health Organization (2002). *National Cancer Control Programme: policies and managerial guidelines*, 2nd edn. Geneva: World Health Organization.

Wright LM, Leahey M (2005). *Nurses and families: a guide to family assessment and intervention* (3rd edn). Philadelphia: FA Davis.

Yampolskya S, Winston N (2003). Hospice care in prison:general principles and outcomes. *Am J Hospice Palliat Care* 20:290–6.

Chapter 5

Current provision of psychosocial care within palliative care

Trevor Friedman

Introduction

The recognition of palliative care as a speciality and the increased awareness of its importance in the management of cancer and other serious diseases have led to a general improvement in the management of this group of patients. At the core management by palliative care services has been recognition of the need to manage all areas of patient care to improve quality of life for patients and their families. There is a general recognition that the provision of psychosocial care and the detection and treatment of the range of psychological disorders is of critical importance in improving patient wellbeing.

This chapter will examine the facts behind the increasing understanding that while a level of psychological distress is understandably associated with the diagnosis of cancer there is also a high level of psychiatric morbidity that, if treated, leads to an improvement in a person's state of mind and their quality of life.

The issues for modern palliative care are no longer, hopefully, making the case for the high incidence of psychological morbidity but the way in which services should be organized to address this problem. These issues include those of screening and the tools that should be used for detection and the management of psychological disorders when they are identified. The role of palliative care services compared with those of specialist psychiatric services and primary care and how services should be best organized to meet the needs of these people in palliative care.

There continues to be a scientific debate as to the relationship between distress, depression, and clinical outcome. There is a widely held belief that among patients and many staff that the presence of a depressive disorder has a negative affect on a prognosis, although there is not good scientific evidence to support this. This finding, however, should not affect the need among staff and patients to be able to feel confident in their management of psychosocial disorders.

There remains an important issue as to the diagnosis of depression in palliative care and this is addressed in another chapter in this book. The importance in terms of provision of care is that the definition of depression in particular can range from a narrow definition based upon international psychiatric criteria to a much wider definition based upon levels of patient distress. The range of depressive disorder identified within patient groups in palliative care varies widely and this is often due to difficulties in definition. In designing psychosocial care it is important to decide upon thresholds and definitions for levels of psychological morbidity and the appropriate interventions required depending upon the different levels and modes of presentation. This is of course particularly in the case where there are limited resources and services have to decide how best to manage these resources to produce the most appropriate benefit.

The nature and prevalence of psychological distress

There is always a particular issue in people with serious or terminal diseases following a diagnosis or changes in their condition where there is acute distress. A decision has to be made between what can be described as normal adjustment disorders, which although distressing and affecting functioning are felt to be proportionate and reasonable, as opposed to reactions that are felt to be pathological and indicative of depression or other disorders in that the response is disproportionate, overwhelming, and too distressing. These latter conditions require some form of intervention.

The prevalence of depression within palliative care varies depending upon the stage of disease, setting, and who is being studied. The range in reported studies varies from 4% to 58% (Swire et al. 1997). In those inpatients with physical impairment at least a quarter of the patients with advanced cancer have treatable depressive illness although probably only a minority of patients receive appropriate pharmacological treatment. There are a number of factors that are well reported relating to the reasons why patients do not report distress and the reasons why staff failed to identify queues indicating the presence of psychological distress.

An early American study, Derogatis et al. (1983) investigated the prevalence of psychiatric disorders in 215 randomly selected adult cancer patients with varying types and stages of disease. As many as 47% of these patients were suffering from a diagnosable psychiatric disorder according to standardized criteria. Approximately 68% of the psychiatric diagnoses consisted of adjustment disorders, with 13% representing major affective disorders. It is important to note that almost 90% of the disorders occurred after the diagnosis of cancer, indicating that they were associated with the illness and its management.

In an early study in the UK, Maguire *et al.* (1978) found in the year following surgery for breast cancer that 25% of the women suffered from clinically significant anxiety and/or depression, and 33% had moderate or severe sexual problems. The same group also found that as many as 81% of a small series of women receiving adjuvant combination chemotherapy for breast cancer developed a psychiatric disorder during treatment (Maguire *et al.* 1980).

A large study by Zabora *et al.* (2001) assessed 4496 patients with differing types and stages of disease. Overall, 35% of the sample was suffering from clinically significant levels of distress, which varied according to cancer type. The level of distress for patients with lung cancer was significantly higher than that for other cancers, with the exceptions of cancer of the brain, liver, pancreas, and head and neck.

In all these studies measuring psychiatric disorder the levels detected depend critically on the tools uses for detecting distress and the criteria used for diagnosis. The use of well validated interviews based upon ICD 10 criteria are preferable but often lacking in this area of research. There is also the difficult issue of deciding whether an individual patient has the symptom of 'depression' in the setting of a serious illness. Self-rating scales similarly have difficulties because many symptoms that are present in depression such as weight loss, lethargy, and lack of future plans may be directed related to the illness process. This explains the range of prevalence of morbidity detected and also is important in understanding the effects of intervention on morbidity; from at one extreme reducing rates of depressive illness based upon international agreed criteria to at the other extreme reductions in self-reported levels of distress.

The determinants of psychological distress

Harrison and Maguire (1994) reviewed predictors of psychological and psychiatric disorders in patients with cancer. They concluded that the following are risk factors: a previous history of mood disturbance, high emotionality, low ego strength, poor performance status ('fitness'), certain types of treatments (e.g. colostomy), lack of social support, passive or avoidant copng, inadequate or inappropriate information, and communication problems. To this we might add the number of unresolved concerns (Worden and Weisman 1984) and the partner's distress level (Anderson and Walker 2002).

Regarding treatment-related distress, it is well known that chemotherapy related side-effects such as nausea, vomiting, alopecia and fatigue are a common cause of distress (Bliss *et al.* 1992; Knobf *et al.* 1998). Considerable morbidity can also be caused by treatments such as radiotherapy (Chaturvedi *et al.* 1996; Greenberg 1998), surgery (Jacobsen and Hann 1998), bone marrow transplantation (Chiodi *et al.* 2000), and the biological response modifiers (Walker *et al.* 1996, 1997).

It is important to recognize that the risk factor of a history of previous psychiatric disorder is of such significance in predicting future disorders that it should be part of a screening process. Other risk factors that are based upon the environment and social factors are amenable to intervention.

Information and support

There has been a general change over the decades in communicating with patients about their diagnosis, treatment, and prognosis. Indeed, regulatory bodies such as the General Medical Council make clear that patients have a right to be aware of their illness and to be consulted about their treatment. Surveys of patients have indicated that they are generally keen to have information about these factors. The increasing use of 'advanced decisions' under the Mental Capacity Act 2005 where people have the right to refuse treatment makes it all the more important that they have pertinent information about their illness, treatment, and prognosis.

There has been recognition of the importance of providing this information and palliative care services should provide training for staff in breaking bad news and communicating these messages. Anecdotal reports suggest that there may have been a move from a reluctance to share information with patients to a sometimes rather brutal and uncaring information giving. This is often by less experienced doctors and staff who believed that they had to tell the patient everything about their illness without first seeking information about what the patient already knows, what information they wished to gain, and how best this should be communicated with the patient.

As part of psychosocial care at assessment patients should be asked about their illness and understanding of their prognosis but there should also be a discussion about how this information was previously given to them. This is important as it may have implications as to how they would accept or are able to ask for such information in the future. The provision of written material describing not only the treatment and management of various cancers, but also psychological responses is probably important. While there has been interest in the use of self-help information booklets in reducing psychological distress following diagnosis and treatment there is not yet good evidence that it is effective in changing outcome. Self-help literature maybe helpful in leading people to be more aware of psychological difficulties, which may lead to them asking for help and assistance. There is less evidence that it leads to an overall reduction in levels of psychological distress and there is always some concern that describing symptoms that people may develop can lead to a preoccupation and possible increase in these symptoms occurring. This has, for example, been shown to be the case in offering routine debriefing and counselling to all people following traumatic experiences, which appears to be detrimental to the majority.

The study by Jenkins *et al.* (2001) of 2027 patients showed that 87% of patients wanted as much information as possible, good or bad, while 5% only wanted good news and 8% wanted to leave the decision to the doctor. Patient were keen to know about all possible side-effects (97%); all possible treatments (94%); chances of cure (95%); week by week progress (91%); whether it is cancer (98%); and the specific medical diagnosis (89%). Men were less likely than women to wish to know about all the possible treatments, and older patients (over 70 years of age) were more likely to say that they preferred to leave disclosure of details to the doctors. In 1961, 90% of doctors did not indicate a preference for giving a diagnosis of cancer but this increased to 97% telling their patients by 1979 (Novack *et al.* 1979).

Ramirez *et al.* (1995) reported that in a survey of non-surgical oncologists in the UK 83% said they had not received enough training. Stress levels were reported as high within this group who had received poor training. These and other findings led to the establishment of training for physicians in this area.

A number of studies have assessed the importance of information in helping patients to cope with the diagnosis and treatment of cancer (Walker 1996). For example, a follow-up study of 117 women attending a gynaecological oncology follow-up clinic indicated that those who were clinically anxious and/or depressed at follow-up were more critical of doctor–patient interaction, particularly regarding the amount of information given (Paraskevaidis *et al.* 1993). It should be borne in mind, however, that this study identified a small group of patients who felt that they would have coped better by having been told less.

It is clear that individuals differ in terms of what they wish to know, when they wish to be told, and from whom they wish to receive the information. Training in breaking bad news should give clinicians the skills to identify how much and in what manner information should be provided. Historically, many patients have felt underinformed leading to the development of information. However, there is evidence that some patients find these of limited value and most prefer information from healthcare professionals who can discuss the implications and answer questions (Farrell 2001). Services such as CancerBACUP have met, and continue to meet, otherwise unmet information needs. In the year 1999–2000, CancerBACUP distributed over 200 000 booklets and their website was visited by over 35 000 people per month.

In a cross-sectional survey, Slevin *et al.* (1996) obtained the views of 431 patients about different sources of support and their satisfaction with these providers. They found that the three most important sources of support were senior registrars (73%), family (73%), and consultant staff (63%). Forty-three per cent said they would definitely use their general practitioner (GP) as a source of support and, of those that had used their GP, 63% were satisfied with the support received. Approximately 80% were satisfied with the support received from senior medical staff, whereas only 42% were satisfied with the support given by the ward nurses.

A study of 49 patients with orofacial cancers showed wide variation in the extent to which patients perceived primary and secondary care teams to be helpful (Broomfield *et al.* 1997). In keeping with the findings of Slevin *et al.* (1996), GPs were seen to be less helpful than family or hospital staff. Whereas 96% found the support received by consultants to be helpful, only 50% reported that they found support from the GP to be helpful; 10% actually said the GPs support had been 'unhelpful', and 4% indicated that it had been 'very unhelpful'.

Randomized controlled trials of psychosocial interventions

It is an essential part of the provision of psychosocial care that if mechanisms and training are initiated to increase the detection of depressive disorder that there are relevant referral pathways to manage these patients. The difficulty if this is not provided is that it leads to staff having the additional burden of having a patient whom they are aware has a psychological disorder requiring treatment but that they have no access for treatment for these people. This leads to increased stress and unhappiness in the staff member and will have a negative impact upon that person wanting to detect illness in the future. The detection of depressive disorder has to be part of a comprehensive management package for this disorder.

Five meta-analyses (of variable quality) have been published (Smith *et al.* 1994; Devine and Westlake 1995; Meyer and Mark 1995; Sheard and Maguire 1999; Luebbert *et al.* 2001), which suggest that a range of psychosocial interventions have beneficial effects on emotional adjustment, function, treatment-related side-effects (especially nausea and vomiting), pain, and global quality of life.

A recent report of the European Association for Palliative Care (Stiefel *et al.* 2001) highlighted that the unresolved issues in staff training in the management of depression and palliative care, in particular, how the transfer of knowledge should be organized given the lack of mental health professionals working in palliative care. The report considers the most effective strategies for training of non-psychiatric staff and who should be the main target of training interventions and what should be their main focus. This group recommended complementing the transfer of knowledge with training and communication skills and that there should be future research on the evaluation and comparison of different comprehensive training interventions. The report highlights the importance of close collaboration with consultation–liaison psychiatric services.

Interventions to reduce distress and improve adaptation in unselected patients

The need for communication skills training would seem essential but the outcomes of such training are complex. Maguire and Faulkner (1988) described a system for improving the counselling skills of doctors and nurses involving cancer care. In a separate study training hospice nurses to elicit patient concerns they show little change in nurses ability to elicit these concerns following training (Heaven and Maguire 1998). In a similar study of cancer nurses, Maguire *et al.* (1996), it was shown that 6 months after such training staff tended to return to behaviour that prevented cancer patients from disclosing their concerns and psychological symptoms.

The general need for communication skills training in oncology has been recognized. A study in the *Lancet* (Fallowfield 2002) of 160 Oncologists from UK cancer centres showed that training led to improvements in doctors' satisfaction and in their ability to ask open questions and obtain appropriate responses.

The issue of training of non-psychiatric health professionals in detecting depression is important and it has proven difficult to show (Kicks 1999) that a brief educational intervention improved doctors' ability to detect depression, although did change their attitudes and knowledge. Other randomized controlled trials of training specialist nurses have shown that this can lead to a sixfold increase in ability to recognize patients with depression with resulting increases in psychiatric referrals and reduction in the incidents of depression (Maguire 1980).

In organizing services it would seem sensible to concentrate on identifying patients exhibiting clinical levels of distress. Trials of psychosocial interventions should also concentrate on this group (Sheard and Maguire 1999; Baider *et al.* 2001). There is also evidence from randomized trials to show that benefit to unselected groups of patients with cancer can be demonstrated.

Maguire *et al.* (1980) randomized 152 women with breast cancer either to specialist counselling from a breast care nurse or to routine practice. Counselling by a specialist nurse did not prevent psychiatric morbidity, although this regular monitoring resulted in the referral of 76% of those who needed psychiatric help to an appropriate agency. Only 15% of the control group whose condition merited referral were recognized and referred. Consequently, at follow-up, the patients who had been randomized to the specialist nurse were less likely to suffer from a psychiatric disorder than those who received standard care (12% versus 39%). Subsequently, Maguire *et al.* (1983) showed that patients randomized to the specialist nurse had improved marital and sexual adjustment; they were more likely to return to work, and they were more satisfied with their prosthesis. The study indicated the importance of detecting the presence of psychiatric disorder and the ineffectiveness of routine counselling for distress.

In another evaluation study of specialist nurses, Watson *et al.* (1988) randomized 40 newly diagnosed breast cancer patients who had undergone mastectomy to routine care, or to routine care plus counselling by a nurse. Although there were some initial advantages for those receiving counselling, there were no significant differences between the two groups 12 months postoperatively. The authors interpret these findings as suggesting that a nurse counselling service can speed up the process of adjustment following surgery.

Spiegel *et al.* (1981) randomized 86 women with metastatic breast cancer to group support or standard care. The groups focused on the problems of terminal illness and associated interpersonal consequences, as well as living as fully as possible in the face of death. Hypnosis and relaxation were also used as appropriate. The data showed that patients receiving group support had fewer maladaptive coping responses and less mood disturbance than those in the standard care arm of the trial.

The effects of a different type of group intervention were evaluated by Fawzy *et al.* (1990). They randomized 68 patients with newly diagnosed malignant melanoma to a brief (once weekly for 6 weeks) psycho-educational intervention consisting of health education, enhancement of problem-solving skills, stress management (including relaxation techniques), and support. When the patients were followed up 6 months later, patients randomized to the intervention showed significantly less depressed mood, fatigue, confusion, and total mood disturbance. They also used more active–behavioural and active–cognitive coping methods than the controls.

Relaxation therapy is widely used in the UK and a number of randomized trials have been reported. Walker *et al.* (1999a) examined the effects of relaxation therapy, with guided imagery (visualizing host defences attacking cancer cells, or in some other way promoting 'healing'), in 96 women receiving combination neoadjuvant (primary) chemotherapy for newly diagnosed locally advanced breast cancer. They found that relaxation and guided imagery were acceptable to most patients. When the data were analysed using an intention-to-treat method, patients randomized to relaxation and guided imagery reported significantly better quality of life during chemotherapy, and they were more relaxed and more easy going as assessed using the Mood Rating Scale. The intervention also reduced emotional suppression. Intriguingly, patient self-rated imagery vividness correlated significantly with clinical response to neoadjuvant chemotherapy. It is interesting to note that there was no significant difference in the incidence of clinically significant depression or anxiety. This again indicates that while such interventions are acceptable and supportive to patients they are nor helpful in treating clinical levels of psychiatric disorder and highlight the importance of detection of these conditions for treatment.

Cunningham *et al.* (1995) addressed the interesting issue of how best to schedule interventions. They compared a brief group psycho-educational programme delivered as 6-weekly 2-hour sessions with a 'weekend intensive'. One hundred and fifty-six patients were randomized. The weekend intensive produced a rapid, large improvement in mood, although the two interventions did not differ with respect to mood after 6 weeks and 19 weeks. At 6 weeks, patients in the 6-week programme had better quality of life, although the difference between the interventions had disappeared by 19 weeks. The authors conclude that the two interventions are broadly comparable. They make the valuable point that there is a 'particular need for ways of bringing the benefits of psychosocial help to a larger population, including people of varying ethnic backgrounds. This will probably mean adapting both the format and the content of programmes to suit consumer's needs, and integrating this adjunctive help more closely into the overall medical treatment scheme.'

Brief, 'low key' interventions have also been shown to be beneficial in unselected patients. McQuellon *et al.* (1998) randomly assigned 150 consecutively referred patients to an oncology outpatient clinic to usual care or to an intervention consisting of a clinic tour, information about the clinic and a question and answer session. At follow-up, those randomized to the intervention programme had lower state anxiety, lower overall distress, and a reduced incidence of depressive symptoms. The patients were also more knowledgeable about clinic procedures and were more satisfied with the care they had received.

Another successful, 'low key' intervention was evaluated by Burton *et al.* (1995) who examined the possible benefits of pre-surgical interventions.

Two hundred women scheduled for mastectomy were randomized to one of four interventions: preoperative interview plus a 30-minute psychotherapeutic intervention, preoperative interview plus a 'chat' (to control for attention), preoperative interview only, and routine care. The preoperative interview covered the discovery of the breast problem, referral, beliefs about the causes of the illness, response to the need for surgery, desire for information, worries about body image support, life events, attitude to the past and the future, etc. A brief structured psychiatric interview was also carried out. Patients receiving a preoperative interview showed less body image disturbance than the patients receiving standard care 3 months, and 12 months, after surgery. Compared with the three intervention groups, patients receiving routine care were more likely to have clinically significant anxiety and depression 12 months after surgery, and they also scored lower on 'fighting spirit'. Interestingly, psychological morbidity was 59% preoperatively and 39% 1 year after surgery. This study highlights the value of a preoperative interview in terms of long-term adjustment.

In addition to improving various aspects of coping and quality of life, psychosocial interventions can also modify various behaviours relevant to treatment outcome. For example, Richardson *et al.* (1990) reported a very interesting study on the effects of three special educational programmes and treatment compliance in 96 patients with haematological malignancies. The educational programmes involved helping the patients to develop a routine for taking medication, educating the patients regarding the importance of treatment compliance and self-care, and a behavioural shaping programme. All three programmes increased treatment compliance (and survival), indicating that treatment compliance can be improved by means of relatively simple interventions.

These studies allow two general conclusions. First, relatively brief, simple interventions, delivered individually or in a group, can reduce distress and improve quality of life in patients who have not been selected because they have clinically significant distress, or who are at high risk of developing such distress. Second, although it may be more difficult to demonstrate between-group differences, it is possible to demonstrate these effects in unselected populations in prospective randomized controlled trials (Walker and Anderson 1999).

Interventions for patients with clinically significant problems

Many studies have shown clear benefits of psychological interventions in patients suffering from various types of treatment-related distress. These have been reviewed recently by Redd *et al.* (2001) who identified 54 studies (not all of which were randomized trials). They concluded that behavioural interventions can effectively control anticipatory nausea and vomiting in adult and paediatric cancer patients undergoing chemotherapy; that they can ameliorate anxiety and distress associated with invasive medical treatments, and that hypnotic-like methods (relaxation, suggestion, and distracting imagery) are helpful for pain management.

To study the effectiveness of preventive intervention in lowering emotional distress and improving coping, Worden and Weisman (1984) assessed 381 newly diagnosed cancer patients. Fifty-nine patients predicted by a screening instrument to be at risk for high levels of emotional distress and poor coping were randomly allocated to one of two interventions designed to enhance problem-solving skills. A non-randomized control group (58 patients) received no intervention. Both interventions reduced emotional distress and improved problem resolution. Although only partially randomized, this influential early study suggests the value of a brief intervention in preventing distress and enhancing coping in high-risk patients.

In a large prospective, randomized controlled trial, Greer *et al.* (1992) evaluated the effect on quality of life of a brief, problem-based, cognitive-behavioural treatment specifically designed for the needs of patients with cancer (adjunctive psychological therapy, APT). One hundred and seventy-four patients who scored above a predetermined cut-off on two measures of psychological morbidity were recruited from 1260 patients who were screened. High scoring patients were randomized to standard care or to APT. At 8 weeks follow-up, compared with the control patients, patients receiving APT were significantly better than control patients on fighting spirit, helplessness, anxious preoccupation, fatalism, anxiety, psychological symptoms, and healthcare orientation. Some of these gains persisted: at 4 months, compared with controls, patients receiving APT were significantly less anxious, had fewer psychological symptoms and had less psychological distress. Clinically, the proportion of severely anxious patients dropped from 46% at baseline to 20% at 8 weeks and 20% at 4 months in the therapy group and from 48% to 41% and to 43% respectively among controls. The proportion of patients with depression was 40% at baseline, 13% at 8 weeks, and 18% at 4 months in the therapy group and 30%, 29%, and 23% respectively in controls. When the patients were followed up after 12 months, patients were less anxious and depressed (Moorey *et al.* 1994). This study shows that, in a mixed group of distressed cancer patients, a brief intervention can improve various key components of quality of life.

A systematic review of the effectiveness of palliative care teams (Hearn and Higginson 1998) in 18 studies indicated improved outcomes in the amount of time spent at home by patients, satisfaction by both patients and their carers, symptom control, a reduction in the number of inpatient hospital days, a reduction in overall cost, and the patients' likelihood of dying where they wished to for those receiving specialist care from a multiprofessional palliative care team. There was evidence that specialist teams in palliative care when compared with conventional care improved satisfaction and identified and dealt with more patient and family needs. Moreover, multiprofessional approaches to palliative care reduce the overall cost of care by reducing the amount of time patients spend in acute hospital settings.

A review of specialist palliative day care provision for adults by Davies and Higginson (2005) of 12 observational studies showed the difficulties of evaluating a service already operating and of recruiting a vulnerable population of patients as they deteriorated. Patients attending seemed a selected group of those already receiving palliative care who were mostly white, aged over 60 years and retired, with needs for emotional and social support and pain control. There were insufficient studies to provide conclusive evidence of improved symptom control or health-related quality of life, but all qualitative studies found patients valued the social support and opportunity to take part in activities that day-care provided. The review concluded there was evidence for high satisfaction among patients selected into day-care but this was not sufficient to judge whether this improves symptom control or health-related quality of life.

Current psychosocial provision

It might be rightly said that psychosocial care is the business of all healthcare professionals who are in contact with patients who have cancer, their carers and relatives. However, across the UK, very little is known about the number and professional backgrounds of healthcare staff that have a particular responsibility for the provision of psychosocial care for patients with cancer and their relatives, in hospital or in the community. In addition, little is known about the training they have had in the provision of psychosocial care, how standards are monitored, and the support that they, themselves, receive to prevent 'burn out' (Ramirez et al. 1995; Wilkinson 1995).

Lloyd-Williams et al. (1999) carried out a survey of psychosocial provision within hospices in the UK. One hundred and sixty hospices were selected and a questionnaire sent to the matron or nurse-in-charge. Ninety-seven (60%) of the questionnaires were returned. The majority (83%) of hospices employed a Chaplain, and all had access to a Chaplain if required. Seventy-five per cent employed a social worker, and all but 6% had access to one. Forty-three per cent employed one or more 'counsellors', although 25% indicated that they did not have access to a counsellor. The most interesting findings, however, are that only 9% employed a full-time, or part time, psychiatrist and only 7%

employed a psychologist. The authors conclude that treatable psychiatric morbidity may go undetected and untreated as a result.

Certainly, outside hospices, increasing numbers of specialist nurses, at least part of whose remit is the provision of psychosocial care, are being employed in hospitals and in the community throughout the UK. For example, the first Macmillan nursing posts were established in 1975. Currently, there are over 2000 Macmillan nurses in posts in almost every local health authority in the UK. In addition, the Medical Services Programme was set up in 1986 to establish Macmillan doctors at all levels and roles, in hospitals, at home and cancer treatment centres and, to date, over 300 Macmillan doctors have been appointed. Macmillan Cancer Relief's contribution to cancer care in the UK is now widely recognized by the public and the NHS.

A widely reported problem with information/support services in the UK is that these services are used disproportionately by middle class women with breast cancer. For example, a survey of clients accessing CancerBACUP, the Macmillan Lynda Jackson Centre, and the Richard Dimbleby Centre found that only 23–29% of those contacting these services were men (Williams *et al.* 2000).

Non-equity of use was also found by Boiudioni *et al.* (2000). They reviewed the sociodemographic data from all 384 clients who had booked an appointment with the Cancer BACUP London Counselling Service during a period of 18 months. The clients were predominantly female, under 50 years of age and from non-manual social classes.

The situation in Germany has been studied by Plass and Koch (2001). One hundred and thirty-two patients attending four oncology outpatient clinics in Hamburg completed a questionnaire to establish their knowledge of institutions offering support, their previous participation in support, their reasons for participation and their evaluation of the support given. Eighty-eight per cent of the respondents were women, and 72% had a history of breast cancer. Twenty-eight per cent of the respondents had participated in some sort of psychosocial support (only 4% of these had attended self-help groups). Those who had participated were younger and scored higher on measures of emotional and physical difficulties. The main reason for non-participation was the presence of adequate support from family, friends, or doctors.

A recent North American study surveyed a randomly selected group of patients with breast, colon, or prostate cancer (Eakin and Strycker 2001). Use of all support and information services (hospital, community, internet) was low (2–8%). The most common reasons for not using the hospital counselling service was adequate support, lack of awareness of the service, and not having been referred. Better educated patients were more likely to use the hospital counselling service. Awareness of the prostate support group was high (90%), although use was low (5%).

Earlier in this chapter, we reviewed some of the evidence demonstrating that individual and group interventions both have beneficial effects on quality of life. However, they may differ markedly in terms of acceptability. Baider *et al.* (2001) reported that 90 of 116 (78%) eligible patients in Jerusalem agreed to participate in their randomized trial of progressive muscular relaxation and guided imagery in groups. Cultural factors may affect acceptability, and group interventions themselves may differ in acceptability, for example, group psycho-educational approaches versus group supportive-expressive methods. Further research is required to clarify these issues.

Example

Leicestershire has developed a specialist psycho-oncology service as part of a wider liaison psychiatry service. This service provides intervention to all areas of oncology, including palliative care. Leicestershire is large central Midlands County with 1 million population, including 30% ethnic minorities (largely from India living in Leicester city).

Like many services the most common presentation is for depression and anxiety. Patients are offered a choice or menu of care including face-to-face psychological work, medication, relaxation (including a formal relaxation programme), and group therapy. A recent innovation is a self-help package, which is a booklet of information, advice, and cognitive-behaviour type therapy. There is also an expert patient programme. In 2005 the service received 228 new referrals and assessed 41 patients on oncology wards and 22 patients from the local hospice. The service provides training and supervision to the range of palliative care services.

Service organization

In organizing a comprehensive service for oncology patients the issue of managing palliative care is obviously essential. The service can be organized by considering the levels of psychiatric disorder and the intervention needed to manage that area.

The most important cases are those patients with acute psychiatric disorders requiring urgent treatment. This includes management of severe depressive disorders, psychosis, and complicated confusional states. It is important to have close links with specialist psychiatric services, ideally a specialist psycho-oncology service or liaison psychiatry service. This service should provide urgent assessments of such people and advice on management.

The next level concerns the detection and management of patients with significant or clinical levels of psychiatric disorder. This includes, in particular, depressive disorder but also anxiety and panic disorders and the range of psychological disorders. Services need to have systems for screening patients at assessment and at other critical periods, such as admission at a hospice. The use of self-rated questionnaires can be helpful but training staff to feel confident in asking simple screening questions about the presence of low mood and depression is probably as effective. It is essential that staff feel supported in detecting psychiatric problems by the presence of effective intervention. The use of antidepressants together with cognitive-behaviour therapy techniques should be routine in such settings. Many palliative care teams have skills in managing these conditions but need access to specialist psychiatric services for advice, supervision, and management of complex cases or those resistant to treatment.

There are then other services and interventions that should also be part of comprehensive psychosocial care. Staff require training in the detection and management of psychiatric disorders. They need advice and support in managing such difficult cases; there are particular issues for specialist practitioners in the community such as Macmillan nurses. There is the need for psychological education to practitioners in oncology, charitable organizations and training in specific areas such as 'breaking bad news' and communication skills. There are often counselling services associated with palliative care and these require supervision and careful agreement about the nature of their intervention. There is evidence that counselling is not helpful in treating clinical levels of psychiatric disorders, such as depressive illness and so there should be screening to detect these conditions. Resources are limited and counselling is probably best organized using brief interventions of six to eight sessions to address particular problems rather than longer-term therapy. Psychological services also have a role in staff support and attendance at joint clinics and other settings is helpful in promoting knowledge and encouraging joint working.

In conclusion, the challenge is how best to organize psychosocial care in order to provide appropriate information and support to all patients (and relatives); to deliver patient-centred care; to prevent psychological morbidity; to improve quality of life; to work in partnership, and to reduce health inequalities.

References

Anderson J, Walker LG (2002). Psychological factors and cancer progression: involvement of behavioural pathways. In Lewis CE, O'Brien R, Barraclough J (ed.). *The psychoimmunology of cancer* (2nd edn). Oxford: Oxford University Press.

Baider L, Peretz T, Hadani PE, Koch U (2001). Psychological intervention in cancer patients: a randomized study. *Gen Hosp Psychiatry* 23:272–7.

Bliss JM, Robertson B, Selby PJ (1992). The impact of nausea and vomiting upon quality of life measures. *Br J Cancer* 66 (Suppl. XIX):S14–23.

Boudioni M, Mossman J, Boulton M, Ramirez A, Moynihan C, Leydon G (2000). An evaluation of a cancer counselling service. *Eur J Cancer* 9:212–20.

Broomfield D, Humphris GM, Fisher SE, Vaughan D, Brown JS, Lane S (1997). The orofacial cancer patient's support from the general practitioner, hospital teams, family, and friends. *J Cancer Educ* 12:229–32.

Burton MV, Parker RW, Farrell A, Bailey D, Connely J, Booth S, Elcombe S (1995). A randomized controlled trial of preoperative psychological preparation for mastectomy. *Psycho-Oncology* 4:1–19.

Chaturvedi SK, Chandra PS, Channabasavanna SM, Anantha N, Reddy BKM, Sharme S (1996). Levels of anxiety and depression in patients receiving radiotherapy in India. *Psycho-Oncology* 5:343–6.

Chiodi S, Spinelli S, Ravera G, Petti AR, Van Lint MT, Lamparelli T, Gualandi F, Occhini D, Mordini N, Berisso G, Bregante S, Frassoni F, Bacigalupo A (2000). Quality of life in 244 recipients of allogeneic bone marrow transplantation. *Br J Haematol* 110:614–19.

Cunningham AJ, Tocco EK (1989). A randomised trial of group psychoeducational therapy for cancer patients. *Patient Care Couns* 14:101–14.

Cunningham AJ, Jenkins G, Edmonds CV, Lockwood GA (1995). A randomised comparison of two forms of a brief, group, psychoeducational program for cancer patients: weekly sessions versus a 'weekend intensive'. *Int J Psychiatry Med* 25:173–89.

Davies E, Higginson J (2005). Systematic review of specialist palliative day care for adults with cacner. *Support Care Cancer* 8:607–27.

Devine EC, Westlake SK (1995). The effects of psychoeducational care provided to adults with cancer: meta-analysis of 116 studies. *Oncol Nurs Forum* 22:1369–81.

Derogatis LR, Morrow GR, Fetting JH, Penman D, Piatsky S, Schmale AM, Henrichs M, Carniche CL (1983). The prevalence of psychiatric disorders amongst cancer patients. *JAMA* 249:751–7.

Eakin EG, Strycker LA (2001). Awareness and barriers to use of cancer support and information resources by HMO patients with breast, prostate, or colon cancer: patient and provider perspectives. *Psycho-Oncology* 10:103–13.

Fallowfield L, Jenkins V, Farewell V, Saul J, Duffy A, Eves R (2002). Efficacy of a Cancer Research UK communication skills training model for oncologists: a randomised controlled trial. *Lancet* 359:650–6.

Farrell C (2001). National Service Framework Assessments No1: NHS Cancer Care in England and Wales. Supporting Paper 1: *There's no system to the whole procedure.* London: Commission for Health Improvement.

Fawzy FI, Cousins N, Fawzy NW, Kemeny ME, Elashoff R, Morton D (1990). A structured psychiatric intervention for cancer patients. I. Changes over time in methods of coping and affective disturbance. *Arch Gen Psychiatry* 47:720–5.

Greenberg DB (1998). Radiotherapy. In: Holland JC (ed.). *Psycho-oncology.* New York: Oxford University Press.

Greer S, Moorey S, Baruch JDR, Watson M, Robertson BM, Mason A, Rowden L, Law MG, Bliss JM (1992). Adjuvant psychological therapy for patients with cancer: a prospective randomised trial. *BMJ* 304:675–80.

Heaven CM, Maguire P (1998). The relationship between patients' concerns and psychological distress in a hospice setting. *Psycho-Oncology* 7:502–7.

Harrison J, Maguire P (1994). Predictors of psychiatric morbidity in cancer patients. *Br J Psychiatry* 165:593–8.

Hearn J, Higginson S (1998). Do specialist palliaticve care teams imprve outcomes for cancer patients? A literature review. *Palliat Med* 12:317–22.

Heaven C, Maguire P (1996). Tranining hospice nurses to elicit patients concerns. *J Adv Nurs* 23:280–6.

Jacobsen PB, Hann DM (1998). Cognitive-behavioural interventions. In: Holland JC (ed.). *Psycho-Oncology*. New York: Oxford University Press.

Jenkins V, Fallowfield L, Saul J (2001). Information needs of patients with cancer: results from a large study in UK cancer centre. *Br J Cancer* 84:48–51.

Kicks D (1999). An educational intervention using the Agency for Health Care Policy and Research Depression Guidelines among internal medicine residents. *Int J Psychiatry Med* 29, 47–61.

Knobf MT, Pasacreta JV, Valentine A, McCorkle R (1998). Chemotherapy, hormone therapy, and immunotherapy. In: Holland JC (ed.). *Psycho-Oncology*. New York: Oxford University Press.

Lloyd-Williams M, Friedman T, Rudd N (1999). A survey of psychosocial service provision within hospices. *Palliat Med* 13:431–2.

Luebbert K, Dahme B, Hasenbring M (2001). The effectiveness of relaxation training in reducing treatment-related symptoms and improving emotional adjustment in acute non-surgical cancer treatment: a meta-analytical review. *Psycho-Oncology* 10:490–502.

Maguire GP (1980). Affects of counselling on the psychiatric morbidity associated with mastectomy. *BMJ* 281:145–146.

Maguire GP, Lee EG, Bevington DJ, Kuchemann CS, Crabtree RJ, Cornell CE (1978). Psychiatric problems in the first year after mastectomy. *BMJ* 1:963–5.

Maguire GP, Tait A, Brooke M, Thomas C, Howat JM, Sellwood RA, Bush H (1980). Psychiatric morbidity and physical toxicity associated with adjuvant chemotherapy after mastectomy. *BMJ* 281:1179–80.

Maguire P, Faulkner A (1988). Improving counselling skills of doctors and nurses in cancer care. *BMJ* 297:847–9.

Maguire P, Tait A, Brooke M, Thomas C, Sellwood R (1980). Effect of counselling on the psychiatric morbidity associated with mastectomy. *BMJ* 281:1454–7.

Maguire P, Brooke M, Tait A, Thomas C, Sellwood R (1983). The effect of counselling on physical disability and social recovery after mastectomy. *Clin Oncol* 9:319–24.

Maguire P, Faulkner A, Booth K, Elliott C, Hillier V (1996). Helping cancer patients disclose their concerns. *Eur J Cancer* 32A:78–81.

McQuellon RP, Wells M, Hoffman S, Craven B, Russell G, Cruz J, Hurt G, DeChatelet P, Andrykowski MA, Savage P (1998). Reducing distress in cancer patients with an orientation program. *Psycho-Oncology* 7:207–17.

Meyer TJ, Mark MM (1995). Effects of psychosocial interventions with adult cancer patients: a meta-analysis of randomized experiments. *Health Psychol* 14:101–8.

Moorey S, Greer S, Watson M, Baruch JDR, Robertson BM, Mason A, Rowden L, Tunmore R, Law M, Bliss JM (1994). Adjuvant psychological therapy for patients with cancer: outcome at one year. *Psycho-Oncology* 3:39–46.

Novack D, Plumer R, Smith R , Ochitill H, Morrow G, Benett J (1979). Changes in physicians attitudes towards telling the cancer patient. *JAMA* 241:897–900.

Paraskevaidis E, Kitchener HC, Walker LG (1993). Doctor-patient communication and subsequent mental health in women with gynaecological cancer. *Psycho-Oncology* 2:195–200.

Plass A, Koch U (2001). Participation of oncological outpatients in psychosocial support. *Psycho-Oncology* 10:511–20.

Ramirez AJ, Graham J, Richards MA, Cull A, Gregory WM, Leaning MS, Snashall DC, Timothy AR (1995). Burnout and psychiatric disorder among cancer clinicians. *Br J Cancer* 71:1263–9.

Redd WH, Montgomery GH, DuHamel KN (2001). Behavioral intervention for cancer treatment side effects. *J Natl Cancer Inst* 93:810–23.

Richardson JL, Shelton DR, Krailo M, Levine AM (1990). The effect of compliance with treatment on survival among patients with hematologic malignancies. *J Clin Oncol* 8:356–64.

Sheard T, Maguire P (1999). The effect of psychological interventions on anxiety and depression in cancer patients: results of two meta-analyses. *Br J Cancer* 80:1770–80.

Slevin ML, Nichols SE, Downer SM, Wilson P, Lister TA, Arnott S, Maher J, Souhami RL, Tobias JS, Goldstone AH, Cody M (1996). Emotional support for cancer patients: what do patients really want? *Br J Cancer* 74:1275–9.

Smith MC, Holcome JK, Stullenbarger E (1994). A meta-analysis of intervention effectiveness for symptom management in oncology nursing research. *Oncol Nurs Forum* 21:1201–10.

Spiegel D, Bloom JR, Yalom I (1981). Group support for patients with metastatic cancer. A randomized outcome study. *Arch Gen Psychiatry* 38:527–33.

Stiefel F, Trill M, Berney A, Olarte J, Razavi D (2001). Depression in palliative care: a pragmatic report from the Expert Working |Group of the European Association for Palliative Care. *Support Care Cancer* 9:477–88.

Swire N, George R (1997). Depression and palliative care. In: Robertson MM, Turner CLE (ed.). *Depression and physical illness*. Chichester: Wiley, pp. 443–64.

Walker LG (1996). Communication skills: when, not if, to teach. *Eur J Cancer* 32A:1457–9.

Walker LG, Anderson J (1999). Testing complementary and alternative medicine within a research protocol. *Eur J Cancer* 35:1614–18.

Walker LG, Wesnes KA, Heys SD, Walker MB, Lolley J, Eremin O (1996). The cognitive effects of recombinant interleukin-2 (rIL-2) therapy: a controlled clinical trial using computerised assessments. *Eur J Cancer* 32A:2275–83.

Walker LG, Walker MB, Heys SD, Lolley J, Wesnes K, Eremin O (1997). The psychological and psychiatric effects of rIL-2: a controlled clinical trial. *Psycho-Oncology* 6:290–301.

Walker LG, Walker MB, Heys SD, Ogston K, Miller I, Hutcheon AW, Sarkar TK, Eremin O (1999a). The psychological, clinical and pathological effects of relaxation training and imagery during primary chemotherapy. *Br J Cancer* 80:262–8.

Watson M, Denton S, Baum M, Greer S (1998). Counselling breast cancer patients: a specialist nurse service. *Couns Psychol Q* 1:25–34.

Wilkinson S (1995). The changing pressures for cancer nurses 1986–93. *Eur J Cancer Care* 4:69–74.

Williams ERL, Ramirez AJ, Richards MA, Young T, Maher EJ, Boudioni M, Maguire P (2000). Are men missing from cancer information and support services? *Psycho-Oncology* 9:364.

Worden JW, Weisman AD (1984). Preventive psychosocial intervention with newly diagnosed cancer patients. *Gen Hosp Psychiatry* 6:243–9.

Zabora J, Brintzenhofenszoc K, Curbow B, Hooker C, Piantadosi S (2001). The prevalence of psychological distress by cancer site. *Psycho-Oncology* 10:19–28.

Chapter 6

Anxiety and adjustment disorders

Steven D. Passik, Kenneth L. Kirsh,
and Mari Lloyd-Williams

Introduction

The many modern advances in oncology are making cancer a survivable, chronic life-threatening illness for many patients (Passik *et al.* 1998). However, cancer is still a high magnitude stressor, and patients experience, at times, catastrophic levels of stress, when confronting the disease and its treatment. How a patient adapts to cancer and its accompanying treatments is key to his or her ongoing quality of life. Moreover, stress can have negative consequences for both physical and mental health. Accordingly, the quality of life of those living with the disease long term, has become a focus of cancer care and research.

It is clear that this inherent stress takes a toll on the lives of cancer patients and their families. In a landmark study of cancer patients, Derogatis *et al.* (1983) found that 50% of patients had a psychiatric diagnosis. This is a much greater percentage than the number of individuals with any psychiatric condition found in the general adult population (22%) (Regier *et al.* 1993), which marks this group as being clearly at risk. Indeed, co-morbidity of psychiatric diagnosis and cancer diagnosis should be viewed as the rule rather than the exception.

Psychological distress

Cancer patients have a high rate of psychiatric co-morbidity. Generally, the psychological complications take the form of adjustment issues, depressed mood, anxiety, impoverished life satisfaction, or loss of self-esteem (Freidenbergs and Kaplan 1993; Molassiotis *et al.* 1995) (see Table 6.1 for overview). However, the making of psychiatric diagnoses and the rapid identification of patients in need of help are difficult for many reasons. One problem is that psychiatric symptomatology may be mimicked by the side-effects of medication or the disease process itself in people with cancer. The shortage of time and emphasis on the physical condition alone during outpatient consultation reinforce the patients' reluctance to report psychosocial problems and can act as barriers to the recognition of

Table 6.1 Key components of the diagnoses of major depression, anxiety disorder, and adjustment disorder

Variable	Major depression	Generalized anxiety disorder	Adjustment disorder
Time course for consideration of the diagnosis:	At least 2 weeks of depressed mood or anhedonia	Anxiety occurring most days for at least 6 months	Symptoms must occur within 3 months of a triggering stressor
Major features: or	There must be some change in either appetite, concentration, weight, sleep, feelings of guilt, suicidal ideation, or psychomotor activity Must affect either social, occupational, or other important areas of functioning	Excessive worry and anxiety that occurs more days than not Person reports that they have difficulty controlling the anxious feelings Symptoms typically include either restlessness, diminished concentration, fatigue, poor sleep, muscle tension, or irritability	Marked by clinically relevant behavioural emotional symptoms in response to an identified psychosocial stressor Reaction causes significant impairment of social or occupational functioning Stressor can be continuous, creating a chronic adjustment disorder
Rule out considerations:	Medication and drug side-effects Bereavement	Medication and drug side effects	All other major psychiatric disorders, including major depression and anxiety disorder Bereavement
Gender prevalence:	Depression is twice as common in women as in men	Approximately 60% of all cases are women, 40% are men	Men and women are equally affected

psychosocial problems (Lawrie *et al.* 2004; Wilson *et al.* 2007). This chapter will focus on the identification and treatment of anxiety and adjustment disorders.

Generalized anxiety disorder

Case study

Thomas was a 65-year-old butcher who had never married. Waking up one morning with acute abdominal pain he was referred to the local hospital where a a laparotomy found advanced cancer of the bowel with multiple liver and lung metastases. Initially, Thomas found that he could cope well at home and was supported by various family members and also past customers.

Three months later, neighbours became increasingly concerned about his behaviour—he could be heard pacing around his house in the early hours of the morning and was agitated whenever anyone asked how he was. His weight dropped dramatically but it was difficult to know if this was his illness or his psychological state. He confessed to one neighbour that he was terrified he would die in the night and of dying alone.

His family eventually persuaded him to see his general practitioner where he was agitated, pacing around the room tearful and distressed. He was tachycardic, short of breath, and had a dry mouth, and was clearly in a high anxiety state.

The above case history shows how patients may present with a complex mixture of physical and psychological symptoms in the context of their frightening reality of having a diagnosis of advanced cancer. Thus the recognition of anxiety symptoms requiring treatment can be challenging. Patients with anxiety complain of tension or restlessness, or they exhibit jitteriness, autonomic hyperactivity, insomnia, distractibility, shortness of breath, numbness, apprehension, worry, or rumination. Often the physical or somatic manifestations of anxiety overshadow the psychological or cognitive ones (Holland 1989). It is always worth considering medical causes in patients who present with anxiety, e.g. uncontrolled pain, thyrotoxicosis, alcohol, or benzodiazepine withdrawl. These symptoms are a cue to further inquiry about the patient's psychological state, which is commonly one of fear, worry, or apprehension regarding the future. Anxious patients, like depressed patients tend to selectively remember the more 'threatening information' given to them and often the process of explanation can be therapeutic in itself. In deciding whether to treat anxiety, the patient's subjective level of distress is the primary impetus for the initiation of treatment as opposed to the patient qualifying strictly for a psychiatric diagnosis (Massie 1989).

Despite the fact that anxiety in patients with advanced cancer commonly results from medical complications, it is equally often related to psychological factors related to existential issues, particularly in patients who are alert and not confused (Holland 1989). Patients frequently fear isolation, estrangement from others, and may have a general sense of feeling like an outcast. Also, financial burdens and family role changes are common stressors.

Treatment of anxiety disorders

Prevention is always better than cure—much anxiety could be prevented by better organization of services for patients with cancer. Informing patients of the results of investigations as soon as possible, ensuring that all information is communicated between primary and secondary care and that those caring for patients with cancer possess good communication skills can all minimize morbidity. The treatment of anxiety in cancer patients involves a combination of psychotherapy and a range of anxiolytic medications. The pharmacotherapy of anxiety in patients with more advanced illness involves the judicious use of the following classes of medications: benzodiazepines, neuroleptics, antihistamines, and antidepressants (Holland 1989; Massie 1989; Miller and Massie 2006).

Benzodiazepines

Benzodiazepines are the mainstay of the pharmacological treatment of anxiety in cancer patients. The shorter-acting benzodiazepines, such as lorazepam, alprazolam, and oxazepam, are safest in this population. The selection of these drugs avoids toxic accumulation due to impaired metabolism in debilitated individuals (Hollister 1986). Lorazepam and oxazepam are metabolized by conjugation in the liver and are therefore safest in patients with hepatic disease. This is in contrast to alprazolam and other benzodiazepines that are metabolized through oxidative pathways in the liver that are more vulnerable to interference with hepatic damage. The disadvantage of using short-acting benzodiazepines is that patients often experience breakthrough anxiety or end of dose distress. Such patients can benefit from switching to longer-acting benzodiazepines, such as diazepam or clonazepam. Common dosage regimens include: lorazepam 0.5–2.0 mg, as required; diazepam 2.5–10 mg, as required; clonazepam 1–2 mg. Clonazepam has been found to be extremely useful, for the treatment of symptoms of anxiety. Patients who experience end of dose failure with recurrence of anxiety on shorter-acting drugs also find clonazepam helpful. Clonazepam is also useful in patients with organic mood disorders who have symptoms of mania, and as an adjuvant analgesic in patients with neuropathic pain (Chouinard et al. 1983; Walsh 1990). Fears of causing respiratory depression should not prevent the clinician from using adequate dosages of benzodiazepines to control anxiety. The likelihood of respiratory depression is minimized when shorter-acting drugs are prescribed and the drug dosages are increased in small increments.

Non-benzodiazepine anxiolytics

Typical and atypical neuroleptics, such as haloperidol, and olanzapine are useful in the treatment of anxiety when benzodiazepines are not sufficient for symptom control. They are also indicated when an organic aetiology is suspected or when psychotic symptoms such as delusions or hallucinations accompany the anxiety. Typically haloperidol 0.5–3 mg, as required, is sufficient to control symptoms of anxiety and avoid excessive sedation. The atypical neuroleptics, such as olanzapine, can control anxiety related to confusional states, delusions, and nausea (Passik and Cooper 1999). Neuroleptics are perhaps the safest class of anxiolytics in patients where there is legitimate concern regarding respiratory depression or compromise. Methotrimeprazine is a phenothiazine with anxiolytic properties that is often used for the treatment of pain and anxiety in the patient with advanced cancer (Oliver 1985). Its side-effects include sedation, anticholinergic symptoms, and hypotension. It can be useful in patients where sedation is desirable. With this class of drugs in general, one must be aware of extrapyramidal side-effects (particularly when patients are taking additional neuroleptics for antiemetic purposes) and the remote possibility of neuroleptic malignant syndrome. Tardive dyskinesia is rarely a concern given the generally short-term usage and low dosages of these medications in this population (Breitbart 1986).

Tricyclic, SSRIs, and heterocyclic antidepressants are the most effective treatment for anxiety accompanying depression and are helpful in treating panic disorder (Liebowitz 1985; Popkin *et al.* 1985). Research (Theobald *et al.* 2002) has shown that Mirtazapine is particularly useful for this use in cancer populations.

Buspirone is a non-benzodiazepine anxiolytic that is useful along with psychotherapy in patients with chronic anxiety or anxiety related to adjustment disorders. The onset of anxiolytic action is delayed in comparison with the benzodiazepines, taking 5–10 days for relief of anxiety to begin. As Buspirone is not a benzodiazepine, it will not block benzodiazepine withdrawal, and so one must be cautious when switching from a benzodiazepine to Buspirone. Owing to its delayed onset of action and indication for use in chronic anxiety states, Buspirone may have limited usefulness to the clinician treating anxiety in the rehabilitation setting with cancer patients.

Non-pharmacological treatment of anxiety disorders

Non-pharmacological interventions for anxiety and distress include supportive psychotherapy and behavioural interventions that are used alone or in combination. Brief supportive psychotherapy is often useful in dealing with both crisis-related issues as well as existential issues (Massie *et al.* 1989). Psychotherapeutic interventions often include both the patient and family, particularly as the patient with cancer becomes increasingly debilitated and less able to interact. The goals of psychotherapy for the anxious patient are to establish a bond that decreases the sense of isolation; to help the patient face cancer with a sense of integrity and self-worth; to correct misconceptions about the past and present; to integrate the present illness into a continuum of life experiences; and to explore issues of separation, loss and the unknown that lies ahead.

Complementary therapies, e.g. aromatherapy and massage, and specific interventions, e.g. hypnosis, relaxation, and imagery may help reduce anxiety and thereby increase the patient's sense of control.

Confusional states interfere dramatically with a patient's ability to focus attention and thus limit the usefulness of these techniques (Breitbart 1989). A typical behavioural intervention for anxiety includes a relaxation exercise combined with some distraction or imagery technique. The patient is first taught to relax with passive breathing accompanied by either passive or active muscle relaxation. Once in such a relaxed state, the patient is taught a pleasant, distracting imagery exercise. In a randomized study comparing a relaxation technique with alprazolam in the treatment of anxiety and distress in cancer patients, both treatments were demonstrated to be quite effective for mild to moderate degrees of anxiety or distress. The drug intervention (alprazolam) was more effective for greater levels of distress or anxiety and had more rapid onset of beneficial effect (Adams *et al.* 1986). Often, such interventions are used in combination, i.e. utilizing relaxation techniques concurrently with anxiolytic medications in highly anxious cancer patients.

Anxiety and agitation during the last few weeks and days of life is distressing for the patient, relatives, and staff. Even the very ill patient can derive great benefit from being encouraged to share their fears and anxieties with others. At this stage there may be concerns over previous experiences or rifts in the family and a visit from a family member who has not visited for months or even years is often found to ease the distress.

Sedation either orally or subcutaneously with a benzodiaspeine (e.g. Midazolam) can calm the patient while still allowing them to work through some of these issues.

Adjustment disorder: definition

Adjustment disorder, according to the fourth edition of the Diagnostic and Statistical Manual of Mental Disorders (DSM-IV) (APA: American Psychiatric Association 1994), is a rather nebulous disorder characterized by a variety of clinically significant behavioural or emotional symptoms that occur as a result of some triggering event or stressor. For diagnostic purposes, there can also be a mixture of the aforementioned subtypes or the disorder may remain unspecified when the symptoms cannot be clearly classified. The onset of adjustment disorder must occur within 3 months of the triggering event and must not be longer than 6 months after the termination of the stressor or its consequences. However, the disorder can be deemed to be chronic, thus lasting more than 6 months, when there is a chronic stressor or when the consequences of the stressor have long-term impact, e.g. advanced cancer. Finally, adjustment disorder can only be diagnosed if the disturbance is identifiable and does not meet the criteria for other identifiable psychiatric disorders, such as major depression or generalized anxiety disorder, and if the symptoms are not a result of bereavement.

The International Classification of Disease-10 (ICD-10) (World Health Organization 1995) also has a similar diagnosis to adjustment disorder, with a few minor exceptions. First, the reaction to the stressor has to occur within a 1-month span of time. Second, the subtypes are different and are labelled separately with names such as brief depressive reaction and disturbance of emotions and conduct. Finally, one of the subtypes, prolonged depressive reaction, may last up to 2 years. Thus, while the disorder is little understood, and some claim that it does not exist (Depue and Monroe 1986; Vinokur and Caplan 1986), there is at least a global attempt to explain the phenomenon.

Differential diagnosis of adjustment disorder

Adjustment disorder is the most prevalent problem associated with cancer. In fact, it is evident in 25–30% of all patients with cancer (Derogatis *et al.* 1983; Dugan *et al.* 1998). Despite this high prevalence, most efforts at screening for psychiatric problems in patients with cancer have focused on major depression rather than so-called minor depression, or adjustment disorder. Moreover, as mentioned earlier, genuine problems in adjustment can be obscured by organic effects of cancer and cancer treatment. Certain drugs used in the treatment of cancer, such as prednisolone, procarbazine, vinicristine, and vinblastine cause depressive symptoms that may be confused with adjustment disorder or mood disorder through their side-effects. Such confounding of the diagnosis can lead to inadequate treatment offered to patients or cause the disorder to be over-looked or explained as a probable drug side-effect.

Adjustment disorder and depression

The relationship between adjustment disorder and major depression may be explained from two main viewpoints. First, one may speculate that adjustment disorder is simply quantitatively different from major depression. This conceptualization as a 'subclinical depression' leads to an approach whereby moderate scores on traditional depression screens are thought to be diagnostic for this disorder (Strain 1998). However, there is no uniform agreement on what cut-offs should be used, if indeed it is a minor or subclinical depression. In other words, adjustment disorder may occupy a niche role somewhere between a major depressive disorder and the normal unhappiness experienced under extreme stress.

An alternative conceptualization of the relationship between adjustment disorder and major depressive disorder is that the two disorders are qualitatively or categorically distinct. According to this point of view, major depression is seen as a symptom-based diagnosis (e.g. anhedonia for more than 2 weeks), whereas adjustment disorder is more function-based (e.g. inability to maintain role functioning).

A study (Passik *et al.* 2001) shows that a traditional depression screen does not adequately identify adjustment disorder in ambulatory oncology patients. Attempts to develop and validate a tool specifically for adjustment disorder have also been disappointing (Kirsch *et al.* 2004).

Adjustment disorder diagnosis as a marker of psychological distress

The underdiagnosis and undertreatment of psychological problems in patients with advanced cancer, and subsequent negative impact in quality of life, remain highly prevalent (Katon and Sullivan 1990; Dugan *et al.* 1998; Zabora 1998). It is clear that persons with psychological distress in general and adjustment disorder in particular are not being diagnosed or recognized by oncology professionals (Razavi *et al.* 1990).

Identification of adjustment disorder

The identification and diagnosis of adjustment disorder is not straightforward. One of the problems with the adjustment disorder diagnosis is that it lacks precise features. The first problem comes in discussing the stressor or triggering event. There are no guidelines or criteria in the DSM-IV for quantifying the stressors leading to adjustment disorder in a given individual (Zilberg *et al.* 1982). It is also difficult to define accurately what constitutes maladaptive behaviour especially under circumstances of monumental stress. There are no universal guidelines and the subjective severity of symptoms or decrement in social function can vary widely within a given individual (Fabrega *et al.* 1987).

There is no doubt that overlap exists between the disorders of major depression, generalized anxiety disorder, and adjustment disorder. However, the diagnosis of adjustment disorder requires that the patient does not qualify for these other diagnoses. Therefore, they can qualify for the diagnosis only if they manifest problems of adapting to the stressor but do not meet criteria for these other diagnoses. The challenge this poses to screening is that there is a need to identify key areas that separate adjustment disorder from major depression in terms of detection. To this end, the notion of coping inflexibility in response to the illness or treatment has been suggested.

It is believed that one of the personality factors that may lead to problems of adjustment is a lack of coping flexibility on the part of the patient regarding illness and illness-related treatment (Rogers and LeUnes 1979; Carson et al. 1989). Those who develop adjustment disorder may be more likely to be rigid in their thinking and determined to address new problems in the manner they did prior to the onset of illness. If previous coping and problem-solving strategies fail, the person may begin to exhibit the emotional reactions (depressed mood and anxiety) associated with adjustment disorder, in contrast to those who have an adaptive style that focuses on being flexible (Lee 1983). This concept has never been formally operationalized for use in assessment and detecting adjustment disorder in cancer patients. Further, there is increasing recognition that a lack of effective, flexible coping is prevalent in cancer patients in distress and that this lack of flexible coping is not being recognized (American Society of Psychosocial and Behavioral Oncology/AIDS 1999).

We conducted a study on the identification of adjustment disorders. The study was specifically an attempt to explore issues related to screening for adjustment disorder. Commonly used scales for depression, anxiety, and quality of life along with two pilot tools were employed for the purpose of detecting patients with psychological distress who met criteria for a diagnosis of adjustment disorder as determined by the structured clinical interview for DSM-IV. Two novel instruments were introduced and piloted during the study to gather initial data and suggestions for items to be included on potential screening tools to undergo a future full psychometric exploration. Both measures exhibited good reliability and overall psychometric properties.

The study results offered some interesting findings. First, none of the scales were significant predictors of adjustment disorder on the structured clinical interview for DSM-IV, although many were able to detect general distress as defined by the presence of any psychological disorder. Thus, a quick and easy method for detecting adjustment disorder remained elusive. Second, having any mental illness (or psychiatric) diagnosis was a good predictor of reduced quality of life. Third, quality of life impact varied with psychiatric diagnosis. Subjects with adjustment disorder had significantly higher quality of life ratings than the comparison group of subjects with either major depression or anxiety, although lower quality of life than those with no psychiatric diagnosis. This provides some initial evidence that, compared with other psychiatric diagnoses or to the absence of psychiatric diagnosis, adjustment disorder may be useful as an independent and identifiable disorder as postulated earlier, with implications for quality of life and well-being that are both different from and less severe than for other psychiatric disorders.

Treatment of adjustment disorder

Patients identified as having adjustment disorder are often associated with being at risk for increased morbidity and even mortality (i.e. suicide) (DeLeo *et al.* 1986). It is important to note, however, that persons with adjustment disorder have been shown to have positive outcomes when they are treated with brief psychotherapy (Sifneos 1989), the usual form of psychotherapy employed by psycho-oncologists. This allows for the possibility of early treatment delivered by nurse specialists, and other staff before a problem worsens to the point of requiring more intensive care and medications. Psychotherapy for adjustment disorder addresses the stressors directly by teaching enhanced coping skills and is focused on immediacy. Establishing social support networks and psychoeducation are also employed (Pollin and Holland 1992; Wise 1994). Informal support groups and more formal group therapy have been shown to be highly effective for improving quality of life and decreasing depression and anxiety symptoms in cancer patients (Speigel 1981; Zabora 1998). The rapid identification of adjustment disorder can prompt early psychological intervention that can help to promote the patient's quality of life, or at the very least, may prevent the further erosion of the patient's ability to function.

The crisis intervention model is the basis for much oncology-related psychotherapy. Crisis intervention is a process for actively influencing psychosocial functioning during a period of disequilibrium. It is directed at alleviating the immediate impact of disruptive stressful events. The aim is to reduce emotional distress while working toward strengthening the patient's psychological and social resources. Generally, crisis therapy is time limited and asserts clear-cut goals (Parad and Parad 1990). Supportive/crisis intervention psychotherapy involves clarifying information and answering questions about the illness and its treatment, correcting misunderstanding, and giving reassurance about the situation. Describing common reactions to illness may help the patient and their family to normalize their experience. Patients' usual adaptive strategies should be explored and their strengths supported as needed in adjustment. The patients should be encouraged to discuss how they feel about their lifestyle modifications, their family role changes, their fears of dependency and abandonment. Themes of loss and anticipatory grief can be useful to discuss. The patients often experience loss of good health, loss of body integrity, loss of self-esteem, along with losses secondary to cancer (e.g. financial, social, and occupational). Therapy should improve a sense of control and morale. When the focus of treatment changes from cure to palliation, it will be extremely important for the patient to know that while curative treatment has ended they will not be abandoned and that their comfort, pain control, and dignity will receive continued attention.

Cognitive-behavioural interventions help patients allay exaggerated fears by encouraging patients to consider different possible outcomes for their situation. Helping the patient focus on what aspects of the disease and its treatment that the patients have control over, and encouraging behaviour modification that will keep them involved and positive, could provide a better quality of life for these patients. Relaxation techniques and imagery may enhance any of these therapeutic interventions. Simple focused breathing exercises, meditation, and progressive muscle relaxation can be used to lessen episodic anxiety that many cancer patients experience. Pleasant imagery, such as visualizing a gentle stream flowing through a beautiful landscape, can also ease tension some patients feel.

Self-help groups and hospice day care useful interventions for cancer patients and family members who are distressed. The professionally run groups will usually use educational, supportive, or cognitive-behavioural methods while the lay groups generally focus on education, practical advice, modelling, and serving as a source of mutual support and advocacy.

Conclusions

Patients with advanced cancer often have co-morbid psychiatric problems including a high frequency of adjustment disorders and anxiety. The identification and management of these disorders can often be accomplished by the oncology staff, but the provision of appropriate mental health staff, e.g. social work, liaison psychiatry, and psychology is invaluable. Working together, the team can enhance quality of life for the patient and family.

References

Adams F, Fernandez F, Andersson B (1986). Emergency pharmacotherapy of delirium in the critically ill cancer patient. *Psychosomatics* 27:33–7.

American Psychiatric Association (1994). *Diagnostic and statistical manual of mental disorders* (4th edn). Washington, DC: APA.

American Society of Psychosocial and Behavioral Oncology/AIDS (1999). *Standards of care for the management of distress in patients with cancer*. New York: American Society of Psychosocial and Behavioral Oncology/AIDS.

Breitbart W (1986). Tardive dyskinesia associated with high dose intravenous metoclopramide. *N Engl J Med* 315:518.

Breitbart W (1989). Psychiatric management of cancer pain. *Cancer* 63:2336–42.

Carson D, Council J, Volk M (1989). Temperament as a predictor of psychological adjustment in female adult incest victims. *J Clin Psychol* 45(2):330–5.

Chouinard G, Young S, Annable L (1983). Antimanic effect of clonazepam. *Biol Psychiatry* 18:451–66.

DeLeo D, Pellagrin C, Cerate L (1986). Adjustment disorders and suicidality. *Psychiatr Rep* 59:355–8.

Depue R, Monroe S (1986). Conceptualization and measurement of human disorder in life stress research: the problem of chronic disturbance. *Psychiatr Bull* 99:36–51.

Derogatis L, Morrow G, Fetting J (1983). The prevalence of psychiatric disorders among cancer patients. *JAMA* 249(6):751–7.

Dugan W, McDonald M, Passik S, Rosenfeld B, Theobald D, Edgerton S (1998). Use of the zung self-rating depression scale in cancer patients: feasibility as a screening tool. *Psycho-Oncology* 7:483–93.

Fabrega H, Mezzich J, Mezzich A (1987). Adjustment disorder as a marginal or transitional illness category in DSM-III. *Arch Gen Psychiatry* 44(6):567–72.

Friedenbergs I, Kaplan E (1993). Cancer. In: Eisenberg M, Glueckauf R, Zaretsky H (ed.). *Medical aspects of disability: a handbook for the rehabilitation professional.* New York: Springer Publishing Company, pp. 105–18.

Holland J (1989). Anxiety and cancer: the patient and family. *J Clin Psychol* 50:20–5.

Hollister L (1986). Pharmacotherapeutic considerations in anxiety disorders. *J Clin Psychol* 47:33–6.

Katon W, Sullivan M (1990). Depression and chronic medical illness. *J Clin Psychol* 51 (Suppl. 6):3–11.

Kirsh KL, McGrew JH, Passik SD (2004). Difficulties in screening for adjustment disorder, Part II: An attempt to develop a novel self-report screening instrument in cancer patients undergoing bone marrow transplantation. *Palliat Support Care* 2:33–41.

Lawrie I, Lloyd-Williams M, Taylor F (2004). How do palliative medicine physicians assess and manage depression. *Palliat Med* 18:234–8.

Lee R (1983). Returning to work: potential problems for mid-career mothers. *J Sex Marital Ther* 9(3):219–32.

Liebowtiz M (1985). Imipramine in the treatment of panic disorder and it's complications. *Psychiatr Clin North Am* 8:37–47.

Massie M (1989). Anxiety, panic and phobias. In: Holland J, Rowland JH (ed.). *Handbook of psychooncology: psychological care of the patient with cancer.* New York: Oxford University Press, pp. 300–9.

Massie M, Holland J, Straker N (1989). Psychotherapeutic interventions. In: Holland J, Rowland JH (ed.). *Handbook of psychooncology: psychological care of the patient with cancer.* New York: Oxford University Press, pp. 455–69.

Miller K, Massie MJ (2006). Depression and anxiety. *Cancer J* 12(5):388–97 (Review).

Molassiotis A, Boughton B, Burgoyne T, Van den Akker O (1995). Comparison of the over-all quality of life in 50 long-term survivors of autologous and allogeneic bone marrow transplantation. *J Adv Nurs* 22(3):509–16.

Oliver D (1985). The use of methotrimeprazine in terminal care. *Br J Clin Pract* 39:339–40.

Passik S, Cooper M (1999). Complicated delirium in a cancer patient successfully treated with olanzapine. *J Pain Symptom Manage* 17:219–23.

Passik S, Dugan W, McDonald M, Rosenfeld B, Theobald D, Edgerton S (1998). Oncologists' recognition of depression in their patients with cancer. *J Clin Oncol* 16:1594–600.

Passik S, Kirsh K, Donaghy K, Theobald D, Lundberg J, Lundberg E (2001). An attempt to employ the zung self-rating depression scale as a lab test to trigger follow-up in ambulatory oncology clinics: criterion validity and detection. *J Pain Symptom Manage* 21(4):273–81.

Pollin I, Holland J (1992). A model for counseling the medically ill: The Linda Pollin Foundation Approach. *Gen Hosp Psychiatry* 14(6S):11–24.

Popkin M, Callies A, Mackenzie T (1985). The outcome of antidepressant use in the medically ill. *Arch Gen Psychiatry* 42:1160–3.

Razavi D, Delvaux N, Farvacques C (1990). Screening for adjustment disorders and major depressive disorders in cancer patients. *Br J Psychiatry* 156:79–83.

Regier D, Narrow W, Rae D (1993). The de facto mental and addictive disorders service system. Epidemiologic catchement area prospective 1-year prevalence rates of disorders and services. *Arch Gen Psychiatry* 50(2):85–94.

Rogers S, LeUnes A (1979). A psychometric and behavioral comparison of delinquents who were abused as children with their non-abused peers. *J Clin Psychology* 35(2):470–2.

Sifneos P (1989). Brief dynamic and crisis therapy. In: Kaplan H, Sadock B (ed.). *Comprehensive Textbook of Psychiatry*, Vol. 2, (5th edn). Baltimore, MD: Williams & Wilkins, pp. 1562–7.

Spiegel D (1981). Group support for patients with metastatic cancer. A randomized outcome study. *Arch Gen Psychiatry* 38:527–33.

Strain J (1998). Adjustment disorders. In: Holland J (ed.). *Psycho-oncology*. New York: Oxford University Press, pp. 509–17.

Theobald DE, Kirsh KL, Holtsclaw E, Donaghy K, Passik SD (2002). An open-label, crossover trial of mirtazapine (15 and 30 mg) in cancer patients with pain and other distressing symptoms. *J Pain Symptom Manage* 23(5):442–7.

Vinokur A, Caplan R (1986). Cognitive and affective components of life events. Their relations and effects on well-being. *Am J Community Psychol* 14:351–71.

Walsh T (1990). Adjuvant analgesic therapy in cancer pain. In: Foley KM, Bonica JJ, Ventafridda V, (ed.). *Advances in Pain Research and Therapy*, Vol. 16, Second International Congress on Cancer Pain. New York: Raven Press, pp. 155–66.

Wilson KG, Chochinov HM, Skirko MG, Allard P, Chary S, Gagnon PR, Macmillan K, De Luca M, O'Shea F, Kuhl D, Fainsinger RL, Clinch JJ (2007). Depression and anxiety disorders in palliative cancer care. *J Pain Symptom Manage* 33(2):118–29.

Wise M (1994). Adjustment disorders and impulse disorders not otherwise classified. In: Talbot J, Hales R, Yudofsky S (ed.). *Textbook of psychiatry*, (2nd edn). Washington DC: American Psychiatric Press.

World Health Organization (1995). *International classification of diseases*, (10th edn). Geneva: World Health Organization.

Zabora J (1998). Screening procedures for psychosocial distress. In: Holland J (ed.). *Psycho-oncology*. New York: Oxford University Press, pp. 653–61.

Zilberg N, Weiss D, Horowitz M (1982). Impact of event scales: cross-validation study and some empirical evidence supporting a conceptual model of stress response syndromes. *J Consult Clin Psychol* 50(3):407–14.

Chapter 7

Diagnosis, assessment, and treatment of depression in palliative care

Hayley Pessin, Yesne Alici Evcimen, Andreas J. Apostolatos, and William Breitbart

Introduction

It is generally accepted practice in the field of palliative care that adequate palliative care must focus beyond a focus on pain and physical symptom control, to include psychiatric, psychosocial, existential, and spiritual domains of care. Therefore, skills in diagnostic assessment of psychiatric disorders in patients with terminal cancer are of increasing importance to palliative care practitioners. Depression is considered the most frequent mental health issue among patients receiving palliative care (Wilson *et al.* 2000). Therefore, the diagnosis and management of depression in patients with advanced cancer is perhaps the most difficult and important psychiatric issue confronting palliative care practitioners.

A number of medical and psychosocial issues such as medication side-effects, physical impairments, dependency, loss of autonomy, anticipatory grief, and family dysfunction, all of which frequently co-occur during a terminal illness, can increase the risk of psychological distress and depressive symptomatology at the end of life (Breitbart *et al.* 1998). Depressed mood and sadness are common, even appropriate responses, for patients who are facing a terminal illness. Yet, despite the common occurrence of feelings of sadness and depression among terminally ill individuals, these symptoms, although often ameliorable, frequently remain unrecognized and untreated, as they are dismissed as 'normal reactions' even in the face of severe affective disturbance. This chapter reviews the prevalence, risk factors, assessment, and management of depression in terminally ill cancer patients. It will provide the tools to effectively recognize, address, and care for patients experiencing depression at the end of life in order to minimize distress and offer a more comprehensive approach to palliative care.

Prevalence of depression in palliative care

There is a wide body of work that attests to the presence of depression among terminally ill populations. In a recent comprehensive review of 64 relevant articles, Solano et al. (2006) concluded that the rate of depression among various terminally ill populations ranged 3–77% (cancer), 10–82% (AIDS), 9–36% (heart disease), 37–71% (chronic obstructive pulmonary disease), and 5–50% (renal disease). a similar analysis of prevalence rates in general advanced disease by Hotopf et al. (2002) noted that between 5% and 26% of patients were depressed when assessed via clinician interviews. With regard to the literature on cancer patients specifically, Massie (2004) reported that between 0% and 38% of cancer patients fit criteria for major depression, while 0–58% were eligible for diagnoses within the full spectrum of depressive syndromes. Furthermore, a number of studies have examined the prevalence of depression in specifically far-advanced cancer patients (Derogatis et al. 1983; Kathol et al. 1990a; Chochinov et al. 1994; Minagawa et al. 1996; Akechi et al. 2004; Lloyd-Williams et al. 2004a; Kadan-Lottick et al. 2005; Wilson et al. 2007). These studies suggest that depression commonly occurs in later stages of cancer, ranging in prevalence from 3.2% to 52% (see Table 7.1), with a median occurrence rate of approximately 21% (Wilson et al. 2007).

Table 7.1 Prevalence of depressive disorders among advanced cancer patients

Study	Population	N	Diagnostic Criteria	Prevalence
Derogatis et al. (1983)	mixed inpatients & outpatients	215	DSM-III	6% major depression 12% adjustment disorder with depression
Bukberg et al. (1984)	mixed inpatients	62	DSM-III (excluded somatic symptoms)	42% major depression
Lansky et al. (1985)	mixed female outpatients & inpatients	505	DSM-III	5% major depression
Evans et al. (1986)	gynecology inpatients	83	DSM-III	23% major depression
Razavi et al. (1990)	mixed inpatients	210	Endicott Criteria/ DSM- III HADS	8% major depression 52% adjustment disorder
Kelsen et al. (1995)	pancreatic cancer	130	BDI	38% major depression
Alexander et al. (1993)	mixed inpatients	60	DSM-III-R	13% major depression 2% dysthymia 17% adjustment disorder with depression

Table 7.1 (continued) Prevalence of depressive disorders among advanced cancer patients

Study	Population	N	Diagnostic Criteria	Prevalence
Power et al. (1993)	palliative care various cancer	98	AMTS DSM III-R	26% depression
Chochinov et al. (1995)	mixed palliative care inpatients	200	RDC	8% major depression 5% minor depression
Minagawa et al. (1996)	palliative care inpatients	109	DSM-III	3.2% major depression 7.5% adjustment disorder
Grassi et al. (1996)	advanced various cancer	86	HADS EORTC-QLQ-C30	45% depression
Chochinov et al. (1997)	advanced terminally ill cancer	197	BDI; VAS semi-structured interview	12.2% depression 7.6% major depression 4.6% minor depression
Breitbart et al. (2000)	mixed palliative care inpatients	92	DSM-IV HDRS	18% major depression
Hopwood and Stephens (2000)	lung cancer	987	HADS quality of life form	33% depression self reported 21% depression and anxiety
Lloyd-Williams et al. (2004a)	mixed palliative care	74	DSM-IV	27% major depression
Akechi et al. (2004)	palliative care mixed cancer	209	DSM-III-R	6.7% major depression 16.3% adjustment disordered
Kadan-Lottick et al. (2005)	advanced cancer mixed	251	Endicott Criteria DSM-IV	6% major depression 7.2% minor depression
Wilson et al. (2007)	palliative care mixed cancer	381	DSM-IV	20.7% depression 13.1% major depression

The broad variation in the reported prevalence of depression in this population is due, in part, to the problems of terminology, methodology, and the application of diagnostic systems not originally intended for use in cancer patients. In addition, differences across settings and clinical populations (e.g. ambulatory, advanced cancer, or hospice patients) may contribute to wide variations across prevalence studies. Methodological issues such as the use of different diagnostic criteria, as well as, the inclusion of adjustment disorder represent a major source of inconsistency. Finally, the sample characteristics and inclusion criteria may impact prevalence rates significantly especially at the end of life where psychiatric comorbidity is highly prevalent.

In summary, the available literature on prevalence of depression in advanced cancer patient suggests that the rate of depression is elevated in cancer as compared with the general population. Furthermore, even when the most stringent criteria are used, about 5–15% of patients with cancer will meet criteria for major depression. Furthermore, another 10–15% of patients present with symptoms that, while less severe, still require treatment. There is good empirical support for the conclusion that at least one-quarter of patients with advanced cancer will present with a significant degree of dysphoria (Massie 2004).

Diagnosis and assessment of depression in palliative care

Criterion-based diagnostic system

A criterion-based diagnostic system includes approaches such as Diagnostic and Statistical Manual of Mental Disorders—Text Revision (DSM-IV-TR; American Psychiatric Association 2000) or its predecessors (DSM-IV; DSM III; DSM-III- R), and the Research Diagnostic Criteria (Endicott and Spitzer 1978). These systems are based on the assumption that depression is a distinct syndromal disorder characterized by a constellation of symptoms, of a certain minimal level of severity and duration, and associated with impairment in functional and social roles. Patients are classified as having a depressive episode based on whether or not they meet these specific criteria.

The symptoms that must be assessed to make the diagnosis of depression are listed in the DSM-IV-TR (see Table 7.2). Utilization of the different diagnostic classification systems, such as the DSM-III, DSM-IV, and Research Diagnostic Criteria, can lead to widely varying rates of detection of depression in patients with life threatening illness. Certainly, the DSM-IV diagnostic criteria for depression are the most widely accepted and best validated tool for diagnosis. Table 7.3 outlines questions used to assess symptoms of depression based on the DSM-IV-TR criteria. In addition, several authors have published more extensive guidelines on how to conduct a more extensive assessment of depression with questions specifically tailored to a palliative care population (Trask 2004; Pessin *et al.* 2005; Block 2006) The assessment of suicide, a particularly important criterion in assessing depression among the terminally ill, will be addressed more fully later.

Assessment of depression

There are several different approaches to assessment procedures, which are categorized into criterion-based diagnostic systems, diagnostic interviews, and

Table 7.2 DSM-IV-TR criteria for major depressive syndrome

A.	At least five of the following symptoms have been persistent for 2 weeks or more (at least one symptom must be #1 or #2)

    1) Depressed mood or dysphoria most of the day, nearly everyday

    2) Loss of interest or pleasure or anhedonia

    3) Sleep disorder, insomnia or hypersomnia

    4) Appetite or weight change

    5) Fatigue or loss of energy

    6) Feelings of worthlessness or guilt

    7) Indecisiveness or poor concentration

    8) Thoughts of death or suicidal ideation

B. The symptoms do not meet criteria for a Mixed Episode

C. The symptoms cause clinically significant social or occupational impairment

D. The symptoms are not due to the direct physiological effects of a substance or a general medical condition.

E. The symptoms are not better accounted for by bereavement

Table 7.3 Questions to assess depressive symptoms in palliative care settings

Cognitive/Emotional Symptom Questions	Symptom
How well are you coping with your cancer? Well? Poorly?	Well-being
How are your spirits since diagnosis? Down? Blue? Do you cry sometimes? How often? Only alone?	Mood
Are there things you still enjoy doing? Have you lost pleasure in things you use to do before you had cancer?	Anhedonia
How does the future look to you? Bright? Black? Do you feel you can influence your care or is your care totally under others' control?	Hopelessness
Do you worry about being a burden to family or friends during treatment for cancer?	Worthlessness
Feel others might be better off without you?	Guilt
Have you had any thoughts of not wanting to live or you would be better off dead?	Suicidal Ideation
Have you stopped taking care of yourself or thought about hurting yourself?	Suicidal Plan

Table 7.3 (continued) Questions to assess depressive symptoms in palliative care settings

Physical Symptoms	Symptom
Do you have pain that isn't controlled?	Pain
How much time do you spend in bed? Do you feel weak? Fatigue easily? Rested after sleep? Any relationship to change in treatment or how you feel otherwise physically?	Fatigue
How is your sleeping? Trouble going to sleep? Awake often?	Insomnia
How is your appetite? Does food taste good? Any change in weight?	Appetite
How is your interest in sex? Has there been a change in how frequently you have sex?	Libido
Do you have problems coming up with thoughts? Have you felt that your thoughts are slower than usual?	Concentration
Have you been moving more slowly than usual?	Psychomotor

self-report measures (see Table 7.4). For research purposes, diagnostic assessments are usually conducted using structured interviews such as the Diagnostic Interview Schedule (Robins *et al.* 1981), the Structured Clinical Interview for DSM-IV (SCID) (First *et al.* 2001) or the Schedule for Affective Disorders and Schizophrenia (SADS) (Endicott and Spitzer 1978). These interviews differ with respect to their degree of structure and in the formats with which the interviewer codes the patient's verbal responses. The DIS is highly structured and designed for use by lay interviewers. The SCID, considered the gold standard in the field, and SADS are semistructured and are intended for use by clinicians. With the DIS and the SCID, the interviewer is required to code specific symptoms as being either present or absent, whereas with the SADS, the interviewer rates the severity of symptoms on ordinal scales. All of these interview protocols have been subjected to extensive checks of their reliability and validity. Typically, investigators administer only the modules within an interview that address depression in order to minimize patient burden.

In addition, the use of self-report measures in assessing depression has recently become more widespread due to their relative ease of use and ability to be scored by non-expert clinicians (Trask 2004). The most commonly used self-report measure in palliative care settings include the Rotterdam Symptom Checklist (SRCL), the Beck Depression Inventory (BDI), the Brief Symptom Inventory-Depression Scale, the Center for Epidemiologic Studies Depression

Table 7.4 Research assessment methods for depression in cancer patients

Criterion-Based Diagnostic Systems
Diagnostic and Statistical Manual DSM-III, III-R, IV
Endicott Substitution Criteria
Research Diagnostic Criteria (RDC)
Structured Diagnostic Interviews
Schedule for Affective and Schizophrenia (SADS)
Diagnostic Interview Schedule (DIS)
Structured Clinical Interview for DSM-III-R (SCID)
Primary Care Evaluation of Mental Disorders (PRIME MD)
Screening Instruments-Self Report
General Health Questionnaire-30
Hospital Anxiety and Depression Scale (HADS)
Beck Depression Inventory (BDI)
Rotterdam Symptom Checklist (RSCL)
Carroll Depression Rating Scale (SDRS)
Brief Edinburgh Depression Scale (BEDS)

Scale (CES-D), the Zung Self-Rating Depression Scale, and the Hospital Anxiety and Depression Scale (HADS). In assessing cancer patients, Trask (2004) notes that the HADS is the most frequently used of these instruments, as it was designed for use with a medically ill patient population. However, it should be noted that there is often debate around the appropriate cut-off score that should be utilized in a palliative care population (Lynch 1995; Trask 2004). If it is set too low there is a risk of increasing false positive diagnosis and too high patients who have significant distress may be missed.

Finally, in addition to more thorough self-report measures, recent efforts have been made to develop short screening tools to either identify cases of depression outright, or to indicate the need for more in-depth psychiatric evaluation (Lloyd-Williams et al. 2003, 2004a, 2006; Arnold 2007), which have obvious utility for palliative care settings due to the brevity. While there is much work to be done in the way of improving the predictive power of these quick, often one-question screening devices, there has been some research that has revealed promising results (Lloyd-Williams et al. 2003, 2004a; Arnold 2007). Another recent study by Mitchell and Coyne (2007), however, suggested that a one-question assessment screening successfully identified only three of every 10 depressed patients in a primary care setting. The authors noted that the addition of subsequent questions improved the predictive power of the screening device. In sum, it seems as though the future of such brief assessment methods might be more in the area of ruling out patients who are not depressed, rather than serving as a basis for full on diagnosis of clinical depression.

Issues in assessment of depression in the terminally ill

The most common diagnostic difficulty that arises in palliative care setting is how to interpret the physical or somatic symptoms patients present with in the context of a possible depression (Pessin *et al.* 2005). The challenge is to determine if these symptoms part of the depression syndrome or a direct biological result of advancing cancer. In answering this question, five different approaches to the diagnosis of major depression in the terminally ill patient have been described (Spitzer *et al.* 1994; Breitbart *et al.* 1995). These approaches are:

- inclusive: includes all symptoms whether or not they may be secondary to illness or treatment)
- exclusive: deletes and disregards all physical symptoms from consideration, not allowing them to contribute to a diagnosis of Major Depressive Syndrome
- aetiological: the clinician attempts to determine if the physical symptom is due to cancer illness or treatment (and so does not include it), or due to a depressive disorder (in which case it is included as a criterion symptom)
- a high diagnostic threshold approach that requires patients have seven (instead of five) criteria symptoms for major depression
- substitutive approach: where physical symptoms of an uncertain aetiology are replaced by other non-somatic symptoms.

The latter approach is best exemplified by the Endicott Substitution Criteria (1984) (see Table 5).

While there are advantages and disadvantages to each of the approaches above, there is not a clear consensus as to which one is the best approach for

Table 7.5 Endicott Substitution Criteria (1984)

Physical/Somatic	Psychological Symptom Substitute
Change in appetite or weight	Tearfulness Depressed appearance
Sleep disturbance	Social withdrawal Decreased talkativeness
Fatigue or Loss of energy	Brooding, Self-Pity Pessimism
Diminished ability to think or concentrate Indecisiveness	Lack of reactivity

accurately diagnosing depression in the terminally ill. Chochinov *et al.* (1994) studied the prevalence of depression in a terminally ill cancer population and compared low versus high diagnostic thresholds, as well as Endicott Substitution Criteria. Interestingly, identical prevalence rates of 9.2% for major depression and 3.8% for minor depression (total = 13%) were found utilizing Research Diagnostic Criteria high threshold criteria and high threshold Endicott criteria.

Unique considerations must be taken into account regarding the presentation of individual depressive symptoms in the terminally ill patient. Pessin *et al.* (2005) offer a comprehensive outline of how extra caution should be used to pin-point whether depressive symptoms are the result of clinical depression *per se*, or if they are an extension of the underlying terminal illness. For typical depressive symptoms such as sleep complications, psychomotor retardation or agitation, and concentration difficulties, it is virtually impossible to rule out the potential influence of the terminal disease itself, or related medication, as the underling cause. Similarly, in assessing anhedonia, clinicians must undergo due diligence to ensure that a patient's desire and motivation for engaging in previously enjoyed activity has been lost, and not that they are simply being constrained by the physical burdens of the illness. In the case of hopelessness and sadness, steps should be taken to ensure that such symptoms present to a degree and frequency that is beyond the general expectation of what is typically experienced by the dying patient. In this regard, the clinician might insure that a patient's suffering from depressed mood represents a significant burden that is dealt with on a near daily basis, and for a substantial period of time. Similarly, hopelessness should be more than a realistic assessment of prognosis but rather a pervasive feeling of futility. It is also common for the very ill to ponder their mortality and contemplate existential issues. However, once these thoughts seem to be better characterized by a frequent preoccupation with a desire for death, the influence of clinical depression may be more relevant. Similarly, with hypochondriasis, while most patients are anxious and seeking clarification as to the cause of symptoms related to their illness, when such concerns are met with obsessive tendencies, or are repeatedly offered without questioning by the clinician, it is more likely that these symptoms are reflective of true depression.

Other depressive disorders

In addition to major depression, there are other DSM-IV diagnoses that commonly present in terminally ill patients that have depressed mood as a central presenting feature. Minor depression is similar to major depression, but requires fewer symptoms in order to qualify for a diagnosis (two to four symptoms in total). Dysthymia, in contrast, is defined as a chronic condition characterized by low-grade depressive symptoms that persist for at least 2 years. Adjustment disorder with depressed mood, on the other hand, describes a relatively short-lived maladaptive reaction to stress. This diagnosis requires that a patient's depressive response to the stressor must be 'in excess of a normal and expectable reaction.' If applied too loosely, the diagnosis of adjustment disorder can pathologize the experience of some patients by applying a psychiatric label on what may be a normal display of grief. Other clinical constructs that have recently received a great deal of attention and may be difficult to distinguish from depression due to a great deal of overlap are demoralization syndrome, characterized by loss of meaning and purpose, hopelessness, existential distress, pessimism, and isolation (Kissane *et al.* 2001) as well as preparatory grief a more common process associated with dying where the patient experiences dysphoria in reaction to the perception of loss in preparation for their death (Kubler-Ross 1997; Periyakoil *et al.* 2005). Differentiating, grief from depression can be quite challenging in palliative care but generally grief is considered more transitory and often diminishes over time (Block 2006; Noorani and Montagni 2007) Therefore, a comprehensive assessment of current and past depressive symptoms is essential in order to distinguish the above syndromes and subsequently determine appropriate treatment.

Risk factors for depression in the terminally ill

Gender

One of the most consistent results across epidemiological studies within the general population has been that women have rates of major depressive disorder that are approximately double those of men (Weissman *et al.* 1996). This finding leads to the hypothesis that women might also be more likely to become depressed in the face of life-threatening illness. In fact, some studies have indeed found higher levels of depressive symptoms and distress among female cancer patients (Stommel *et al.* 1993; Wilson *et al.* 2007), including patients at an advanced terminal stage. However, Lloyd-Williams *et al.* (2004a) note that the majority of relevant research has reported equal rates of depression among terminally ill men and women. Although gender is perceived to be a major risk for depression, it should be treated with caution among the terminally ill, as men may be more vulnerable to depression in this population.

Age

Epidemiological studies suggest that depressive disorders are more common among younger adults (i.e. under age 45 years) than older adults. However, the expectation that this would translate into higher rates of depression among younger cancer patients must be tempered by the fact that cancer is a disease that predominantly afflicts people in their older years. Nevertheless, a number of studies, have identified the same trend, and found that younger cancer patients do indeed show higher rates of diagnosed depressive disorders (Levine *et al.* 1978; Kathol *et al.* 1990b; Wilson *et al.* 2000) or self-reported distress. Factors that can contribute to the higher prevalence of depression in younger patients may include the feeling that life has been cut short and ambitions have not been realized, concerns about the welfare of one's dependants, and also the methodological issue that younger people may be more willing to acknowledge psychological symptoms.

Prior history of depression

There is a growing recognition that for some individuals, depression can be a chronic or recurrent disorder. Within the general population, a prior episode of depression appears to be one of the stronger risk factors that predict the onset of new episodes. A number of studies have also found that patients with cancer who are currently depressed are more likely to report prior episodes from earlier periods in their lives (Hughes 1985; Wilson *et al.* 2000). In this context, the struggle with life-threatening illness is clearly a major stressor that may precipitate an episode of depression in individuals who are particularly vulnerable (Harrison and Maguire 1994).

Social support

In studies of the general population, deficits in the adequacy of one's social support network have often been related to clinical depression (Bruce and Hoff 1994). The experience of social support is also thought to play a role in the psychological adjustment of patients with serious medical illness and has been found to be associated with depression in the terminally ill. The physical and psychosocial stressors associated with cancer are likely to result in a greater need for all forms of support. The provision of support may depend on family members, who are under considerable strain, as they attempt to cope with the life-threatening illness of a loved one. Furthermore, many patients with good relationships hesitate to add to their family's burden and avoid discussing their emotional state, which can intensify the sense of isolation. This cycle of isolating events can cause the patient to withdraw, and become depressed.

Functional status

Decreasing physical ability is correlated with measures of depression or distress (Kaasa *et al.* 1993; Williamson and Schulz 1995; Lloyd-Williams *et al.* 2004b).

Of course, functional ability is likely to decrease with the progression of the disease, so patients with more advanced illness appear to have the greatest risk for a number of psychiatric disorders. As patients receiving palliative care lose functional abilities, a sense of helplessness, dependency, deterioration, and confrontation with their own inevitability may fuel depressive symptomatology.

Pain

There is now a considerable body of evidence indicating that studies of patients with cancer have found an association between increased pain and reports of depression, and such a link is indeed reliable across a range of settings and methods of assessment (Chochinov et al. 1995; Glover et al. 1995; Chen et al. 2000; Wilson et al. 2000). While the magnitude of the correlations are not especially high, on the order of $r = 0.25$–36, the clinical implications are substantial. Research has shifted from merely demonstrating that there is an association between pain and depression, to considering more precisely what the nature of the causal link might be. Uncontrolled pain may not only increase depression, but depression may result in an amplification of the pain experience (Spiegel and Bloom 1983).

Cancer and treatment-related factors

Specific types of cancers themselves, the subsequent disease process, as well as treatment-related side-effects may induce depressive symptoms. With regard to cancer diagnosis, Massie (2004) reports that oropharyngeal, pancreatic, breast, and lung cancers are more associated with depression, while lower rates of depression are seen in patients with lymphoma, colon, and gynaecological cancers. Some sites of cancer are associated with depression, beyond the level of the expected reactive symptoms. Tumours that originate in or metastasize to the central nervous system have the potential to cause depressive symptoms (Brown and Parakevas 1982). Pancreatic cancer is also associated with depression (Shakin and Holland 1988). Metabolic complications such as hypercalcaemia, most often associated with cancer of the breast and lung. These remote effects may be due to several factors, including toxins secreted by the tumour, autoimmune reactions, viral infections, nutritional deficits, and neuroendocrine dysfunction (McDaniel et al. 1995). Problems such as weight loss, fatigue, sleep disturbance, and poor concentration are common symptoms of the disease process in cancer, and they can also be associated with the toxic side-effects of treatment. These treatments include corticosteroids (Stiefel et al. 1989), as well as various chemotherapy medications, and radiotherapy protocols. More recently treatment with cytokine interferon α treatments has been shown to induce symptom of depression as well (Mussleman *et al.* 2000). These risk factors are summarized in Table 7.6.

Existential concerns

The recognition that one is facing a life-threatening crisis may bring with it a greater focus on existential concerns regarding unfulfilled ambitions, past regrets, meaning in life, and the maintenance of dignity and self-control, as well as social concerns about the welfare of one's family (Breitbart 2002). In a study of sources of distress among patients with cancer, Noyes *et al.* (1990) found that items related to a loss of meaning showed higher correlation with depression than physical symptoms, medical treatment, or social isolation. In contrast, maintaining a sense of meaning and purpose has been found to be protective against depression and desire for death (Breitbart *et al.* 2000; Nelson *et al.* 2002; Block 2006). The relationship of existential distress to depressive syndromes among patients who are terminally ill is worthy of further investigation in future research (Breitbart *et al.* 2000).

Suicide and desire for hastened death in the terminally ill

Occasional thoughts of suicide are quite common in patients in palliative care settings and appear to act as a 'steam valve' for patients to cope with their feelings (Breitbart *et al.* 1993). However, persistent suicidal ideation is relatively infrequent and limited to patients in the context of psychiatric complications, such as depression. Patients with advanced cancer are at highest vulnerability because they are most likely to have such cancer complications as pain, depression, delirium, lost of autonomy, as well as, strong feelings of

Table 7.6 Medical causes of depression in patients with advanced cancer

Uncontrolled pain
Metabolic abnormalities
hypercalcemia, sodium or potassium imbalance, anemia, deficiencies in vitamins B_{12} or folate
Endocrinological abnormalities
hyper- or hypothyroidism, adrenal insufficiency
Medications
glucocorticosteroids, interferon and interleukin-2, methyldopa, reserpine, barbituates, propranolol, some antibiotics (amphotericin B), some chemotherapeutic agents (vincristine, vinblastine, procarbazine, L-asparaginase)

helplessness and hopelessness. A review of the consultations done at Memorial Sloan–Kettering Cancer Center demonstrated that 30% of suicidal cancer patients had a major depression, 50% were diagnosed with adjustment disorder at the time of evaluation, and about 20% suffered from a delirium (Breitbart 1987).

Understanding why some patients with a terminal illness wish or seek to hasten their death remains an important element in both the physician-assisted suicide debate as well as the practice of palliative care. Although euthanasia and physician-assisted suicide have been distinguished legally and ethically from the administration of high-dose pain medication intended to relieve pain, there still are numerous questions to investigate such as understanding clearly the underlying wish and intent in expressing such demands as well as the factors associated with a patient's expression of a desire to die (Rosenfeld *et al.* 2000). Despite the continued legal prohibitions against assisted suicide in most places, a substantial number of patients think about and discuss those alternatives with their physicians, family, and friends.

Desire for hastened death, the construct underlying requests for assisted suicide, euthanasia, and suicidal thoughts, remains an important element in the practice of palliative care. Recent research has focused on physical and psychological concerns, such as depression that may give rise to a desire for hastened death (Cassem 1987). Several studies have demonstrated that depression plays a significant part in the terminally ill patient's desire for hastened death. Breitbart *et al.* (2000) demonstrated in a sample of terminally ill cancer patients that both depression and hopelessness, characterized as a pessimistic cognitive style rather than an assessment of one's poor prognosis, appear to be independent determinants of desire for hastened death.

Assessment of suicide risk

Assessment of suicide risk and appropriate intervention are critical in palliative care settings. Furthermore, the myth that asking about suicidal thoughts put the 'idea into their head' is one that should be dispelled. In fact, patients often reconsider the idea of suicide when the legitimacy of these feelings and the patients need for a sense of control over death is acknowledged. A comprehensive evaluation, which includes a thorough history and inquiry into the patients' specific suicidal thought, plans, and intentions, is required for any patient expressing interest in suicide or the related constructs of desire for hastened death and physician-assisted suicide (see Table 7.7). A clinician's ability to establish a report is essential, as they conduct a thorough evaluation includes an assessment of risk, degree of intent, relevant history, quality of internal and external control, as well as the meaning behind the

Table 7.7 Evaluation of suicidal patients in palliative care*

Establish rapport using empathetic approach
Obtain patient's understanding of patient's illness and symptoms
Assess mental status
Assess vulnerability, pain control
Assess support system
Assess for history of alcohol/substance abuse
Inquire about recent losses/deaths
Obtain prior psychiatric history
Obtain family history
Obtain history of prior attempts or threats
Assess suicidal thinking, intent and plans (see below)
Evaluate need for one on one observation in hospital or at home
Formulate treatment plan, short term and long term

Questions to Assess for Suicide

Open with a statement such as: **"Most patients with cancer have passing thoughts about suicide, such as 'I might do something if things get bad enough'"**...

Question	Rational
Have you ever had thoughts like that?	Normalize
Any thoughts of not wanting to live or that it would be better if you were dead?	Ideation
Do you have any thoughts of suicide? Plans?	Intent
Have you thought about how you would do it?	Plan

*Adapted from Breitbart W. Cancer pain and suicide. In Foley K, Bonica JJ, Ventafridda V (Eds.) *Advances in Pain Research and Therapy, vol 16*. New York, Raven Press, 1990, p. 409.

suicidal thoughts. In addition, mental status and adequacy of pain and symptom control should be determined. When assessing risk for suicide, Rudd and Joiner (1999) have recommended evaluating the following factors: predisposition to suicidal behaviour (i.e. history of suicidal behaviour, psychiatric diagnosis, and demographic risk factors), precipitators or stressors, symptomatic presentation (i.e. depression, anger, and agitation), nature of suicidal thinking (frequency, intensity, duration, specificity of plans, availability of means, and explicitness of intent), hopelessness, previous suicide behaviour (frequency, method, lethality, and outcome), impulsivity, and lack of protective factors (social support, problem-solving skills, and mental health treatment.

Management of the suicidal patient

The response of a clinician to a patient's expression of desire for death, suicidal ideation, or request for assisted suicide has important and obvious implications on all aspects of care that impact on the patient, the patient's family, and staff. Once the setting has been made secure, these issues must be addressed both rapidly and thoughtfully, offering the patient a non-judgemental willingness to engage in a discussion of the factors that contribute to the suffering and despondency that leads patients to express such a desire for death. Most palliative care clinicians believe that effective management of physical and psychological symptoms will naturally prevent expressions of distress or requests for assisted suicide. Pharmacological interventions, including antidepressants, analgesics, or narcoleptics should be utilized to treat symptoms of depression, and any accompanying symptoms of anxiety, agitation, psychosis, or pain. The mobilization of the patients' support system may be highly effective as well. Furthermore, clinical interventions may need to be developed to more specifically address hopelessness and related constructs such as loss of meaning, demoralization, and spiritual distress that are especially prevalent near the end of life. Ultimately the palliative care clinician may not be able to prevent all suicides in all terminally ill patients. Prolonged suffering caused by poorly controlled symptoms can lead to such desperation, and it is the appropriate role of the palliative care team to provide effective management of physical and psychological symptoms as an alternative to desire for death, suicide or request for assisted suicide by patients.

Management of depression in palliative care

General principles

Once a depressive disorder has been identified in a terminally ill patient, the relationship with the primary medical caregiver and or the mental health practitioner is the most important component of support for many patients with a serious illness. Optimally, these relationships are based on mutual trust, respect, and sensitivity. The ability to acknowledge the patients distress, see the patient as 'whole persons', and respond to them on the basis of their own individual personal style and needs, tends to work best. Perhaps, more than in any other clinical setting, maintaining on going contact with the depressed terminally ill patient is of critical importance. This not only ensures that patients will be continually re-evaluated, but also provides reassurance to patients that they will not be abandoned, and care will be forthcoming and available throughout their terminal course.

Psychosocial interventions

Depression in cancer patients is optimally managed utilizing a combination of supportive psychotherapy, cognitive-behavioural techniques, antidepressant medication, as well as patient and family education (Maguire *et al.* 1985; Block 2006). For patients with cancer suffering from major depression, adjustment disorder, or dysthymia, there are a variety of psychosocial interventions with proven efficacy. These include individual psychotherapy, group psychotherapy, hypnotherapy, psycho-education, relaxation training and biofeedback, and self-help groups. Psychotherapy and cognitive-behavioural techniques are useful in the management of psychological distress in cancer patients, and have been applied to the treatment of depressive and anxious symptoms related to cancer and cancer pain. Furthermore, cognitive-behavioural interventions are especially favourable due to their ability to be catered to the specific psychological state of each patient, such as differential needs to address symptom control and quality of life issues (Jacobsen and Hann 1998). An additional focus in these types of therapeutic regimens is to help the patient recognize what depressive symptoms might represent a normal emotional response to a cancer diagnosis (Bailey *et al.* 2005). Psychotherapeutic interventions, either in the form of individual or group counselling, have been shown to effectively reduce psychological distress and depressive symptoms in cancer patients (Spiegel and Wissler 1987). Cognitive-behavioural interventions, such as relaxation and distraction with pleasant imagery, have also been shown to decrease depressive symptoms in patients with mild to moderate levels of depression (Spiegel *et al.* 1981; Massie and Holland 1990). Owing to the time limited nature of treatment for the terminally ill, supportive psychotherapy however, is a useful treatment approach to depression in the terminally ill patient. Finally, psychotherapy in conjunction with pharmacological treatment may be the quickest, most effective, and comprehensive way to address patients' symptoms and distress near the end of life.

Pharmacological treatment of depression

Pharmacotherapy is the mainstay for treating terminally ill cancer patients meeting diagnosis criteria for major depression, as it often provides symptom reduction most quickly. Factors such as prognosis and the timeframe for treatment may play an important part in determining the type of pharmacotherapy for depression. A depressed patient with several months of life expectancy can afford to wait the 2–4 weeks it may take to respond to an antidepressant, such as SSRIs. The depressed dying patient with less than 3 weeks to live may do best with a more rapidly acting psychostimulant. However, a recent meta-analysis of 28 randomized controlled trials has yielded encouraging findings demonstrating symptomatic improvement in depression by the end of first week of treatment with SSRIs (Taylor *et al.* 2006). Finally, patients who are within hours to days of death and in distress are likely to benefit most from the use of sedatives or narcotic analgesic infusions.

There are a number of controlled studies of antidepressant drug treatment for depressive disorders in cancer patients in general, fewer that focus on the terminally ill. The efficacy of antidepressants in the treatment of depression in cancer patients has been well established (Costa *et al.* 1985). However, a survey of antidepressant prescribing in the terminally ill found that out of 1,046 cancer patients, only 10% received antidepressants, 76% of whom did not receive them until the last 2 weeks of life (Lloyd-Williams *et al.* 1999). However, a more recent survey among 381 patients receiving palliative cancer care presents a more encouraging picture in that 22.6% of the total sample was prescribed antidepressants, which included 39.8% of those diagnosed with a mental disorder. It is important to note that 60% of those with a disorder were not being treated with antidepressants (Wilson *et al.* 2007). As discussed earlier, depressive symptoms are estimated to be present in a quarter of cancer patients. Therefore, it can be concluded that many depressed patients with advanced cancer never receive appropriate pharmacological treatment or receive them only in the final 2 weeks of life, when it is too late for a treatment response. Table 7.8 outlines the antidepressant medications used in advanced cancer patients. The choice of antidepressant depends on the patient's medical history, concomitant medical problems, prior responses to antidepressants, possible drug–drug interactions, and the side-effects associated with the medications. The clinicians should target the specific distressing symptoms of depression such as insomnia, fatigue, and anorexia.

Selective serotonin re-uptake inhibitors (SSRIs)

SSRIs are commonly the first line of treatment in advanced cancer patients with an estimated life span of few weeks or longer, because of their safety and low side-effect profile. It is good practice 'to start low and go slow' in cancer patients in order to reduce gastrointestinal side-effects of nausea and transient weight loss. The SSRIs are safe with chemotherapeutic agents, but should be avoided in patients receiving procarbazine for management of some haematological malignancies, as procarbazine is a monoamine oxidase inhibitor.

The SSRIs have a number of features that are advantageous for cancer patients. They have a very low affinity for adrenergic, cholinergic, and histamine receptors, thus accounting for negligible orthostatic hypotension, urinary retention, memory impairment, sedation, or reduced awareness. They do not require therapeutic drug level monitoring and have not been found to

Table 7.8 Antidepressant medications used in palliative care settings

Drug	Therapeutic Daily Dosage mg (PO)
Psychostimulants	
Dextroamphetamine	2.5-30
Methylphenidate	2.5-30
Modafinil	50-400
Serotonin selective reuptake inhibitors	
Fluoxetine*	10-60
Paroxetine	10-40
Citalopram*	10-40
Escitalopram*	5-20
Fluvoxamine	50-300
Sertraline*	25-200
Newer Antidepressants	
- Serotonin/norepinephrine reuptake inhibitors	
Venlafaxine	37.5-225
Duloxetine	20-60
- 5-HT2 antagonists/serotonin/norepinephrine reuptake inhibitors	
Nefazodone	100-300
Trazodone	50-300
- Norepinephrine/dopamine reuptake inhibitor	
Buproprion	75-450
- α-2 antagonist/5-HT2/5HT3 antagonist	
Mirtazapine	7.5-45
Tricyclic antidepressants	
Secondary Amines	
Desipramine	25-200
Nortriptyline*	10-150
Tertiary Amines	
Amitriptyline	10-150
Doxepin*	25-300
Imipramine	10-200
Monoamine oxidase inhibitors	
Phenelzine	15-60
Tranylcypromine	10-40

*Available in liquid formulations.

cause clinically significant alterations in cardiac conduction and are generally favourably tolerated along with a wider margin of safety than the tricyclic antidepressants in the event of an overdose.

Most of the side-effects of SSRIs result from their selective central and peripheral serotonin reuptake properties. These include increased intestinal motility, diarrhoea, nausea, vomiting, insomnia, headaches, and sexual dysfunction. Some patients may experience anxiety, tremor, restlessness, and akathisia. These side-effects tend to be dose related and may be problematic for patients with advanced disease. However, most disappear with continued use of the medication (Masand and Gupta 1999). Initially, adding a benzodiazepine with the SSRI helps to prevent the common side-effects of anxiety, restlessness, and akathisia. Use of SSRIs has been associated with an increased risk of gastrointestinal bleeding, especially when used in combination with non-steroidal anti-inflammatory drugs (de Abajo *et al.* 2006). Syndrome of inappropriate antidiuretic hormone secretion has also been associated with SSRI use (Grover *et al.* 2007). SSRIs may interact with other serotonergic drugs (i.e. opioid analgesics) resulting in serotonin syndrome. Symptoms of serotonin syndrome include restlessness, hyperreflexia, myoclonus, tremor, and autonomic dysfunction (Boyer and Shannon 2005).

Currently, there are six SSRIs available in the market including sertraline, fluoxetine, paroxetine, citalopram, escitalopram, and fluvoxamine. With the exception of fluoxetine, whose elimination half-life is 2–4 days, the SSRIs have an elimination half-life of about 24 hours. Fluoxetine is the only SSRI with a potent active metabolite—norfluoxetine—whose elimination half-life 7–14 days. Fluoxetine can cause mild nausea and a brief period of increased anxiety as well as appetite suppression that usually lasts for a period of several weeks. Some patients can experience transient weight loss, but weight usually returns to baseline level. This has not been a limiting factor in the use of fluoxetine in cancer patients. Fluoxetine and norfluoxetine do not reach a steady state for 5–6 weeks, compared with 4–14 days for paroxetine, fluvoxamine, and sertraline. These differences are important, especially for the terminally patient in whom a switch from an SSRI to another antidepressant is being considered. If a switch to a monamine oxidase inhibitor is required, the washout period for fluoxetine will be at least 5 weeks, given the potential drug interactions between these agents. Paroxetine, fluvoxamine, citalopram, escitalopram, and sertraline on the other hand require considerably shorter washout periods (10–14 days) under similar circumstances. SSRIs with a short half-life, such as paroxetine, have occasionally been associated with flu-like withdrawal symptoms if stopped abruptly, so slow taper is recommended if the medicine is to be stopped.

An important aspect that distinguishes between SSRIs is the cytochrome P450-related metabolism. Fluoxetine and paroxetine both are metabolized by and inhibit the 2D6 pathway. Citalopram, escitalopram, and sertraline are all metabolized through the 3A4, 2C19, and 2D6 pathways, but they have a low likelihood of drug–drug interactions possibly due to their low protein binding (Miller *et al.* 2006). Fluvoxamine has been shown in some instances to elevate the blood levels of propranolol and warfarin by as much as twofold, and should thus not be prescribed together with these agents.

For advanced cancer patients, SSRIs can be started at approximately half the usual starting dose used in a healthy patient. Titration of fluoxetine, can begin as 5 mg (available in liquid form) given once daily (preferably in the morning) with a range of 10–40 mg per day; given its long half-life, some patients may only require this drug every second day. Paroxetine can be started at 10 mg once daily (either morning or evening) and has a therapeutic range of 10–40 per day. Fluvoxamine, which tends to be somewhat more sedating, can be started at 25 mg (in the evenings) and has a therapeutic range of 50–300 mg. Sertraline can be initiated at 50 mg, morning or evening and titrated within a range of 50–200 mg per day. Citalopram can be initiated at 10 mg in the morning and titrated within a range of 10–40 mg per day. Escitalopram can be started at 5–10 mg daily and may be titrated up to 20 mg a day. If patients experience activating effects on SSRIs, the medication can be given earlier in the day. An additional advantage is that liquid formulations are available for most SSRIs for patients with difficulty swallowing pills.

Newer antidepressants

This category of antidepressants, namely, venlafaxine, duloxetine, nefazodone, trazodone, mirtazapine, and bupropion display a wide range of therapeutic mechanisms.

Serotonin-norepinephrine reuptake inhibitors (SNRI)

Venlafaxine and duloxetine are the only antidepressants in this class. They are potent inhibitors of neuronal serotonin and norepinephrine reuptake and appear to have no significant affinity for muscarinic, histamine or α_1-adrenergic receptors. They are generally well-tolerated with a relatively benign side-effect profile similar to SSRIs. However, norepinephrine reuptake inhibition may result in palpitations and hypertension. Therefore blood pressure monitoring is recommended for patients on an SNRI. Venlafaxine mostly inhibits serotonin uptake at low doses, its norepinephrine reuptake inhibition is seen at doses higher than 150 mg a day. Duloxetine shows serotonin and norepinephrine reuptake inhibition at starting doses. Both medications have low

P450 inhibition and moderate plasma protein binding (Dugan and Fuller 2004). Venlafaxine and duloxetine are preferably used for patients with comorbid depression and neuropathic pain.

Bupropion

Bupropion acts primarily on the dopamine system and may have mild stimulant effect, which can be beneficial for patients with fatigue and psychomotor retardation. It is generally not associated with weight gain or sexual dysfunction and has an additional application for use in the pharmacotherapy of smoking cessation. It is generally tolerated well. Bupropion is associated with an increased risk of seizures at higher doses and should be avoided in patients with central nervous system or seizure disorders. Single doses of bupropion should not exceed 150 mg, a dose increase should not be greater than 100 mg of bupropion per day, and the dose increases should be gradual.

Nefazodone

Nefazodone and trazodone are chemically related antidepressants that block post-synaptic 5-HT$_2$ receptors. Nefazodone is much less sedating than trazodone but more likely to cause gastrointestinal activation. Nefazodone does not have any sexual dysfunction side-effects. Nefazodone is a potent inhibitor of cytochrome P450 3A4 isoenzyme. Nefazodone has received a blackbox warning for cases of hepatic failure, therefore is now rarely prescribed by psycho-oncologists.

Trazodone

If given in sufficient doses (100–300 mg/day), trazodone can be an effective antidepressant. However, in addition to its blockade of post-synaptic 5-HT$_2$ receptors, it also has considerable affinity for α_1-adrenoceptors and may thus predispose patients to orthostatic hypotension and its problematic sequelae (i.e. falls, fractures, and head injuries). Trazodone is very sedating and in low doses is helpful in the treatment of the depressed cancer patient with insomnia. Sedation and weight gain are additional common and useful side-effects in patients with insomnia and anorexia. Lack of anticholinergic side-effects with these medications is helpful in treating patients prone to delirium and cognitive dysfunction. Rare side-effects include priapism and cardiac arrhythmias.

Mirtazapine

Mirtazapine enhances central noradrenergic and serotonergic activity with blockade of central presynaptic α_2 inhibitory receptors and postsynaptic serotonin 5-HT$_2$ and 5-HT$_3$ receptors. It compares favourably with amitriptyline and trazodone, with further studies needed to compare the clinical efficacy of mirtazapine with serotonin reuptake inhibitors. Mirtazapine improves appetite resulting in weight gain, which is desirable in cancer patients. In addition, the marked sedative effect of this medication proves quite useful in patients with insomnia. It also has antiemetic properties (Nutt 2002). At lower doses the sedating effects are greater, at doses higher than 30 mg a day the sedating effect is less pronounced and the antidepressant effect is more prominent. It is available in a dissolvable tablet form that is particularly useful for patients who have difficulty swallowing, and for patients with nausea and vomiting. Mirtazapine has rarely been implicated in producing severe blood dyscrasias, such as agranulocytosis.

Tricyclic antidepressants

The application of TCAs specifically to cancer patients requires a careful risk–benefit ratio analysis, especially when used in patients with advanced cancer. Although nearly 70% of patients treated with a tricyclic for non-psychotic depression can anticipate a positive response, their side-effect profile can be troublesome for cancer patients. Tricyclics are effective antidepressants but require monitoring of cardiac function and drug levels in patients who are prone to toxicity and side-effects. Constipation and dry mouth are undesirable in cancer patients, especially those on opioids. Other anticholinergic side-effects such as urinary retention, blurred vision, orthostatic hypotension, and arrhythmias make tricyclics less desirable. The tricyclics are well proven to be effective analgesic agents, especially for neuropathic pain and are more affordable, as compared with other antidepressants. Their multiple pharmacodynamic actions accounting for these side-effects include blockade of muscarinic cholinergic receptors, α-adrenoceptors and H_1 histamine receptors. The tertiary amines (amitriptyline, doxepin, and imipramine) have a greater propensity to cause side-effects than do secondary amines (nortriptyline, desipramine). The anticholinergic actions of TCAs can cause serious tachycardia. Their quinidine-like effects can lead to arrhythmias by delaying the conduction through the His–Purkinje system.

In addition, TCAs are highly protein bound and are metabolized primarily by the liver. Serum levels may vary from person to person due to differences in the rate of metabolism. Desipramine and nortriptyline are metabolized through cytochrome P450 2D6 pathway, the tertiary amines use the 1A2, 3A4, and 2C19 pathways. About 5–10% of Caucasians have a recessive gene that results in a deficient 2D6 activity. About 20% of Asians are deficient in the 2C19 pathway. These genetic differences may result in wide variation in blood levels of TCAs (Nelson 2004).

Therefore, TCAs should be started at low doses (10–25 mg qhs) and increased in 10–25 mg increments every 2–4 days, until a therapeutic dose is attained or side-effects become a dose-limiting factor. Depressed cancer patients often achieve a therapeutic response at significantly lower doses of TCAs (25–125 mg) than are necessary in the physically well (150–300 g). The choice of which specific TCA to use depends on a variety of factors including the nature of the underlying medical condition, the characteristics of the depressive episode, past responses to antidepressant therapy and the specific drug side-effect profile. For depressed cancer patients, the choice of TCA is made on the basis of a side-effect profile, which will be least incompatible with the patients' overall medical condition. Most tricyclics are available as rectal suppositories for patients who are no longer able to take medication orally. Most importantly, therapeutic response to TCAs, has a latency period of 3–6 weeks.

Monoamine oxidase inhibitors

In general MAOIs are rarely used in the cancer settings, including palliative care facilities. Patients who receive MAOIs must avoid foods rich in tyramine, sympathomimetic drugs (amphetamines, methylphenidate) and medications containing phenylpropanolamine and pseudoephedrine (Breitbart and Mermelstein 1992). The combination of these agents with MAOIs may cause a potentially fatal hypertensive crisis. MAOIs in combination with opioid analgesics have also been reported to be associated with myoclonus and delirium, and must therefore be used together cautiously (Breitbart 1988). MAOIs can also cause considerable orthostatic hypotension.

The reversible inhibitors of monoamine oxidase-A (RIMAs) may reduce some of the problems associated with the older MAOIs. Moclobemide, a RIMA available in the Canadian market, appears to be loosely bound to the MAO-A receptor and is thus relatively easily displaced by tyramine from its binding site. It has a very short half-life, which further reduces the possibility of any prolonged adverse effects, e.g. hypertensive crisis. Dietary restrictions avoidant of tyramine-containing foods are thus not required. The side-effect profile of moclobemide is far more favourable than non-selective MAOIs and tends to be well tolerated. Although the risk of hypertensive crisis is significantly reduced, it is not entirely eliminated and MAOIs are likely to remain second-line antidepressants.

Selegiline transdermal formulation has recently been approved by the US Food and Drug Administration. It may have a particular value in the treatment of depressed cancer patients who are not able to take any oral medications; however, it has not been evaluated for use in cancer patients.

Selegiline is a non-selective MAOI. Because the medication is transdermal, it theoretically bypasses the gut wall, significantly reducing the medication's effect on the MAO-A in the digestive tract. Selegiline is also thought to inhibit MAO-B preferentially at low doses. However, it is important to consult with a psychiatrist before considering selegiline for a depressed cancer patient due to its potential side-effects and multiple drug–drug interactions.

Psychostimulants

Psychostimulants used in cancer patients include methylphenidate, dextroamphetamine, and modafinil, the so-called 'wakefulness promoting agent'. Pemoline has been withdrawn from the market due to risk of hepatic failure associated with its use. All psychostimulants have a rapid onset of action. Psychostimulants exert dopaminergic effects. They have been shown to be rapidly effective antidepressants especially in the cancer setting (Bruera *et al.* 1987; Fernandez *et al.* 1987; Breitbart and Mermelstein 1992; Burns and Eisendrath 1994; Olin and Masand 1996). Several investigators have demonstrated the efficacy of methylphenidate in the treatment of depression in advanced cancer patients, reporting rapid onset of action (1–3 days) and response rates as high as 85%.

In relatively low doses, psychostimulants stimulate appetite, promote a sense of well-being, and improve feelings of weakness, fatigue, and concentration in cancer patients. Treatment with dextroamphetamine or methylphenidate usually begins with a dose of 2.5 mg at 08.00 hours and at noon. The dosage is slowly increased over several days until a desired effect is achieved or side-effects (anxiety, insomnia, paranoia, and confusion) intervene. Patients are usually maintained on methylphenidate for 1–2 months, and approximately two-thirds will be able to be withdrawn from methylphenidate without recurrence of depressive symptoms. Tolerance will develop and adjustment of dose may be necessary. An additional benefit of stimulants is that they have been shown to reduce sedation secondary to opioid analgesics and provide adjuvant analgesics in cancer patients (Bruera *et al.* 1987). Common side-effects of stimulants include anxiety, mild increase in blood pressure and pulse rate, anorexia, insomnia, irritability, and tremor. Rare side-effects include dyskinesias or motor tics, psychotic symptoms or exacerbation of an underlying and unrecognized confusional state. However, side-effects are not common at low doses and can be avoided by slow titration.

Modafinil

Modafinil is known as a wakefulness-promoting agent. The predominant mode of action of modafinil is that of inhibition of GABA. This inhibition appears to allow release of dopamine, norepinephrine, and serotonin. Modafinil increases Fos expression in tuberomamillary nuclei and orexin neurons; activation of these neurons may be an essential component of the wakefulness-promoting action (Prommer 2006). Although further controlled studies are required, early reports suggest its efficacy as an antidepressant. Most studies assessing the role of modafinil in the treatment of depression have been limited to augmentation studies in healthy individuals (Fava *et al.* 2005). Modafinil is safe to use in patients with depression. It appears to be useful in rapidly improving fatigue, and sleepiness associated with depression or antidepressants. It produces increased alertness, wakefulness, and energy. Modafinil should be given in the morning and can be started at a dose of 100 mg for most patients. Starting at 50 mg is advisable for elderly or frail patients. The dose can then be titrated upwards. Side-effects may include anxiety, restlessness, and insomnia.

Electroconvulsive therapy

Electroconvulsive therapy is an effective treatment modality for depressed patients. Occasionally, it is necessary to consider electroconvulsive therapy for depressed cancer patients who have depression with psychotic features or in whom treatment with antidepressants poses unacceptable side-effects (Wilson *et al.* 2000). Although generally a safe treatment for medically ill patients, the use of electroconvulsive therapy is often impractical in a palliative care setting and therefore rarely utilized.

Conclusions

Depression is a common complication among patients receiving end of life care that continues to be under-recognized and remains a source of considerable suffering. The underdiagnosis and undertreatment of depression has a substantial impact on the quality of the last weeks of life for the terminally ill patient. Awareness of the risk factors associated with depression, as well as, the utilization of methods of accurate assessment depression can increase the likelihood of identifying these patients. Both pharmacological and non-pharmacological treatments for depression are often highly effective in patients with advanced disease and should be readily utilized. The amelioration of depression is essential in order to provide effective and comprehensive palliative care, as it will minimize prolonged suffering, maximize the potential for a meaningful existence, and help provide a higher quality of life for patients near the end of life.

References

de Abajo FJ, Montero D, Rodriguez LA, Madurga M (2006). Antidepressants and risk of upper gastrointestinal bleeding. *Basic Clin Pharmacol Toxicol* 98(3):304–10.

Akechi T, Okuyama T, Sugawara Y, Nakano T, Shima Y, Uchitomi Y (2004). Major depression, adjustment disorders, and post-traumatic stress disorder in terminally ill cancer patients: associated and predictive factors. *J Clin Oncol* 22:1957–65.

Alexander PJ, Dinesh N, Vidyasagar MS (1993). Psychiatric morbidity among cancer patients and its relationship with awareness of illness and expectations about treatment outcome. *Acta Oncol* 32(6):623–6.

American Psychiatric Association (2000). *Diagnostic and Statistical Manual of Mental Disorders, 4th edition-TR*. Washington DC: American Psychiatric Association.

Arnold RM (2007). Screening for Depression in Palliative Care #146. *J Palliat Med* 10(2):484–5.

Bailey RK, Geyen DJ, Scott-Gurnell K, Hipolito MMS, Bailey TA, Beal JM (2005). Understanding and treating depression among cancer patients. *Int J Gynecol Cancer* 15:203–8.

Block SD (2006). Psychological issues in end-of-life care. *J Palliat Med* 9(3):751–72.

Boyer EW, Shannon M (2005). The serotonin syndrome. *N Engl J Med* 352(11):1112–20.

Breitbart W (1987). Suicide in cancer patients. *Oncology* 1:49–53.

Breitbart WS (1988). Psychiatric complications of cancer. In: Brain MC (ed.). *Current Therapy in Hematology Oncology*, Vol. 3. Toronto: BC Decker, Inc., pp. 268–74.

Breitbart W (2002). Spirituality and meaning in supportive care: spirituality and meaning-centered group psychotherapy interventions in advanced cancer. *Support Care Cancer* 10:272–80.

Breitbart W, Mermelstein H (1992). Pemoline. An alternative psychostimulant for the management of depressive disorders in cancer patients. *Psychosomatics* 33(3):352–6.

Breitbart W, Bruera E, Chochinov H, Lynch M (1995). Neuropsychiatric syndromes and psychological symptoms in patients with advanced cancer. *J Pain Symptom Manage* 10(2):131–41.

Breitbart W, Levenson JA, Passik SD (1993). Terminally ill cancer patients. In: Breitbart W, Holland JC (ed.). *Psychiatric aspects of symptom management in cancer patients*. Washington DC: American Psychiatric Press, pp. 192–4.

Breitbart W, Chochinov HM, Passik S (1998). Psychiatric aspects of palliative care. In: Doyle D, Hanks GEC, McDonald N (ed.). *Oxford textbook of palliative medicine*, pp. 933–54. New York: Oxford University Press.

Breitbart W, Rosenfeld B, Pessin H et al. (2000). Depression, hopelessness, and desire for hastened death in terminally ill patients with cancer. *JAMA* 284(22):2907–11.

Brown JH, Paraskevas F (1982). Cancer and depression: cancer presenting with depressive illness: an autoimmune disease? *Br J Psychiatry* 141:227–32.

Bruce ML, Hoff RA (1994). Social and physical health risk factors for first-onset major depressive disorder in a community sample. *Soc Psychiatry Psychiatr Epidemiol* 29(4):165–71.

Bruera E, Chadwick S, Brenneis C, Hanson J, MacDonald RN (1987). Methylphenidate associated with narcotics for the treatment of cancer pain. *Cancer Treat Rep* 71:67–70.

Bukberg J, Penman D, Holland JC (1984). Depression in hospitalized cancer patients. *Psychosom Med* 46(3):199–212.

Burns MM, Eisendrath SJ (1994). Dextroamphetamine treatment for depression in terminally ill patients. *Psychosomatics* 35:80–3.

Cassem NH (1987). The dying patient. In: Hackett TP, Cassem NH (ed.). *Massachusetts general hospital handbook of general hospital psychiatry*. Littleton, MA: PSG Publishing, pp. 332–52.

Chen M, Chang H, Yeh C (2000). Anxiety and depression in Taiwanese cancer patients with and without pain. *J Adv Nurs* 32:944–51.

Chochinov HM, Wilson KG, Enns M, Lander S (1994). Prevalence of depression in the terminally ill: effects of diagnostic criteria and symptom threshold judgments. *Am J Psychiatry* 151(4):537–40.

Chochinov HM, Wilson KG, Enns M, Lander S, Levitt M, Clinch JJ (1995). Desire for death in the terminally ill. *Am J Psychiatry* 152(8):1185–91.

Chochinov HM, Wilson KG, Enns M, Lander S (1997). 'Are you depressed?' Screening for depression in the terminally ill. *Am J Psychiatry* 154:674–6.

Costa D, Mogos I, Toma T (1985). Efficacy and safety of mianserin in the treatment of depression of women with cancer. *Acta Psychiatr Neurol Scand Suppl* 320:85–92.

Derogatis LR, Morrow GR, Fetting J, Penman D, Piasetsky S, Schmale AM, Henrichs M, Carnicke CL Jr. (1983). The prevalence of psychiatric disorders among cancer patients. *JAMA* 249(6):751–7.

Dugan SE, Fuller MA (2004). Duloxetine: a dual reuptake inhibitor. *Ann Pharmacother* 38:2078–85.

Endicott J (1984). Measurement of depression in patients with cancer. *Cancer* 53:2243–8.

Endicott J, Spitzer RL (1978). A diagnostic interview: the schedule for affective disorders and schizophrenia. *Arch Gen Psychiatry* 35(7):837–44.

Evans DL, McCartney CF, Nemeroff CB, Raft D, Quade D, Golden RN, Haggerty JJ Jr, Holmes V, Simon JS, Droba M, *et al.* (1986). Depression in women treated for gynecological cancer: clinical and neuroendocrine assessment. *Am J Psychiatry* 143(4):447–52.

Fava ME, Thase M, DeBattista C (2005). A multicenter, placebo-controlled study of modafinil augmentation in partial responders to selective serotonin reuptake inhibitors with persistent fatigue and sleepiness. *J Clin Psychiatry* 66:85–93.

Fernandez F, Adams F, Holmes VF, Levy JK, Neidhart M (1987). Methylphenidate for depressive disorders in cancer patients. An alternative to standard antidepressants. *Psychosomatics* 28(9):455–61.

First M, Spitzer R, Gibbon M, Williams J (2001). *Structured clinical interview for DSM-IV-TR Axis I Disorders, Research Version (SCID)*. New York: Biometrics Research, New York State Psychiatric Institute.

Glover J, Dibble SL, Dodd MJ, Miaskowski C (1995). Mood states of oncology outpatients: does pain make a difference? *J Pain Symptom Manage* 10(2):120–8.

Grassi L, Rosti G, Albertazzi L, Marangolo M (1996). Depressive symptoms in autologous bone marrow transplant (ABMT) patients with cancer: an exploratory study. *Psychooncology* 5:305–10.

Grover S, Biswas P, Bhateja G, Kulhara P (2007). Escitalopram-associated hyponatremia. *Psychiatry and Clinical Neurosci* 61:132–3.

Harrison J, Maguire P (1994). Predictors of psychiatric morbidity in cancer patients [see comments]. *Br J Psychiatry* 165(5):593–8.

Hopwood P, Stephens RJ (2000). Depression in patients with lung cancer: prevalence and risk factors derived from quality-of-life data. *J Clin Oncol* 18:893–903.

Hotopf M, Chidgey J, Addington-Hall J, Ly KL (2002). Depression in advanced disease: a systematic review Part 1. Prevalence and case finding. *Palliat Med* 16:81–97.

Hughes JE (1985). Depressive illness and lung cancer. I. Depression before diagnosis. *Eur J Surg Oncol* 11:15–20.

Jacobsen PB, Hann DM (1998). Cognitive-behavioral interventions. In: Holland JC (ed.). *Psycho-oncology*. New York: Oxford University Press, pp. 717–29.

Kaasa S, Malt U, Hagen S, Wist E, Moum T, Kvikstad A (1993). Psychological distress in cancer patients with advanced disease. *Radiother Oncol* 27(3):193–7.

Kadan-Lottick NS, Vanderwerker LC, Block SD, Zhang B, Prigerson HG (2005). Psychiatric disorders and mental health service use in patients with advanced cancer. *Cancer* 104:2872–81.

Kathol RG, Mutgi A, Williams J, Clamon G, Noyes R, Jr. (1990a). Diagnosis of major depression in cancer patients according to four sets of criteria. *Am J Psychiatry* 147(8):1021–4.

Kathol RG, Noyes R, Jr., Williams J, Mutgi A, Carroll B, Perry P (1990b). Diagnosing depression in patients with medical illness. *Psychosomatics* 31(4):434–40.

Kelsen DP, Portenoy RK, Thaler HT, Niedzwiecki D, Passik SD, Tao Y, Banks W, Brennan MF, Foley KM (1995). Pain and depression in patients with newly diagnosed pancreas cancer. *J Clin Oncol* 13(3):748–55.

Kissane DW, Clarke DM, Street AF (2001). Demoralization syndrome—A relevant psychiatric diagnosis for palliative care. *J Palliat Care* 17:12–21.

Kubler-Ross E (1997). *On Death and Dying*. New York: Simon & Schuster.

Lansky SB, List MA Hermann CA, Ets-Hokin EG, DasGupta TK, Wilbanks GD, Hendrickson FR. (1985). Absence of major depressive disorders in female cancer patients. *J Clin Oncol* 3(11):1553–60.

Levine PM, Silberfarb PM, Lipowski ZJ (1978). Mental disorders in cancer patients: a study of 100 psychiatric referrals. *Cancer* 42(3):1385–91.

Lloyd-Williams M, Friedman T, Rudd N (1999). A survey of antidepressant prescribing in the terminally ill. *Palliat Med* 13(3):243–8.

Lloyd-Williams M, Spiller J, Ward J (2003). Which depression screening tools should be used in palliative care? *Palliat Med* 17:40–43.

Lloyd-Williams M, Dennis M, Taylor F (2004a). A prospective study to compare three depression screening tools in patients who are terminally ill. *Gen Hosp Psychiatry* 26:384–9.

Lloyd-Williams M, Dennis M, Taylor F (2004b). A prospective study to determine the association between physical symptoms and depression in patients with advanced cancer. *Palliat Med* 18:558–63.

Lloyd-Williams M, Shiels C, Dowrick C (2006). The development of the Brief Edinburgh Depression Scale (BEDS) to screen for depression in patients with advanced cancer. *J Affect Disord* 99:259–64.

Lynch ME (1995). The assessment and prevalence of affective disorders in advanced cancer. *J Palliat Care* 11:10–18.

Maguire P, Hopwood P, Tarrier N, Howell T (1985). Treatment of depression in cancer patients. *Acta Psychiatr Scand Suppl* 320:81–4.

Masand PS, Gupta S (1999). Selective serotonin-reuptake inhibitors: an update. *Harv Rev Psychiatry* 7:69–84.

Massie MJ (2004). Prevalence of depression in patients with cancer. *J Natl Cancer Inst Monogr* 32:57–71.

Massie MJ, Holland JC (1990). Depression and the cancer patient. *J Clin Psychiatry* 51(Suppl.):12–17, discussion 18–19.

McDaniel JS, Musselman DL, Porter MR, Reed DA, Nemeroff CB (1995). Depression in patients with cancer. Diagnosis, biology, and treatment. *Arch Gen Psychiatry* 52(2):89–99.

Miller KE, Adams SM, Miller MM (2006). Antidepressant medication use in palliative care. *Am J Hospice Palliat Care* 23(2):127–33.

Minagawa H, Uchitomi Y, Yamawaki S, Ishitani K (1996). Psychiatric morbidity in terminally ill cancer patients. A prospective study. *Cancer* 78(5):1131–7.

Mitchell AJ, Coyne JC (2007). Do ultra-short screening instruments accurately detect depression in primary care? *Br J Gen Pract* 57:144–51.

Musselman DL, Lawson DH, Gumnick JF (2000). Paroxetine for the prevention of depression induced by high dose interferon alfa. *N Engl J Med* 344(13):961–6.

Nelson C, Rosenfeld B, Breitbart W, Galietta M (2002). Spirituality, depression, and religion in the terminally ill. *Psychosomatics* 43:213–20.

Nelson JC (2004). Tricyclic and heterocyclic drugs. In: Schatzberg AF, Nemeroff CB (ed.). *The American psychiatric publishing textbook of psychopharmacology*, (3rd edn). Washington DC: American Psychiatric Publishing, pp. 207–30.

Noorani NH, Montagnini M (2007). Recognizing depression in palliative care patients. *Palliat Med* 10(2):58–64.

Noyes R Jr, Kathol RG, Debelius-Enemark P, Williams J, Mutgi A, Suelzer MT, Clamon GH (1990). Distress associated with cancer as measured by the illness distress scale. *Psychosomatics* 31(3):321–30.

Nutt DJ (2002). Tolerability and safety aspects of mirtazapine. *Human Psychopharmacol* 17(Suppl. 1):S37–41.

Olin J, Masand P (1996). Psychostimulants for depression in hospitalized cancer patients. *Psychosomatics* 37:57–62.

Periyakoil VS, Kraemer HC, Noda A, Moos R, Hallenbeck J, Webster M, Yesavage JA (2005). The development and initial validation of the Terminally Ill Grief or Depression Scale (TIGDS). *Int J Methods Psychiatr Res* 14(4):202–12.

Pessin H, Olden M, Jacobson C, Kosinski A (2005). Clinical assessment of depression in terminally ill cancer patients: a practical guide. *Palliat Support Care* 3(4):319–24.

Power D, Kelly S, Gilsenan J et al. (1993). Suitable screening tests for the cognitive impairment and depression in the terminally ill—a prospective prevalence study. *Palliat Med* 7:213–18.

Prommer E (2006). Modafinil: is it ready for prime time? *J Opioid Manage* 2(3):130–6.

Razavi D, Delvaux N, Farvacques C, Robaye E (1990). Screening for adjustment disorders and major depressive disorders in cancer in-patients. *Br J Psychiatry* 156:79–83.

Robins LN, Helzer JE, Croughan J, Ratcliff KS (1981). National Institute of Mental Health Diagnostic Interview Schedule. Its history, characteristics, and validity. *Arch Gen Psychiatry* 38(4):381–9.

Rosenfeld B, Krivo S, Breitbart W, Chochinov HM (2000). Suicide, assisted suicide, and euthanasia in the terminally ill. In: Chochinov HM, Breitbart W (ed.). *Handbook of psychiatry in palliative medicine.* New York: Oxford University Press, pp. 51–62.

Rudd MD, Joiner T (1999). Assessment of suicidality in outpatient practice. In: VandeCreek L, Jackson T (ed.). *Innovations in clinical practice: a sourcebook*, Vol. 17. Sarasota, FL: Professional Resource Press, pp. 101–17.

Shakin EJ, Holland J (1988). Depression and pancreatic cancer. *J Pain Symptom Manage* 3(4):194–8.

Solano JP, Gomes B, Higginson IJ (2006). A comparison of symptom prevalence in far advanced cancer, AIDS, heart disease, chronic obstructive pulmonary disease and renal disease. *J Pain Symptom Manage* 31:58–69.

Spiegel D, Bloom JR (1983). Pain in metastatic breast cancer. *Cancer* 52(2):341–5.

Spiegel D, Wissler T (1987). Using family consultation as psychiatric aftercare for schizophrenic patients. *Hosp Community Psychiatry* 38(10):1096–9.

Spiegel D, Bloom JR, Yalom I (1981). Group support for patients with metastatic cancer. A randomized outcome study. *Arch Gen Psychiatry* 38(5):527–33.

Spitzer RL, Williams JB, Kroenke K *et al.* (1994). Utility of a new procedure for diagnosing mental disorders in primary care. The PRIME-MD 1000 study. *JAMA* 272(22):1749–56.

Stiefel FC, Breitbart WS, Holland JC (1989). Corticosteroids in cancer: neuropsychiatric complications. *Cancer Invest* 7(5):479–91.

Stommel M, Given BA, Given CW, Kalaian HA, Schulz R, McCorkle R (1993). Gender bias in the measurement properties of the Center for Epidemiologic Studies Depression Scale (CES-D). *Psychiatry Res* 49(3):239–50.

Taylor MJ, Freemantle N, Geddes JR, Bhagwager Z (2006). Early onset of selective serotonin reuptake inhibitor antidepressant action: systematic review and meta-analysis. *Arch Gen Psychiatry* 63(11):1217–23.

Trask PC (2004). Assessment of depression in cancer patients. *J Natl Cancer Inst Monogr* 32:80–92.

Weissman MM, Bland RC, Canino GJ *et al.* (1996). Cross-national epidemiology of major depression and bipolar disorder. *JAMA* 276(4):293–9.

Williamson GM, Schulz R (1995). Activity restriction mediates the association between pain and depressed affect: a study of younger and older adult cancer patients. *Psychol Aging* 10(3):369–78.

Wilson KG, Chochinov HM, de Faye BJ, Breitbart W (2000). Diagnosis and management of depression in palliative care. In: Chochinov HM, Breitbart W (ed.). *Handbook of psychiatry in palliative medicine.* New York: Oxford University Press, pp. 25–49.

Wilson KG, Chochinov HM, Skirko *et al.* (2007). Depression and anxiety disorders in palliative cancer care. *J Pain Symptom Manage* 33(2):118–29.

Chapter 8

Psychotherapeutic interventions in palliative care

Friedrich Stiefel and Mathieu Bernard

Introduction

Patients in palliative care are confronted with a limited future, a situation that often stimulates them to look back on their lives, to establish links between past and present, to think about the relationships with significant others, and to search for meaning. Psychotherapy focuses exactly on such issues and can thus be of help for psychologically distressed patients with a limited life expectancy. As palliative care aims to treat patients comprehensively, psychotherapy, as one of the main approaches to relieve psychological suffering, has therefore an important part to play in the palliative care setting.

The aim of this chapter is to introduce the definitions and the theoretical and practical concepts of the established psychotherapeutic approaches and to present their clinical relevance and associated scientific evidence for the palliative care setting. Finally, the role of unspecific factors, of relational and technical aspects of psychotherapy, as well as the integration of psychotherapy in palliative care are discussed.

Definition of psychotherapy

A general definition, which covers the field of psychotherapy—reads as follow: 'Psychotherapy is a relation among persons, engaged in by one or more individuals defined as needing special assistance to improve their functioning as persons, together with one or more individuals defined as able to render such special help' (Orlinsky *et al.* 2004).

Franck and Frank (1991) identified four dimensions shared by all psychotherapeutic approaches: (1) a relationship in which the patient has confidence that the therapist is competent and cares about his welfare; (2) a practice setting that is socially defined as a place of healing; (3) a rationale or 'myth' that explains the patient's suffering and how it can be overcome; (4) a set of procedures that requires the active participation of the patient and the therapist and of which both believe to be means of restoring the patient's health. Psychotherapy can therefore be viewed as part of the general treatments of disorders as proposed by Franck and Frank (1991):

> Attempts to relieve suffering and disability are usually labeled treatment. Treatment typically involves a personal relationship between healer and sufferer. Certain types of therapy are primarily based on the healer's ability to mobilize healing forces in the sufferer by psychololgical means. These forms of treatment may be generically termed psychotherapy.

Is any approach, which 'mobilizes healing forces in the sufferer by psychological means' a psychotherapeutic treatment? Can 'being nice with a patient' be considered as a psychotherapeutic intervention? The inclusion of a given intervention in a general definition does not guarantee its appropriateness or effectiveness, and does not mean its provider is competent. In analogy, the above-mentioned general definitions are sensitive enough to include all psychotherapeutic interventions, but they lack the specificity to identify an included approach as a psychotherapeutic intervention.

Because of this lack of specificity, authors, such as Wampold (2001) or Lambert and Ogles (2004) insist that psychotherapy, as a form of personal help, is a professional activity or service that implies a certain level of skills. The expertise in helping skills must be formally recognized by training institutes and licensing bodies. Moreover, Wampold (2001) considers as a psychotherapeutic intervention only a treatment, which is anchored in a *psychological* theory and based on a recognized *psychological conceptualization*. Consequently, treatments based on 'occult, indigenous peoples' cultural beliefs about mental health and behavior, New Age ideas, and religion' are not psychotherapeutic interventions.

A psychotherapeutic treatment is not only based on a sound theoretical framework, and, if possible, supported by scientific evidence, it is provided by mental health specialists, who undergo training, acquire specific skills, knowledge, and clinical experience, and who benefit from regular supervision and continuous postgraduate education. In many countries, psychotherapeutic treatments can therefore only be provided by psychiatrists and psychologists who receive certified, additional training. The status of being a psychotherapist is usually accorded by professional societies and approved by regulating bodies.

In the following, we will present the four most often used psychotherapeutic approaches: the psychodynamic psychotherapies, the systemic psychotherapies, the cognitive and behavioural psychotherapies, and the experiential psychotherapies. All of them share the common feature, that they have a long history of theoretical and conceptual development, they have gained an important body of evidence confirming their effectiveness, they provide specialized and certified training programs and they allow a large clinical application. Their theoretical background is presented, followed by a discussion of their clinical relevance for palliative care and, where possible, the associated scientific evidence of their effectiveness in this setting.

Psychotherapeutic interventions in palliative care

Psychodynamic psychotherapy

Theoretical background

Psychodynamic psychotherapies are based on ego psychology derived from Freud's work, object relation theory derived from Klein's and Winnicott's work, and self-psychology derived from Sullivan's interpersonal work (Lewin 2005). Psychodynamic techniques are intended to develop self-understanding and insight into recurrent problems with others. During the therapeutic process, symptoms and interpersonal difficulties are identified and interpreted based on the concept that this insight and the experiences in the therapeutic relationship can be transferred to 'the world outside the therapeutic setting' (Kaplan and Sadock 1998).

Psychodynamic psychotherapies share some key assumptions, such as (1) the existence of an unconscious, which colours our thoughts, emotions, and behaviours; (2) the influence of early human development on later stages of life; (3) the organization of the psyche by the ego, which has the capacity to reason and to anticipate, the id, which is a source of sexual and aggressive drives, and the superego, which contains these drives and which is generally called 'guilty conscience'; (4) the protection of the individual's equilibrium by (unconscious) defence mechanisms, such as rationalization, projection, or denial, which are triggered by threatening emotions or thoughts; and (5) the observation, that unresolved issues of the patient are re-enacted in the therapeutic setting, where they can be interpreted, discussed, and thus be modified.

The different types of psychodynamic psychotherapy reach from the **insight-oriented psychotherapy**, which uncovers repressed, unconscious material and to gain autonomy to **supportive psychotherapy**, which aims to suppress anxiety-provoking, unconscious material and to foster ego functions and adaptive defences (Lewin 2005). As therapists of the other psychotherapeutic approaches discussed in this chapter, psychodynamically oriented psychotherapists work within a consistent theoretical framework, but are flexible with regard to its clinical application. Usually working in a two persons setting and skilled to identify significant events of the patient's past, psychodynamically oriented therapists, where indicated, also focus on the 'here and now' or involve significant others in the treatment.

Psychodynamic psychotherapy in palliative care

Different forms of psychodynamic psychotherapies are used in the palliative care setting. **Supportive psychotherapy** is most often indicated, as for most of the patients, the goal is to enhance adaptation, to diminish dysfunctional coping, to decrease psychological distress and to restore psychological well-being (Stiefel *et al.* 1998; Rodin and Gillies 2000; Guex *et al.* 2000).

Insight-oriented therapy, is suitable for less vulnerable patients with intact ego functions, who are motivated to explore their thoughts and feelings in order to develop a broader range of reactions when facing adverse events (Rodin and Gillies 2000). A special form of psychodynamic psychotherapy is **the psychodynamic life narrative**, which can be understood as a psychodynamic intervention, but also as a way to conceptualize human responses to physical illness. This intervention is particularly indicated for individuals whose psychological equilibrium has been disrupted by a physical illness. The psychodynamic life narrative aims to help the patient to understand their current psychological reactions to illness by linking them to important elements of their life trajectory. This type of therapy offers the patient an opportunity to enhance a sense of control and coherence in a situation, which beforehand has been perceived as chaotic (Viederman 2000).

While there are only few clinical trials, which evaluated the effectiveness of psychodynamic therapies in the physically ill (Ando *et al.* 2007), several single cases studies were published over the last years (Lacy and Higgins 2005; Redding 2005; Tepper *et al.* 2006).

The current quest in medicine for scientific evidence has also reached the domain of the psychotherapeutic treatments of the physically ill. Two major confusions arise from this development: (1) approaches, which have not been evaluated scientifically may be perceived as 'not effective', and (2) there is a tendency to spend a lot of time and energy developing and evaluating 'new and specific treatment modalities' for the palliative care setting. One has to be reminded that all of the four main psychotherapeutic approaches are well established and proved to be effective (Luborsky *et al.* 1999; Wampold 2001; Lambert and Ogles 2004; Zimmermann *et al.* in press); but there are differences with regard to scientific evidence. For example psychodynamically oriented psychotherapists have struggled for a long time to evaluate their treatments, while cognitive-behavioural therapists easily accepted scientific investigations. However, to conclude that cognitive-behavioural approaches are more effective is an error.

With regard to the second point, we consider that the invention of 'new, specific treatment modalities for the palliative care setting' is not appropriate. As mentioned above, the four main psychotherapeutic approaches are applied with flexibility and adapted to the patient's needs; it is well known that they all have their strengths and weaknesses, but most important, they show different effectiveness for different psychological problems and psychiatric disturbances. Instead of 'inventing new and specific' therapies, which often lack a sound theoretical framework and clinical concept and thus losing the rich heritage of psychotherapy, it would be more important to identify which patients respond best to one of the four established psychotherapeutic approaches and for what indication.

Systemic psychotherapy

Theoretical background

Systemic psychotherapy is based on general systems theory, which allows a system, such as the family, to be understood as an organized system. The main principle implies to understand not only the functions of the different elements of a system, but their interrelations. Systemic psychotherapy views the family or other forms of social coexistence as a complex and integrated whole, which is greater than the sum of its parts (Sameroff 1983; Minuchin 1988). Family therapists utilize special techniques for family interviews and focus on variables, such as family cohesion and hierarchy or on family roles and rules (Bressoud *et al.* 2007). In a recent report on the evidence of systemic family therapy, Stratton (2005) indicated that family systemic therapy started with a common basis of systems thinking, but has since grown in various directions over the last 50 years. Indeed, different approaches are associated to the systemic therapy, with the most significant belonging to the work of Bateson and the Palo Alto team (Jackson 1968a,b), the family structural therapy derived from Minuchin (1974), the strategic family therapy developed by Haley (1976) and Madanes (1981), and the work of Selvini Palazzoli and the Milan team (1978, 1991).

Being a systemic therapist does not imply that clinical care is restricted to social systems; a systemic therapist also treats individual patients, but is probably more sensitive to systemic aspects of the patient's problem and tries to gain a comprehensive view of intergenerational and intrafamilial problems and resources.

Systemic psychotherapy in palliative care

Of the different forms of systemic therapies, all can be beneficial in the palliative care setting. We present in the following, as an example, one type of systemic therapy, which has been scientifically evaluated.

The **family-focused grief therapy (FFGT)**, a preventive intervention for high-risk families (Kissane 2006), is based on the assumption that the family is the primary provider of care for the terminally ill patient and that the type of functioning of the family is essential for the patient (Kissane *et al.* 1996a,b). The aim of FFGT is to optimize family functioning and to facilitate the share of grief in order to minimize psychosocial morbidity. The FFGT is a time-limited intervention (four to eight sessions of 90 minutes duration), planed with flexibility over a 9–18-month period. A manual with specific guidelines and clinical illustrations has been developed by Kissane *et al.* (2006). In 2006 they published the results of a randomized controlled trial, which indicated that the overall impact of FFGT was modest, with a reduction of family distress 13 months after the patient's death. The authors concluded, that families with a dysfunctional or intermediate class of functioning, based on the Family Environment Scale (Moos and Moos 1981), were more suitable for preventive intervention with FFGT.

Beside the patient-oriented work, systemic therapist are specially skilled for team supervision, which is an important tool for the palliative care setting.

Cognitive and behavioural psychotherapy

Theoretical background

Cognitive-behavioural therapy is a general term for several forms of therapies with similar characteristics, such as cognitive therapy, rational behaviour therapy, rational living therapy, schema focused therapy, dialectical behaviour therapy, and rational emotive behaviour therapy. Cognitive and behavioural interventions are based on the assumption that conscious thoughts and behaviours are most relevant variables in the aetiology and maintenance of psychological disorders. The interventions, often completed by homework assignments, intend to reduce psychological distress and enhance adaptive coping by modifying maladaptive thoughts and behaviours, and by providing new skills (Hollon and Beck 2004).

According to **cognitive theory** (Beck 1991), maladaptive thoughts are part of an integrated knowledge structure (schema), which influences the way judgements are built. In cognitive therapy, patients are invited to systematically evaluate their beliefs, judgements, and information processes and to challenge them with alternative views provided by the therapist (Beck *et al.* 1979). Various forms of cognitive therapies exist, such as self-control therapy (Rehm 1977), psychoeducational (Lewinsohn *et al.* 1986) or problem-solving therapy. **Behavioural interventions** focus on overt behaviour and strategies to modify them. They are based on classical stimulus–response theory, founded by Pavlov and Gantt (1928), and subsequent theorists, such as Thorndike (1932) who developed the 'law of effect', Skinner (1961) who added complementary concepts, such as operant behaviour and reinforcement, and Watson and Watson (1949) who focused on behaviours of people and their reactions in given situations.

The first therapeutic approach was developed by Ellis (1959) in reaction to psychoanalysis and based on the stoic philosophers who claimed that men were not disturbed by things, but by how they perceived them. In the 1960s clinical therapists, such as Beck (1991) and Maultsby (1971) contributed to the development of cognitive-behavioural interventions. Since 1980, cognitive-behavioural therapies are influenced by the work of Burns (1999) and Freeman *et al.* (2004).

Cognitive or behavioural interventions are not only efficient to modify thoughts and behaviours, but the therapeutic relationship is always also part of the treatment. Thoughts, emotions, and behaviour are modulated by different factors, such as coping, defences, social support, personality, or biography, which influence each other; most cognitive-behavioural therapists include these factors in their treatment.

Cognitive and behavioural psychotherapy in palliative care

Cognitive and behavioural interventions in the medically ill are especially mentioned with regard to symptom control, such as pain, especially non-cancer pain (Turk and Feldman 2000), with a few studies evaluating these approaches in the palliative care setting (Graffam and Johnson 1987; Sloman 1995). While cognitive-behavioural techniques are optimal in a one-to-one professional/patient relationship, in most medical settings the lack of time implies that these methods are provided by means of written or audio-taped material. Cluver *et al.* (2005) evaluated the feasibility of remote cognitive psychotherapy in 10 cancer patients with six sessions alternating between face-to-face settings and remote sessions provided by videophone. Patients reported positive perceptions and acceptance after therapy sessions, regardless of the method utilized. Recently, Anderson *et al.* (2006) conducted a randomized clinical trial to test the efficacy of cognitive-behavioural approaches (positive mood intervention, relaxation, and distraction) for pain management with 59 cancer patients under medication. Patients in the relaxation and distraction group indicated a decrease of pain after listening the tapes. Differences between groups after 2-week follow-up was not significant for pain, or self-efficacy. A few other studies evaluated the effectiveness of cognitive-behavioural interventions to control cancer pain (Kolcaba and Fox 1999; Redd *et al.* 2001; Jacobsen *et al.* 2002; Dalton *et al.* 2004).

Several studies confirmed that focusing on positive states of mind (Seligman and Csikszentmihalyi 2000) through the acquisition of stress-management skills with cognitive-behavioural interventions can have a positive impact on improving quality of life in cancer patients (Penedo *et al.* 2004; Penedo *et al.* 2006). Highlighting the advantages of brief behavioural treatment due to an easier implementation in the medical context, Hopko *et al.* (2005), in a preliminary study of a brief behavioural activation treatment for depression, showed positive results in reducing symptoms of depression and outcomes, such as quality of life, patient compliance and satisfaction (Lejuez *et al.* 2002 for the comprehensive protocol). Owing to a small sample and the lack of a control group, a generalization of these results is not possible.

Experiential psychotherapy

Theoretical background

Experiential psychotherapies are part of humanistic psychology. Humanistic psychology emerged in the 1950s in reaction to both behaviourism and psychoanalysis and is concerned with the human dimension of psychology and the human context for the development of psychological theory. The main principles of humanistic psychology are summarized by five postulates developed by Bugental (1964): (1) human beings cannot be reduced to components; (2) human beings belong to a unique human context; (3) human consciousness includes the awareness of oneself in the context of other people; (4) human beings have choices and responsibilities; and (5) human beings are intentional, they seek meaning, value, and creativity. The relevant types of experiential psychotherapy are the person-centred and Gestalt therapy, the process-experiential and the focusing-oriented psychotherapy, and existential therapy. Experiential-interpersonal methods of authors, such as Yalom (1995) and Schmid (1998) have also been grouped under the 'experiential umbrella' (Greenberg *et al.* 1994, 1998). All these approaches share some common theoretical assumptions, of which the most important is that they consider human nature as 'inherently trustworthy, growth-oriented, and guided by choices' (Elliott *et al.* 2004).

Experiential psychotherapy is probably very attractive to palliative care professionals, as it places the patient in the human context, it provides a comprehensive view of the individual and it deals with existential issues. This is illustrated by the recent revival of existential or meaning-centred therapy in palliative care (see below). However, the fact that a certain type of psychotherapy focuses on issues, which are emerging in a given clinical context, does not imply that they are suitable or especially efficient in this setting. For example, the fact that psychoanalytic psychotherapy focuses on the biography does not imply that it is most effective in patients who have been severely traumatized in their development.

Experiential psychotherapy in palliative care

According to Richman (1995), **existential psychotherapy** with the terminally ill should be based on the view that every life is worth living to the very end. Objectives of the treatment are to enrich the last days of life, to deal with unfinished business, to increase social and family cohesion, and to prepare for a 'good' death. Over the last years, psychological concepts in palliative care have increasingly focused on spirituality and meaning as important resources for coping with difficult issues at the end of life. Existential psychotherapy emerged as an outgrowth of existentialism based on the work of philosophers, such as Nietzsche, Kirkegaard, or Schopenhauer. Several psychotherapists have contributed to the conceptualization of different therapeutic modalities based on existential philosophy (Yalom 1995; Spira 2000).

More recently, Miller *et al.* (2005), developed a group intervention from the 'spirituality' dimension of the psychosocio–spiritual framework (Mc Skimming *et al.* 1997). This group intervention, entitled **Life-Threatening Illness Supportive-Affective Group (LTI-SAGE)**, is designed as 'a group sharing and learning experience that focuses on the spiritual, emotional/psychological, and relational dimension of the living well while dying' (Miller *et al.* 2005, p. 334). The intervention (maximum of 12 sessions over a 12-month period) was evaluated by means of a randomized trial, in which measures of depression, anxiety, spiritual well-being, and death-related distress of the LTI-SAGE group were compared with a control group. The removal of non-compliant patients improved the outcomes concerning depression and religious spiritual well-being.

One of the most frequently used form of existential therapy is Viktor Frankel's **logotherapy** (1997), which is based on his experience as a prisoner in a Nazi concentration camp during the Second World War. *Logos*, which means 'meaning', indicates that this therapy is concerned with the search for meaning. Frankel considered that men perceive meaning in three main domains: in creativity, in relationships, and in a broader sense of existence surpassing the individual's experience of being. Greenstein (2000) and Greenstein and Breitbart (2000), for example, described the format and the process of an intervention based on meaning-centred psychotherapy for patients with advanced cancer. Recently, Noguchi *et al.*(2006), based on Frankel's existential therapy, also suggested to focus on spirituality and negative thoughts in patient under existential threat and underlined the various possibilities logotherapy offers with regard to spiritual care. However, no clinical trial evaluating the potential benefits of logotherapy has been conducted and they have not been compared with traditional psychotherapeutic interventions.

Complementary and alternative medicine

While complementary and alternative medicine can not be viewed as psychotherapeutic interventions, we will briefly review some of the data, which concern psychological outcome in the palliative care setting. These data also illustrate that unspecific factors (discussed below), inherent in any forms of psychotherapy, may have a beneficial effect on psychological distress.

Complementary and alternative medicine has been defined as 'diagnosis, treatment and/or prevention, which complements mainstream medicine by contributing to a common whole, by satisfying a demand not met by orthodoxy or by diversifying the conceptual frameworks of medicine' (Ernst *et al.* 1995). Today a whole range of complementary and alternative medicine has been integrated in end-of-life care, such as acupuncture, meditation, aromatherapy, enzyme therapy, homeopathy, hypnotherapy, massage, reflexology, relaxation techniques, or art or music therapy.

With regard to **massage and meditation**, Lafferty *et al.* (2006) reviewed 27 clinical trials and concluded that 26 studies showed improvements in symptoms such as anxiety, emotional distress, discomfort, and pain. The limitations of these studies concern essentially the design and sample size of the trials. Although double-blinding is impossible in massage and meditation studies, the authors encourage future researchers to at least separate data collection and intervention.

Two articles (Rajasekaran *et al.* 2005; Liossi 2006) review **hypnotherapy** with oncology patients and came to divergent conclusions. According to Rajasekaran, the relatively poor quality of the studies and the important heterogeneity of the populations considerably limited the validity of the results. On the other hand, Liossi in her general review of the use of hypnotherapy in paediatric and adult oncology selected studies with a rigorous methodology and design (randomized trials). She explored different outcomes (pain, effects of chemotherapy, quality of life, immune response) and concluded that the use of hypnosis decreased patients' distress in a number of studies.

Art therapy aims to stimulate awareness and expression of personal experience and deep affects. Most research evaluating the impact of art therapy on quality of life and well-being is based on either single case studies or studies with very small sample sizes (Favara-Scacco *et al.* 2001; Gabriel *et al.* 2001; Walsh *et al.* 2004). Recently a quasi-experimental design using pre/postmethodology evaluated immediate symptom change after one therapy session (Nainis *et al.* 2006) and indicated a reduction of symptoms such as pain, tiredness, depression, anxiety, drowsiness, or appetite.

Music therapy has been evaluated by qualitative research or case studies (Daveson 2000; Hilliard 2001; Magill 2001; Krout 2003). Gallagher *et al.*

(2006) reported on 15 studies based on quantitative measurement to test the effectiveness of music therapy with cancer patients (two hundred patients, prospective pre/post-design). Music therapy showed positive results with regard to anxiety and depression, reduction of pain, enhanced verbalization, and an increase of body movement and facial expression. As for art therapy, the duration of the effects of music therapy were not recorded.

Unspecific elements, technique, relational aspects, and outcome of psychotherapy

Unspecific elements

Beside technical skills and familiarity with the method, unspecific elements have been identified to influence outcome. Unspecific elements refer to factors, which are common to all psychotherapies. Among these factors are, for example, 'learning factors', which refer to the fact that human beings learn from experience. More specifically, learning is based on self-development mediated by interpersonal relations and depends on the capability to establish links (i.e. between emotions and cognitions), integration of skills and working through separation experiences to achieve autonomy. Learning factors are thus largely based on interpersonal relationships, but also on cognitive-behavioural elements, such as information processing.

Technique and relational aspects in psychotherapy

Another relevant issue with regard to psychotherapy concerns the question whether technique or relational aspects are more important for outcome. In clinical practice, both technical skills (such as the analysis and feedback concerning material provided by the patient, adequate identification of the patient's capacity and limits for growth) and relational aspects (such as empathy, authenticity, flexibility, and open-mindness) are important. Moreover, technique and relational competencies are interrelated (Chambless *et al.* 2006) and an adequate psychotherapeutic intervention requires both technical and relational skills. The importance of unspecific and relational aspects are also illustrated by the placebo effect.

Variance of psychotherapy outcome

Recent psychotherapy research (Lambert and Ogles 2004; Chambless *et al.* 2006) indicates that an important part (50%) of outcome variance remains unexplained. Different factors contributing to the remaining outcome variance: psychopathology or severity of the symptoms of the patient (about 25%), relational aspects (about 10%), variables related to the therapist (about 10%), and technical skills (about 5%) (Beutler *et al.* 2004). These findings do not imply that technique and specific skills can be replaced by 'sympathy'. Technical skills and theoretical knowledge are important tools allowing a therapist to understand and thus be able to develop fully the relational aspects, such as empathy, which greatly depends on the comprehension of a given situation. However, studies on outcome somehow challenge the ideology of psychotherapeutic 'schools', but also the constant reinventions of 'new' psychotherapeutic approaches, especially prevalent in palliative care.

Who provides psychotherapy and who benefits from psychotherapy?

Who should provide psychotherapy? Lambert and Ogles (2004) specifies that psychotherapeutic interventions 'are offered in modern urban societies, as a professional service, by persons whose expertise in helping skills has been formally recognized by training institutes, licensing bodies, and professional reputation'. Indeed, as any other treatment, which involves vulnerable patients, psychotherapy requires training, specific skills, theoretical knowledge, and regular supervisions. One has to remember that psychotherapy is a powerful tool with an efficacy similar to psychopharmacological treatments (Casacalenda *et al.* 2002; Gray 2004).

Who should benefit from psychotherapy? A psychotherapeutic intervention cannot be imposed on a patient. Usually, patients who seek psychotherapy have a 'diagnosable form of suffering or disability' (Franck and Frank 1991) and are unhappy with their lives, their relationships, and themselves. Some patients may also feel pressured to 'accept' psychotherapeutic support; this should not be the case, as alternative approaches to relieve distress, such as social support or psychopharmacological treatment, exists.

On the other hand, of those who are psychologically distressed and motivated to accept psychological support, not all of them qualify for psychotherapeutic treatment. Psychotherapy is not a magic method with an immediate effect; it demands active participation of the patient, a motivation to confront and communicate his distress and clarify painful thoughts, feelings and interpersonal difficulties and the ability to establish a trusting relationship. In addition, psychotherapy is provided within a defined setting, which demands from the patient that he is able to tolerate frustration between sessions and to accept the therapist's limits with regard to time and attention he is able to provide. With other words, psychotherapy is a challenging endeavour. This is the reason why some patients do not enter psychotherapy, quit psychotherapy, or prefer to try other approaches.

Perspectives

The literature on psychotherapy is growing and increasing evidence of its effectiveness in the palliative care setting exists. This is not surprising, as psychotherapeutic interventions have already been proven to be effective in the medically ill (Huyse and Stiefel 2006). While randomized clinical trials demonstrate effectiveness in general psychotherapy research (Lambert and Ogles 2004), and in psychotherapy research with the medically ill (Stiefel *et al.* in press), such trials are difficult to realize in palliative care due to recruitment difficulties, high dropout rates, ethical problems related to randomization to name but a few.

From our point of view, more important than trying to introduce randomized controlled trials or to invent so-called specifically designed psychotherapeutic intervention for the palliative care setting, we believe is to evaluate which patients and psychological problems respond best to different, well established psychotherapeutic interventions. This requires a clear and rigorous working definition of psychotherapy and of the therapists' qualification; otherwise one risks to lose the characteristics and strengths of psychotherapy and to deprive palliative care from interventions known to reduce psychological suffering. Moreover, a clear definition of what is called psychotherapy and who can provide psychotherapy allows a continuous reflexive approach on the psychological aspects of the severely ill and provides a theoretical framework and meaning for those who work with these psychologically often vulnerable patients.

While it is certainly true that psychotherapeutic interventions have to be adapted to the needs of the severely ill and that psychotherapists ought to be flexible when working in palliative care (Guex *et al.* 2000), it is also a fact that there is a body of clinical, theoretical, conceptual, and scientific evidence of over a hundred years of psychotherapeutic work, which should not be disregarded. Human beings differ from each other and differ when facing severe illness, death, and dying. However, the similarities between humans beings and between the physically healthy and the medically ill are much more important than the differences. Therefore, psychotherapy, especially the established psychotherapeutic approaches—the psychodynamic, systemic, experiential, and cognitive-behavioural therapies—can easily be adapted to the needs of the palliative care setting.

References

Anderson KO, Cohen MZ, Mendoza TR, Guo H, Harle MT, Cleeland CS (2006). Brief cognitive-behavioral audiotape intervention for cancer-related pain: immediate but not long-term effect. *Cancer* 107:207–14.

Ando M, Tsuda A, Morita T (2007). Life review interview on the spiritual well-being of terminally ill cancer patients. *Support Care Cancer* 15:225–31.

Beck AT (1991). Cognitive therapy: a 30-year retrospective. *Am Psychol* 46:368–76.

Beck AT, Rush AJ, Shaw B, Emery G (1979). *Cognitive therapy of depression*. New York: Guilford Press.

Beutler LE, Malik M, Alimohamed S et al. (2004). Clinicians variables. In: Lambert MJ (ed.). *Bergin and Garfield's handbook of psychotherapy and behavior change* (5th ed). New York: Wiley, pp. 227–306

Bressoud A, Real del Sarte O, Stiefel F, Mordasini P, Perey L, Bauer J, Leyvraz PF, Leyvraz S (2007). Impact of family structure on long-term survivors of osteosarcoma. *Suppor Care Cancer* 15, 525–31.

Bugental JFT (1964). The third force in psychology. *J Humanistic Psychol* 4:19–25.

Burns DD *(1999). The feeling good handbook,* (revised edn). *New York: Plume/Penguin Books.*

Casacalenda N, Perry JC, Looper K (2002). Remission in major depressive disorder: a comparison of pharmacotherapy, psychotherapy, and a control condition. *Am J Psychiatry* 159, 1354–60.

Chambless DL, Crits-Christoph P, Wampold BE (2006). What should be validated ? In: Norcross JC, Beutler LE, Levant RF (ed.). *Evidence-based practice in mental health: debate and dialogue of the fundamental questions.* Washington: Wiley, pp. 191–256.

Cluver JS, Schuyler D, Frueh BC, Brescia F, Arana GW (2005). Remote psychotherapy for terminally ill cancer patients. *J Telemed Telecare* 11:157–9.

Dalton JA, Keefe FJ, Carlson J, Yougbood R (2004). Tailoring cognitive-behavioral treatment for cancer pain. *Pain Manage Nurs* 5:3–18.

Daveson BA (2000). Music therapy in palliative care for hopitalized children and adolescents. *J Palliat Care* 16:35–8.

Elliott R, Greenberg LS, Lietaer G (2004). Research on experiential psychotherapies. In: Lambert MJ (ed). *Bergin and Garfield's handbook of psychotherapy and behavior change* (5th edn). New York: Wiley, pp. 493–539.

Ellis A (1950). What is psychotherapy? *Ann Psychother* 1:1–57.

Ernst E, Resch KL, Hill S (1995). Referrals between GPs and Complementary practitioners. *Br J Gen Pract* 46:(409):494.

Favara-Scacco C, Smirne G, Schiliro G, Di Cataldo A (2001). Art therapy as support for children with leukemia during painful procedures. *Med Pediatr Oncol* 36:474–80.

Franck JD, Frank JB (1991). *Persuasion and healing: a comparative study of psychotherapy.* Baltimore, MD: John Hopkins University Press.

Frankel VF (1997). *Man's search for ultimate meaning. New York: Plenum Press.*

Freeman A, Mahoney MJ, DeVito P, Martin D *(2004). Cognition and psychotherapy* (2th edn). *New York: Springer Publishing Co.*

Gabriel B, Bromberg E, Vandenbovenkamp J (2001). Art therapy with adult bone marrow transplant patients in isolation. *Psycho-oncology* 10:114–23.

Gallagher LM, Lagman R, Walsh D, Davis MP, Legrand SB (2006). The clinical effects of music therapy in palliative medicine. *Support Care Cancer* 14:859–66.

Graffam S, Johnson A (1987). A comparison of two relaxation strategies for the relief of pain and its distress. J Pain Symptom Manage 2:*229–321.*

Gray GE (2004). *Evidence-based psychiatry.* Washington: American Psychiatric Publishing.

Greenberg LS, Elliott R, Lietaer G (1994). Research on humanistic and experiential psychotherapies. In: Bergin AE, Garfield SL (ed.). *Handbook of psychotherapy and behavior change* (4th edn). New York: Wiley, pp. 509–39.

Greenberg LS, Watson J, Lietaer G (1998). *Handbook of experiential psychotherapy. New York: Guilford Press.*

Greenstein (2000). The house that's on fire: Meaning-centered psychotherapy pilot group for cancer patients. *Am J Psychother* **54**,501–511.

Greenstein and Breitbart (2000). Cancer and the experience of meaning: A group psychotherapy program for people with cancer. *Am J Psychother* **54**:486–500.

Guex P, Stiefel F, Rousselle I (2000). Psychotherapy for the patient with cancer. Psychother Rev 2:269–73.

Haley J (1976). *Problem-solving therapy: new strategies for effective family therapy.* San Francisco, CA: Josey Bass.

Hilliard RE (2001). The use of music therapy in meeting the multidimensional needs of hospice patients and families. *J Music Ther* 17:161–6.

Hollon SD, Beck AT (2004). Cognitive and cognitive behavioral therapies. In: Lambert MJ (ed.). *Bergin and Garfield's handbook of psychotherapy and behavior change* (5th edn). New York: Wiley, pp. 447–542.

Hopko DR, Bell JL, Armento MEA, Hunt MK and Lejuez CW (2005). Behavior therapy for depressed cancer patients in primary care. *Psychother Theory Res Pract Train* 42:236–43.

Huyse F, Stiefel F (ed.) (2006). *Integrated care for the complex medically ill.* The Medical Clinics of North America. New York: Elsevier.

Jackson DD (1968a). *Human communication, t.1: communication, family and marriage.* Palo Alto, CA: Science and Behavior Books.

Jackson DD (1968b). *Human communication, t.2: communication, family and marriage.* Palo Alto, CA: Science and Behavior Books.

Jacobsen PB, Meade CB, Stein KD, Chirikos TN, Small BJ, Ruckdeschel JC (2002). Efficacy and costs of two forms of stress management training for cancer patients undergoing chemotherapy. *J Clin Oncol* 20:2851–62.

Kaplan HI, Sadock BJ (1998). *Kaplan and Sadock's synopsis of psychiatry: behavioral sciences/clinical psychiatry* (8th edn). *Baltimore, MD: Williams and Wilkins.*

Kissane DW, Bloch S (2002). *Family focused grief therapy: a model of family-centered care during palliative care and bereavement.* Buckingham: Open University Press.

Kissane DW, Bloch S, Dowe DL, Snyder RD, Onghena P, McKenzie DP, Wallace CS (1996a). The Melbourne Family Grief Study, I: perceptions of family functioning in bereavement. *Am J Psychiatry* **153**:650–8.

Kissane DW, Bloch S, Dowe DL, Snyder RD, Onghena P, McKenzie DP, Wallace CS (1996b). The Melbourne Family Grief Study, II: psychosocial morbidity and grief in bereaved families. *Am J Psychiatry* **153**:659–66.

Kissane DW, McKenzie M, Bloch S, Moskowitz C, McKenzie DP, O'Neill I (2006). Family Focused Grief Therapy: a randomized, controlled trial in palliative care and bereavement. *Am J Psychiatry* **163**:1208–18.

Kolcaba F, Fox C (1999). The effects of guided imagery on comfort of women with early stage breast cancer undergoing radiation therapy. *Oncol Nurs Forum* **26**:67–72.

Krout RE (2003). Music versus distraction for procedural pain and anxiety in patients with cancer. *Am J Hospice Palliat Care* **20**:129–34.

Lacy TJ, Higgins MJ (2005). Integrated medical-psychiatric care of a dying patient: a case of dynamically informed 'practical psychotherapy'. *J Am Acad Psychoanal Dynamic Psychiatry* **33**:619–36.

Lafferty WE, Downey L, McCarty RL, Standish LJ, Patrick DL (2006). Evaluating CAM treatments at the end of life: a review of clinical trials for massage and meditation. *Complementary Ther Med* **14**:100–12.

Lambert MJ, Ogles BM (2004). The efficacy and effectiveness of psychotherapy. In: Lambert MJ (ed.). *Bergin and Garfield's handbook of psychotherapy and behavior change*, (5th edn). New York: Wiley, pp. 139–93.

Lejuez CW, Hopko DR, Lepage J, Hopko SD, McNeill W *(2002). The Brief behavioral activation treatment for depression (BATD): a comprehensive patient guide. Boston, MA: Pearson Custom Publishing.*

Lewin K (2005). The theoretical basis of dynamic psychiatry. In: Gabbard GO (ed.) *Psychodynamic psychiatry in clinical practice: the DSM-IV edition*. Washington: American Psychiatric Press, pp. 29–63.

Lewinsohn PM, Munoz RF, Yougreen MA, Zeiss AM (1986). *Control your depression.* Englewoods Cliff, NJ: Prentice Hall.

Liossi C (2006). Hypnosis in cancer care. *Hypnosis* **23**:47–57.

Luborsky L, Diguer L, Luborsky E, Schmid KA (1999). The efficacy of dynamic versus other psychotherapies: is that true that 'everyone has won and all must have prize'?: an update. In: Janowsky DS (ed.). *Psychotherapy indications and outcomes*. Washington: American Psychiatric Press, pp. 3–22.

Madanes C (1981). *Strategic family therapy*. San Francisco, CA: Josey Bass.

Magill L (2001). The use of music therapy to adress the suffering in advanced cancer pain. *J Palliat Care* **17**:167–72.

Maultsby MC (1971). Systematic, written homework in psychotherapy. Psychother Theory Res Pract **8**:*195–8.*

Mc Skimming SA, Super A, Driever MJ, Schoessler M, Franey SG, Fonner E (1997). Living and healing during life-threatening illness. Supportive care of the dying: a coalition for the compassionate care. *J Palliat Med* **8**:333–43.

Miller DK, Chibnall JT, Videen SD, Duckro PN (2005). Supportive-affective group experience for persons with life-threatning illness: reducing spiritual, psychological, and death-related distress in dying patients. *J Palliat Med* **8**:333–43.

Minuchin P (1988). Relationships within the family: a systems perspective on development. In: Hinde RA, Stevenson-Hinde J (ed.). *Relationships within families: mutual infleuences.* New York: Wiley, pp. 7–26.

Minuchin S (1974). *Families and family therapy*. Cambridge, MA: Harvard University Press.

Moos RH, Moos BS (1981). *Family environment scale manual*. Stanford, CA: Consulting Psychologists Press.

Nainis N, Paice JA, Ratner J, Wirth JH, Lai J, Schott S (2006). Relieving symptoms in cancer: innovative use of art therapy. *J Pain Symptom Manage* **31**:162–9.

Noguchi W, Morita S, Ohno T, Aihara O, Tsujii H, Shimozuma K, Matsushima E (2006). Spiritual needs in cancer patients and spiritual care based on logotherapy. *Support Care Cancer* 14:65–70.

Orlinsky DE, Ronnestad MH, Willutzky U (2004). Fifty years of psychotherapy process-outcome research: continuity and change. In: Lambert MJ (ed.). *Bergin and Garfield's handbook of psychotherapy and behavior change* (5th edn). New York: Wiley, pp. 307–89.

Pavlov IP, Gantt WH *(1928)*. Lectures on conditioned reflexes: twenty-five years of objective study of the higher nervous activity (behaviour) of animals. *New York: Liverwright Publishing Corporation.*

Penedo FJ, Dahn JR, Molton I, Gonzalez JS, Kinsinger D, Roos BA, Carver CS, Schneiderman N, Antoni MH (2004). Cognitive-behavioral stress management improves stress management skills and quality of life in men recovering from treatment of prostate carcinoma. *Cancer* 100:192–200.

Penedo FJ, Molton I, Dahn JR, Shen BJ, Kinsinger D, Traeger L, Siegel S, Schneiderman N, Antoni M (2006). A randomized clinical trial of group-based cognitive behavioral stress management in localized prostate cancer: development of stress management skills improves quality of life and benefit finding. *Ann Behav Med* 31:261–70.

Rajasekaran M, Edmonds PM, Higginson IL (2005). Systematic review of hypnotherapy for treating symptoms in terminally ill adult cancer patients. *Palliat Med* 14:100–12.

Redd WH, Montgomery GH, Duhamel KN (2001). Behavioral intervention for cancer treatment side effects. *J Natl Cancer Inst* 93:810–23.

Redding KK (2005). When death becomes the end of an analytic treatment. *Clin Work Soc J* 33:69–79.

Rehm LP (1977). A self-control model of depression. *Behav Ther* 8:787–804.

Richman J (1995). From despair to integrity: an eriksonian approach to psychotherapy for the terminally ill. *Psychotherapy* 32:317–22.

Rodin G, Gillies LA (2000). Individual psychotherapy for the patient with advanced disease. In: Chochinov HM, Breitbart W GO (ed.). *Handbook of psychiatry in palliative medicine.* New York: Oxford University Press, pp. 189–96.

Sameroff AJ (1983). Developmental systems: context and evolution. In: Mussen PH, Kessen W (ed.) 4. *Handbook of child psychology: history, theory, and methods.* New York: Wiley, pp. 237–94.

Schmid, PF (1998). 'Face to face': the art of encounter. In: Thorne B, Lambers E (ed.). *Person-centred therapy: a European perspective.* Thousand Oaks, CA: Sage Publications, pp. 74–90.

Seligman MEP, Csikszentmihalyi M (2000). Positive psychology: an introduction. *Am Psychol* 55:5–14.

Selvini Palazzoli M (1978). *Self starvation: from the individual to family therapy.* New York: Aronson.

Selvini Palazzoli M (1991). Team consultation: an indispensable tool for the process of knowledge. *J Fam Ther* 13:31–53.

Skinner BF *(1961)*. Cumulative record, enlarged edn. *East Norwalk, CT: Appleton-Century-Crofts.*

Sloman R (1995). Relaxation and the relief of cancer pain. Nurs Clin North Am 30:*697–709.*

Spira JL (2000). Existential psychotherapy in palliative care. In: Chochinov HM, Breitbart W GO (ed). *Handbook of psychiatry in palliative medicine.* pp. 197–214. New York: Oxford University Press.

Stratton P (2005). *Report on the evidence base of systemic family therapy.* Association for Family Therapy.

Stiefel F, Guex P, Real O (1998). An introduction to psycho-oncology with special emphasis to its historical and cultural context. In: Bruera E, Portenoy R (ed.). *Topics in palliative care,* Vol. 3. New York: Oxford University Press, pp. 175–89.

Stiefel F, Zdrojewski C, Bel Hadj F, Boffa D, Dorogi Y, So A, Ruiz J, de Jonge P. Effects of a Multi-Faceted Psychiatric Intervention Targeted at the Complex Medically Ill: a Randomized Controlled Trial. *Psychother Psychosom* (in press).

Tepper MC, Dodes LM, Wool CA, Rosenblatt LA (2006). A psychotherapy dominated by separation, termination, and death. *Harv Rev Psychiatry* 14:257–67.

Thorndike EL (1932). *The fundamentals of learning.* New York: Teachers College Bureau of Publications.

Turk DC, Feldman CS (2000). A cognitive-behavioral approach to symptom management in palliative care: augmenting somatic interventions. In: Chochinov HM, Breitbart W GO (ed). *Handbook of psychiatry in palliative medicine.* New York: Oxford University Press, pp. 215–22.

Viederman M (2000). The supportive relationship, the psychodynamic life narrative, and the dying patient. In: Chochinov HM, Breitbart W GO (ed). *Handbook of psychiatry in palliative medicine.* New York: Oxford University Press, pp. 215–22.

Walsh SM, Martin SC, Schmidt LA (2004). Testing the efficacy of a creative-arts intervention with family caregivers of patients with cancer. *J Nurs Scholarship* 36:214–19.

Wampold BE (2001). *The great psychotherapy debate: models, methods and findings.* Mahwah, NJ: Lawrence Erlbaum Associates.

Watson JB, Watson RR (1949). Conditioned emotional reactions. In: *Wayne D (ed.). Readings in general psychology. New York: Prentice-Hall.*

Yalom ID (1995). *The theory and practice of group psychotherapy,* (4th edn). New York: Basic Books.

Zimmermann M, de Rothen Y, Despland JN. Efficacy. Cost-effectiveness and appropriateness of psychotherapy: a review. *Swiss Arch Neurol Psychiatry* (in press).

Chapter 9

Complementary therapies

Edzard Ernst

Complementary therapies are a heterogeneous array of interventions that are not commonly used in conventional medicine. Even though they originate from different traditions and represent fundamentally different approaches to healthcare, they have several common characteristics that unite them:

+ the emphasis on holistic healthcare,
+ the claim of being natural and safe,
+ the high degree of individualization of treatments,
+ the emphasis on the self-healing properties of our body,
+ the fact that most have been in use for centuries,
+ the fact that most have to be paid for privately.

The role of complementary therapies in cancer is complex. The interventions in question are used in at least three fundamentally different ways:

+ for cancer prevention,
+ for treatment of cancer,
+ in supportive and palliative cancer care.

There is some encouraging evidence suggesting that several therapies that might be considered as complementary might decrease cancer risks. For instance, the regular intake of allium vegetables (e.g. garlic) or green tea seems to reduce the risk of gastrointestinal cancers, regular physical exercise minimizes the risk of colon and breast cancer, and the consumption of tomato products (leucopene) reduces the risk of prostate cancer (Ernst *et al.* 2006).

There is, however, very little evidence to suggest that any of the many 'alternative cancer cures' (alternative treatments promoted to change the natural history of cancers) are effective. On the contrary, some may be harmful. The very concept of an 'alternative cancer cure' has the potential to bar swift access to effective treatments, which can hasten the death of cancer patients (Ernst *et al.* 2006).

In palliative and supportive care the situation is fundamentally different again. Here complementary therapies have a considerable potential for doing more good than harm. Thus they enjoy increasing acceptance from both patients and healthcare professionals (Risberg *et al.* 2004). Many surveys have been published investigating the prevalence of use of complementary therapies. The results show a large degree of variation, but generally speaking their prevalence is high (Ernst 2006).

In this chapter I will review the evidence for or against complementary therapies in cancer palliation. I will do this by first considering the most relevant modalities in turn. Subsequently, I will focus on two symptoms that are of particular importance to palliative and supportive care.

Treatments

Acupuncture

Acupuncture can be defined as 'a practice in Chinese medicine in which the skin, at various points along the meridians, is punctured with needles to remove energetic blockages and stimulate the flow of qi' (Jonas 2005). Several variations of the theme exist: stimulation by heat (moxibustion), pressure (acupressure), electrical current (electroacupuncture), etc. In cancer patients it is used mostly for pain control, for alleviation of chemotherapy-induced nausea and vomiting to treat radiation-induced xerostomia, and to reduce vasomotor symptoms (Ernst *et al.* 2006).

Nausea and vomiting

Different techniques are used to stimulate the pericardium 6 (P6 or neiguan) acupuncture point thought to be useful in the management of chemotherapy-induced nausea and vomiting (Ezzo *et al.* 2005): manual stimulation with the insertion of fine needles (Streitberger *et al.* 2003), electrostimulation through needles (Shen *et al.* 2000) or percutaneously (Roscoe *et al.* 2002), and non-invasive pressure on the skin (Roscoe *et al.* 2003). The potential benefits and limitations of these approaches are illustrated by two of the larger randomized clinical trials (RCTs):

- Low-frequency electroacupuncture was evaluated in an RCT with 104 women suffering from breast cancer. They received the active intervention, mock electrostimulation, or no intervention in addition to antiemetic pharmacotherapy and highly emetogenic chemotherapy (Shen *et al.* 2000). The number of emesis episodes occurring during the 5 days was significantly lower for patients receiving electroacupuncture compared with those receiving the mock procedure or antiemetic pharmacotherapy alone (median number of episodes, 5, 10, and 15, respectively). During the 9-day follow-up period no significant differences were observed between groups, suggesting that the observed effect is short-lived.

◆ A lack of benefit from acupuncture was suggested in an RCT with 80 patients undergoing high-dose chemotherapy with autologous haematopoietic stem cell transplantation. They received ondansetron plus either acupuncture at P6 or non-skin penetrating placebo acupuncture (Streitberger *et al.* 2003). There were no significant differences between the groups in the rate of emesis or retching, nausea, or use of rescue antiemetics.

With this level of contradiction, one is best advised to consider the totality of the available trial data. A systematic review evaluated the results from 11 RCTs with 1247 cancer patients (Ezzo *et al.* 2005). Overall, acupuncture-point stimulation significantly reduced the proportion of patients with acute vomiting (31% versus 22%). However, the mean number of emetic episodes was not significantly decreased and no effect in the control of delayed emesis was noted. Electrostimulation through acupuncture needles appeared to be the most effective modality.

Pain control

Although some studies have suggested that acupuncture might be useful in ameliorating cancer pain, our systematic review in 2005 of the totality of the reliable RCT data concluded that the value of acupuncture has not been established (Lee *et al.* 2005). More recent RCTs have been contradictory and the overall picture remains inconclusive.

Vasomotor symptoms

Preliminary evidence suggests a potential benefit of acupuncture for the treatment of vasomotor symptoms in men receiving gonadotrophin analogues for prostate cancer. In one pilot study, electroacupuncture for 30 minutes twice weekly for 2 weeks followed by once weekly for 10 weeks resulted in a significant decrease in the number of hot flushes per day for the six men who continued therapy for more than 2 weeks (7.9 at baseline compared with 2.5 after 10 weeks of treatment) (Hammar *et al.* 1999).

Hypnotherapy

Hypnotherapy is 'the practice of using hypnosis for the treatment of illness' (Jonas 2005). Several (mostly small) RCTs have demonstrated the usefulness of hypnotherapy in palliative cancer care for controlling pain and nausea/vomiting (Mills 1992, Jacknow *et al.* 1994). Hypnotherapy may be particularly useful for reducing the anticipatory emesis associated with chemotherapy (Redd *et al.* 2001). It can also be useful in children for preventing anxiety and pain due to procedures, such as lumbar puncture or bone marrow aspiration (Richardson *et al.* 2006).

The use of hypnotherapy has been evaluated as an adjunct to radiation therapy in an RCT, with 69 patients undergoing curative radiotherapy for a variety of cancers (Stalpers *et al.* 2005). There was no effect on anxiety and quality of life, although patients reported an improved sense of both overall and mental well-being.

It is unclear to what extent the alleged positive effects of hypnotherapy are due to specific or non-specific (placebo) effects. A review that summarized all published clinical trials of hypnotherapy concluded that there is encouraging, albeit not compelling evidence to suggest that hypnotherapy is helpful for controlling anxiety and pain as well as nausea and vomiting in cancer patients (Genuis 1995).

Behavioural interventions

Behavioural interventions encompass a range of techniques which have been applied separately or in combination. In an RCT with 115 patients, a structured multidisciplinary programme, including cognitive, emotional, physical, social, and spiritual interventions proved to be useful in patients receiving radiation therapy for advanced cancer (Rummans *et al.* 2006). Those receiving the active therapy were able to maintain their quality of life during the 4-week treatment period, while the control group who did not receive this adjunctive treatment had a significant decrease in quality of life. Six months after the intervention the quality of life was similar in both groups. Thus the effects seem to be short-lasting and therefore perhaps of debatable clinical value.

Relaxation therapy

Relaxation techniques such as imagery (Syrjala *et al.* 1992; Sloman *et al.* 1994; Walker *et al.* 1999), breathing exercises (Sloman *et al.* 1994), manual massage (Sims 1986; Ernst and Fialka 1994; Ahles *et al.* 1999; Cassileth and Vickers 2004), music therapy (Beck 1991), art therapy (Nainis *et al.* 2006), and reflexology (Ernst and Köder 1997; Stephenson *et al.* 2000) have been used to reduce symptoms and increase the quality of life in cancer patients (Beck 1991; Syrjala *et al.* 1992; Sloman *et al.* 1994; Walker *et al.* 1999). In one RCT, 96 women receiving chemotherapy for newly diagnosed breast cancer were assigned to receive either regular relaxation training and imagery or standard care only (Walker *et al.* 1999). The experimental group experienced a better quality of life than the control group.

Manual massage therapy conveys relaxation to both the body and the mind (Ernst and Fialka 1994; Ahles *et al.* 1999; Cassileth and Vickers 2004). In a retrospective series of 1290 cancer patients in which pain, fatigue, anxiety, and nausea were assessed before and after massage therapy, moderate to severe symptoms decreased by approximately 50% (Cassileth and Vickers 2004). Therapeutic benefits persisted for at least 48 hours in outpatients.

Aromatherapy

Aromatherapy is the 'controlled use of essential oils to promote the vitality and health of spirit, mind and body' (Jonas 2005). Aromatherapists use aromatic plant-based oils, often in conjunction with gentle massage. Evidence from small trials suggested that it may have some benefit in relieving self-reported symptoms (Fellowes *et al.* 2004). More recently, aromatherapy massage was assessed in a multicentre trial in which 282 cancer patients were randomly assigned to aromatherapy weekly for 4 weeks or to a control group receiving no such adjunctive treatments (Wilkinson *et al.* 2007). No benefits were present at 10 weeks after treatment, the primary endpoint of the trial. Although patients experienced improvement 2 weeks after treatment these benefits were no longer present at 6 weeks after therapy.

Supplements

Ginseng for fatigue

A beneficial effect of ginseng on chemotherapy-induced fatigue was noted in a small pilot RCT of 20 patients who were assigned to ginseng supplements or placebo (Younus *et al.* 2003). The patients receiving ginseng had significantly less fatigue and a better sense of overall health and quality of life. This was an extremely small study and independent confirmation is needed before firm conclusions can be drawn.

Fish oil for symptom control

Fish oil, which contains omega-3 fatty acids, has been studied as a treatment for cancer-related anorexia/cachexia. The results are mixed and far from convincing (Jonas 2005).

Sixty patients with a variety of cancers were randomly assigned to fish oil capsules or placebo in addition to their conventional treatments (Bruera *et al.* 2003). Among the patients who both began and completed 2 weeks of their allotted therapy (27 dropped out during treatment because they could not tolerate the regimen), supplemental fish oil did not influence appetite, fatigue, nausea, weight loss, caloric intake, nutritional status, or sense of well-being.

Symptoms

In addition to the evidence derived directly from palliative care setting there is indirect evidence for treating problems such as anxiety or depression, which does not originate from palliative care settings. However, as both symptoms are prominent issues in palliative care, they seem relevant in the context of this chapter.

Anxiety

Anxiety is an important reason for patients to consider using complementary and alternative medicine (CAM). Most CAM treatments are perceived as relaxing and many have been submitted to controlled clinical trials to test their anxiolytic properties. These studies have generated encouraging evidence for a wide range of approaches (Ernst *et al.* 2006):

◆ acupuncture
◆ aromatherapy
◆ autogenic training
◆ biofeedback
◆ guided imagery
◆ hypnotherapy
◆ massage therapy
◆ meditation
◆ music therapy
◆ relaxation training.

Treatments that have been tested in controlled clinical trials but have failed to generate positive results, include homeopathy, flower remedies, and chiropractic (Ernst *et al.* 2006). In addition, a range of herbal remedies have been demonstrated to have anxiolytic effects, e.g. German camomile, kava, lemon balm, and passionflower. By far the best evidence exists for kava (Ernst *et al.* 2006), but unfortunately it has been associated with serious liver damage and was therefore banned in the UK and several other countries.

Depression

Several CAM treatments have been tested in controlled clinical trials for their antidepressive effects. Generally speaking, results were mixed (Ernst *et al.* 2006). Encouraging findings have emerged for the following interventions (Ernst *et al.* 2006).

◆ autogenic training
◆ regular exercise (arguably not CAM)
◆ massage therapy
◆ music therapy
◆ relaxation training
◆ yoga.

For other treatments the results are contradictory or inconclusive because of a lack of independent confirmation: acupuncture, guided imagery, and mindfulness-based stress reduction. In addition, a range of herbal remedies have been tested: ginkgo biloba, lavender, saffron, and St Johns wort (Ernst *et al.* 2006). The evidence is conclusively positive only for the latter; about 40 randomized clinical trials have tested its antidepressant properties and their vast majority indicates that it reliably and safely alleviates mild to moderate depression (Linde *et al.* 2005). If combined with other drugs, it can, however, cause important herb–drug interactions. St John's wort stimulates the cytochrome P450 enzymes and thus significantly reduces the plasma levels of drugs metabolized by this pathway (Mills *et al.* 2004).

Safety issues

While many complementary therapies for cancer are associated with minimal or no risk, this is not true for all. Potential safety issues include direct toxicity of medications and procedures, indirect effects due to interactions of supplements with other medications, and the risk to the patient who uses such treatments to avoid or delay established, effective treatment in the management of malignant disease (Markman 2002).

Direct toxicity of medications and procedures

A variety of herbal remedies may produce serious adverse effects. Quality control of these preparations can be a major concern. Pertinent issues include variability in biological potency in different crops, the possibility of fungal or bacterial contamination, the use of incorrect plant species, and consumer fraud (Murch *et al.* 2000). One of the most severe examples of the potential for harm with herbal preparations is the development of renal failure and urothelial cancer in individuals who thought they were using the herbal preparation *Stephania tetrandra* for weight loss, but who actually received the Chinese herb *Aristolochia fangchi* because of a manufacturing error (Nortier *et al.* 2000; Lord *et al.* 2001). Numerous examples of potential adverse effects associated with commonly used herbal remedies exist (Ernst *et al.* 2006).

Adverse effects of acupuncture include transmission of an infectious agent through needle insertion, broken, forgotten, or misapplied needles, pneumothorax, transient hypotension, minor bleeding, contact dermatitis, and pain (Kaptchuk 2002). Therapeutic massage can result in haematoma, particularly in anticoagulated or thrombocytopenic patients, and other serious complications have been reported (Ernst 2003).

Interactions

Herbal medicines and other supplements are pharmacologically active, raising concerns about potential interactions with conventional therapy.

- St John's wort induces CYP3A4 (Budzinski *et al.* 2000), which can lead to subtherapeutic levels of chemotherapeutic agents that are metabolized by CYP3A4 (e.g. taxanes, irinotecan, imatinib).

- Essiac consists of multiple biologically active ingredients that may act synergistically with chemotherapeutic agents by its inhibition of CYP3A, or through the cytotoxic or immunosuppressive activities of anthraquinones present in this mixture (Dy *et al.* 2004).

- The polyphenols in green tea inhibit multiple cytochrome P450 enzymes, which are important in drug metabolism, and induce other drug-metabolizing enzymes.

- Because it can inhibit the cytochrome P450 system, milk thistle has the potential to decrease the metabolism of some cytotoxic agents such as paclitaxel (Zuber *et al.* 2002; Werneke *et al.* 2004) and doxorubicin (Kivisto *et al.* 1995).

- Panax ginseng and ginkgo biloba increase the functional activity of several drug-metabolizing enzymes of the CYP family, and should be avoided in patients receiving cytotoxic agents metabolized by CYP3A4 or CYP2C19 (Sparreboom *et al.* 2004).

- Pretreatment of cancer cells with some botanical agents (e.g. berberine, a constituent of huanglian) reduces the sensitivity of these cells to chemotherapy-induced apoptosis (Lin *et al.* 1999).

Indirect risks

The use of complementary therapies may result in a significant delay in instituting conventional treatment that is of documented benefit for a specific condition (Coppes *et al.* 1998; Ernst 2001; Brienza *et al.* 2002; Davis *et al.* 2006). Furthermore, some complementary therapists recommend that only natural substances be used for the duration of the treatment, as non-natural products are alleged to negate the benefit of the therapy (Anon 1993). This strategy can lead to the rejection of effective medical therapies, such as opioid analgesics, regardless of the severity of pain (Markman 2002).

Conclusions

Several complementary therapies seem to have considerable potential in palliative cancer care. Similarly, there is promising evidence for treating anxiety or depression with a range of CAM modalities. The challenge for the future is to conduct rigorous systematic research to identify those that are best under given circumstances.

References

Ahles TA, Tope, DM, Pinkson B (1999). Massage therapy for patients undergoing autologous bone marrow transplantation. *J Pain Symptom Manage* 18:157–63.

Anon (1993). Questionable methods of cancer management: 'nutritional' therapies. *CA Cancer J Clin* 43:309–19.

Beck SL (1991). The therapeutic use of music for cancer-related pain. *Oncol Nurs Forum* 18:1327–37.

Brienza RS, Stein MD, Fagan MJ (2002). Delay in obtaining conventional healthcare by female internal medicine patients who use herbal therapies. *J Womens Health Gender-Based Med* 11:79–87.

Bruera E, Strasser F, Palmer JL *et al.* (2003). Effect of fish oil on appetite and other symptoms in patients with advanced cancer and anorexia/cachexia: a double-blind, placebo-controlled study. *J Clin Oncol* 21:129–34.

Budzinski JW, Foster BC, Vandenhoek S, Arnason JT (2000). An in vitro evaluation of human cytochrome P450 3A4 inhibition by selected commercial herbal extracts and tinctures. *Phytomedicine* 7:273–82.

Cassileth BR, Vickers AJ (2004). Massage therapy for symptom control: outcome study at a major cancer center. *J Pain Symptom Manage* 28:244–9.

Coppes MJ, erson RA, Egeler RM, Wolff JEA (1998). Alternative therapies for the treatment of childhood cancer. *N Engl J Med* 339:846–7.

Davis GE, Bryson CL, Yueh B, McDonnell MB, Micek MA, Fihn SD (2006). Treatment delay associated with alternative medicine use among veterans with head and neck cancer. *Head Neck* 28:926–31.

Dy GK, Bekele L, Hanson LJ, Furth A, Mandrekar S, Sloan JA, Asjei AA. (2004). Complementary and alternative medicine use by patients enrolled onto phase I clinical trials. *J Clin Oncol* 22:4810–15.

Ernst E (2001). Intangible risks of complementary and alternative medicine. *J Clin Oncol* 19:2365–6.

Ernst E (2003). The safety of massage therapy. *Rheumatology* 42:1101–6.

Ernst E (2006). Prevalence surveys: to be taken with a pinch of salt. *Comp Ther Clin Pract* 12:272–5.

Ernst E, Fialka V (1994). The clinical effectiveness of massage therapy—a critical review. *Forsch Komplementarmedizin* 1:226–31.

Ernst E, Köder K (1997). An overview of reflexology. *Eur J Gen Pract* 3:52–7.

Ernst E, Pittler MH, Wider B, Boddy K (2006). *The desktop guide to complementary and alternative medicine*, (2nd edn). Edinburgh: Elsevier Mosby.

Ezzo J, Vickers A, Richardson MA, Allen C, Dibble SL, Issell B, Lao L, Pearl M, Ramirez G, Roscoe JA, Shen J, Shivnan J, Streitberger K, Treish I, Zhang G (2005). Acupuncture-point stimulation for chemotherapy-induced nausea and vomiting. *J Clin Oncol* 23, 7188–98. Review.

Fellowes D, Barnes K, Wilkinson S (2004). Aromatherapy and massage for symptom relief in patients with cancer. *Cochrane Database Syst Rev* Issue 3. Art No. CD002287

Genuis ML (1995). The use of hypnosis in helping cancer patients control anxiety, pain, emesis: a review of recent empirical studies. *Am J Clin Hypn* 37:316–326.

Hammar M, Frisk J, Grimas O, Hook M, Spetz AC, Wyon Y (1999). Acupuncture treatment of vasomotor symptoms in men with prostatic carcinoma: a pilot study. *J Urol* 161:853–7.

Jacknow DS, Tschann JM, Link MP, Boyce WT (1994). Hypnosis in the prevention of chemotherapy-related nausea and vomiting in children: a prospective study. *J Dev Behav Pediatr* 15:258–64.

Jonas WB (2005). *Mosby's dictionary of complementary and alternative medicine*. St Louis, MO: Elsevier Mosby.

Kaptchuk TJ (2002). Acupuncture: theory, efficacy and practice. *Ann Intern Med* 136:374–83.

Kivisto KT, Kroemer HK, Eichelbaum M (1995). The role of human cytochrome P450 enzymes in the metabolism of anticancer agents: implications for drug interactions. *Br J Clin Pharmacol* 40:523–30.

Lee H, Schmidt K, Ernst E (2005). Acupuncture for the relief of cancer-related pain – a systematic review. *Eur J Pain* 9:437–44.

Lin HL, Liu TY, Wu CW, Chi CW (1999). Berberine modulates expression of mdr1 gene product and the responses of digestive track cells to Paclitaxel. *Br J Cancer* 81:416–422.

Linde K, Mulrow C, Berner M, Egger M (2005). St John's wort for depression. *Cochrane Database of Systematic Rev* 2005, Issue 2. Art No. CD000448.

Lord GM, Cook T, Arlt VM, Schmeiser HH, Williams G, Pusey CD (2001). Urothelial malignant disease and Chinese herbal nephropathy. *Lancet* 358:1515–16.

Markman M (2002). Safety issues in using complementary and alternative medicine. *J Clin Oncol* 20:39–41S.

Mills E, Montori VM, Wu P, Gallicano K, Clarke M, Guyatt G (2004). Interaction of St John's wort with conventional drugs: systematic review of clinical trials. *BMJ* 329:27–30.

Mills GK (1992). Comments on Syrjala *et al.*, Pain 48 (1992):137–46. *Pain* 50 137–46.

Murch SJ, KrishnaRaj S, Saxena PK (2000). Phytopharmaceuticals: problems, limitaitons, solutions. *Sci Rev Altern Med* 4:33–7.

Nainis N, Paice JA, Ratner J, Wirth JH, Lai J, Shott S (2006). Relieving symptoms in cancer: innovative use of art therapy. *J Pain Symptom Manage* 31:162–9.

Nortier JL, Martinez MC, Schmeiser HH, Arlt VM, Bieler CA, Petein M, Depierreux MF, De Pauw L, Abramowicz D, Vereerstraeten P, Vanherweghem JL (2000). Urolethial carcinoma associated with the use of a Chinese herb (Aristolochia fangchi). *N Engl J Med* 342:1686–92.

Redd WH, Montgomery GH, DuHammel KN (2001). Behavioral intervention for cancer treatment side effects. *J Natl Cancer Inst* 93:810–23.

Richardson J, Smith JE, McCall G, Pilkington K (2006). Hypnosis for procedure-related pain and distress in pediatric cancer patients: a systematic review of effectiveness and methodology related to hypnosis interventions. *J Pain Symptom Manage* 31:70–84.

Risberg T, Kolstad A, Bremnes Y, Holte H, Wist EA, Mella O, Klepp O, Wilsgaard T, Cassileth BR (2004). Knowledge of and attitudes toward complementary and alternative therapies; a national multicentre study of oncology professionals in Norway. *Eur J Cancer* 40:529–35.

Roscoe JA, Morrow GR, Bushunow P, Tian L, Matteson S (2002). Acustimulation wristbands for the relief of chemotherapy-induced nausea. *Altern Ther Health Med* 8:56–63.

Roscoe JA, Morrow GR, Hickok JT, Bushunow P, Pierce HI, Flynn PJ, Kirshner JJ, Moore DF, Atkins JN. (2003). The efficacy of acupressure and acustimulation wrist bands for the relief of chemotherapy-induced nausea and vomiting. A University of Rochester Cancer Center Community Clinical Oncology Program multicenter study. *J Pain Symptom Manage* 26:731–42.

Rummans TA, Clark MM, Sloan JA, Frost MH, Bostwick JM, Atherton PJ, Johnson ME, Gamble G, Richardson J, Brown P, Martensen J, Miller J, Piderman K, Huschka M, Girardi J, Hanson J (2006). Impacting quality of life for patients with advanced cancer with a structured multidisciplinary intervention: a randomized controlled trial. *J Clin Oncol* 24:635–42.

Shen J, Wenger N, Glaspy J, Hays RD, Albert PS, Choi C, Shekelle PG (2000). Electroacupuncture for control of myeloablative chemotherapy-induced emesis: a randomized controlled trial. *JAMA* 284:2755–61.

Sims S (1986). Slow stroke back massage for cancer patients. *Nurs Times* 82:47–50.

Sloman R, Brown P, Aldana E, Chee E (1994). The use of relaxation for the promotion of comfort and pain relief in persons with advanced cancer. *Contemporary Nurse* 3:6–12.

Sparreboom A, Cox PG, Achiron A, Figg WD (2004). Herbal remedies in the United States: potential adverse interactions with anticancer agents. *J Clin Oncol* 22:2489–503.

Stalpers LJ, da Costa HC, Merbis MA, Fortuin AA, Muller MJ, van Dam FS (2005). Hypnotherapy in radiotherapy patients: a randomized trial. *Int J Radiat Oncol Biol Phys* 61:499–506.

Stephenson NL, Weinrich SP, Tavakoli AS (2000). The effects of foot reflexology on anxiety and pain in patients with breast and lung cancer. *Oncol Nurs Forum* 27:67–72.

Streitberger K, Friedrich-Rust M, Bardenheuer H, Unnebrink K, Windeler J, Goldschmidt H, Egerer G (2003). Effect of acupuncture compared with placebo-acupuncture at P6 as additional antiemetic prophylaxis in high-dose chemotherapy and autologous peripheral blood stem cell transplantation: a randomized controlled single-blind trial. *Clin Cancer Res* 9:2538–44.

Syrjala KL, Cummings C, Donaldson GW (1992). Hypnosis or cognitive behavioral training for the reduction of pain and nausea during cancer treatment: a controlled clinical trial. *Pain* 48:137–46.

Walker LG, Walker MB, Ogston K, Heys SD, Ah-See AK, Miller ID, Hutcheon AW, Sarkar TK, Eremin O (1999). Psychological, clinical and pathological effects of relaxation training and guided imagery during primary chemotherapy. *Br J Cancer* 80:262–8.

Werneke U, Earl J, Seydel C, Horn O, Crichton P, Fannon D (2004). Potential health risks of complementary alternative medicines in cancer patients. *Br J Cancer* 90:408–13.

Wilkinson SM, Love SB, Westcombe AM, Gambles MA, Burgess CC, Cargill A, Young T, Maher EJ, Ramirez AJ. (2007). Effectiveness of aromatherapy massage in the management of anxiety and depression in patients with cancer: a multicenter randomized controlled trial. *J Clin Oncol* 25:532–9.

Younus J, Collins A, Wang X (2003). A double-blind, placebo-controlled pilot study to evaluate the effects of ginseng on quality of life in adult chemotherapy-naïve cancer patients. *Proc Am Soc Clin Oncol* 22:733a.

Zuber R, Modriansky M, Dvorak Z *et al.* (2002). Effect of silybin and its congeners on human liver microsomal cytochrome P450 activities. *Phytother Res* 16:632–8.

Chapter 10

Spiritual care

Mark Cobb

Introduction

The mortal nature of life presents many challenges to the sciences and practices related to the human body and its biology. Life-threatening conditions also confront us with profound questions about the meaning of illness, about the nature of suffering, about the fragility of being human, and about death. Michael Mayne, wrote of his experience of living with and dying from cancer of the jaw, in his posthumously published book *The Enduring Melody* (Mayne 2006). He recognizes the subtle distinction, noted by others, between illness and disease with their subjective and objective connotations. The clinical disease leads to a focus on the 'bits and pieces', whereas the personal experience of cancer for Mayne is that of the 'apparent disintegration of my life.' Consequently, he considers that we can fail to distinguish between treating the disease and the patient as a person: 'To treat a disease is to inhibit it and hopefully help the body to destroy or control it: to treat a patient is to observe, foster, nurture and listen to a life.' (p. 236).

Spiritual care is in part a way of listening to those who lives are profoundly challenged; it is a way of attending to the spiritual assault of an illness and it provides a space in which the spiritual dimensions of human experience can be expressed, explored, and nurtured. Listening to a life from a spiritual perspective therefore requires a sensitivity and discernment towards the beliefs, values, and connections that shape the way people make sense and find meaning in their lives. When a life journey is disrupted or threatened with disintegration a person's spiritual orientation may become significant to understanding how the individual and those they relate to cope with the illness, respond to care, make decisions about treatment, and face dying and death. Spirituality may therefore provide a significant perspective to all those involved in the care of people living with terminal conditions in fostering the humanity of the whole person and in connecting people to sources of meaning, value, and hope even when life is drawing towards its end.

Spiritual issues towards the end of life

This chapter is concerned with the spiritual dimension, and specifically how it applies to palliative care practice. Spirituality as a concept is not without its problems and difficulties (Cobb 2001) but it has always had a place in the hospice movement and it continues to be a challenging presence in palliative care (Wright 2001). The term has strong religious roots in the Judaeo-Christian tradition (Sheldrake 2007) but it is also used in palliative care to refer to an intrinsic characteristic of personhood that can exist without necessary reference to a faith tradition or external body of beliefs. Contemporary spirituality therefore has rich and varied meanings across a spectrum from the traditional to the non-traditional, and from the individual to the collective. Rather than provide a systematic or comparative account of the varieties of spirituality we will consider four aspects that have a particular relevance to the context of palliative care: faith and beliefs, practice, suffering, and death.

Faith and beliefs

People take different stances towards illness and death and these depends upon the way they make sense of their lives and the world view they inhabit, or to put it another way, their beliefs. In dialogue with the social and cultural context, life history, and the way reality is conceived these beliefs provide a dependable framework of meaning within which people understand and respond to experiences and events. When this meaning extends beyond a materialistic account and includes a transcendent reality then we are dealing with matters of faith (Cottingham 2003). The language of faith refers to that which is fundamentally important or real to people, and transcendent reality is traditionally associated in the Western context with terms such as God, the Holy, and the Eternal. The major religious traditions have their own descriptions of ultimate reality (Hick 1999) and these provide the basis for beliefs around which people can structure and direct their lives. However, a person who does not hold to any particular faith tradition may still adopt a spiritual orientation and inhabit a world view that includes the transcendent. Spirituality is therefore not simply an intellectual proposition but consists of cognitive, emotional, and behavioural components (Argyle 2000) that contribute to defining the person and to the way life is experienced.

When people have to contemplate their own death, they have to contemplate the end of themselves and their non-existence in the world as they know it. A diagnosis of terminal illness signals that life is not inviolable and that the frail and fragile body through which we experience and live in the world will fail us. Mortality is a challenge to life and it is a challenge to the beliefs we hold about life. From the questions of 'why me?' to those about life beyond death, beliefs will shape the way people respond to their ailing health and eventually to their death. Beliefs can develop over a lifetime but significant foundations are laid in our childhood when we form our sense of faith, hope, and love.

Children are naturally sensitive to the spiritual dimensions of life but by about the age of 12 a child's spiritual awareness, experience, and expression starts to become inhibited as a result of social forces and if unsupported and unnourished will not develop further (Hay and Nye 2006). When someone is trying to make sense of disruptions to the life journey latent or childhood beliefs may come into focus. For this reason it can be helpful to explore the spiritual autobiography or history (Puchalski and Romer 2003) of a person who is struggling with an incongruity between beliefs and experience and who ask the question of why 'bad' things are happening to a 'good' person.

Spiritual beliefs can have an important relevance in palliative care in that they may contribute to the way in which a person copes with a terminal illness. For example, in a study of patients with malignant melanoma, those who rated high religious and spiritual beliefs often used active-cognitive means of coping. The researchers suggested that beliefs may provide patients with a sense of connection, involvement, and meaning that helps them to accept their illness (Holland *et al.* 1999). However, while for some people beliefs contribute to coping, for others they may be ineffective or even problematic. Stressful life events challenge a person's world view and they can put a strain on beliefs. Negative aspects of coping may result when there is a disintegration of beliefs evident in doubts, confusion, conflict, and distress. It should be noted that what may be interpreted as problematic to a clinician may to a patient be an opportunity to wrestle with beliefs and to reappraise them (Pargament *et al.* 1998). What this suggests is that learning what it means to be dying may involve spiritual growth and enrichment.

Spiritual beliefs can give meaning to experience, but more practically they can provide the basis upon which patients respond to care, choose treatment options, and face their death. What may seem to be abstract spiritual beliefs are therefore situated in a personal context that is related to a wider social and cultural network. Spiritual beliefs may be consistent both within this network and with the philosophy of a palliative care service. However, there may be discord between differing beliefs that impinge directly on decisions affecting care and treatment (Hamel and Lysaught 1994). Issues concerning quality of life, the nature and meaning of pain, the need to fulfil end of life tasks, and accepting the finality of life may all throw into relief differences in belief that may require some accommodation or resolution. Discrepancy in views, and particularly negative or uncertain attitudes, may signal to a patient a disinterest by healthcare professionals or discrimination against such beliefs.

Practices

Beliefs and faith are seldom just philosophical concepts for they relate to being human and living meaningfully. Spirituality has practical, social, and material expressions and manifestations (Smart 1996). The practical aspects of spirituality may involve activities such as rituals, prayer, meditation, the reading of sacred texts, sacramental rites, and pilgrimage. Spirituality also exists in social forms, most notably through religious communities and in the values, beliefs, and ethics that they express. Spirituality is therefore embodied in people's lives and actions as well as in concrete material forms. Chapels, temples, mosques, icons, rosaries, holy books, and art can all be considered material expressions of the spiritual. It is therefore important when approaching spiritual issues that we consider their form as well as their content and the implications this has for the resources we may need to support people.

Patients may have practices and rituals that they wish to maintain and observe because of their faith and beliefs. Illness and its consequences can interfere with the routines of life and the habits through which people sustain meaning. Faith practices can be interrupted by healthcare commitments and patients can be easily dislocated from their faith communities and the people who support them in their religious beliefs and customs. In particular people from minority faith traditions may find it difficult to access the support they need (Gilliat-Ray 2001). The obligations of being a patient or the limitations of illness can also restrict the access of patients who currently have no connection to a faith community but want to return to a former community or explore new connections.

People who observe faith practices, rituals, festivals, and ceremonies do so for a range of reasons, but they may find them affirming and sustaining, particularly in the face of change and uncertainty. Faith practices may help to maintain a sense of personal identity as well as connectedness to a faith community. For this reason beliefs and practices cannot be separated from the social dynamic of culture. Faith practices are not generic and ignorance, stereotyped assumptions, or the rigid categorization of practices can obscure the actual needs of individuals. When a patient has a clearly identified religious faith then specific practices may be identified. However, people of nominal or no expressed religious commitment may still employ faith practices, such as prayer or meditation, and they may wish to participate in religious ritual. Research suggests a relationship between positive religious coping methods and improved quality of life (Tarakeshwar *et al.* 2006) and patients involved with a faith community may benefit from ongoing social support and care.

Finally, in considering rituals and faith practices in the context of palliative care we have to take account of those that concern the dead. Rituals around death underscore the transition from life to death and place the event of an individual within a wider collective context. Many faith traditions have a span

of ritual practice that begins when a person is approaching death and continues through to acts of remembrance and calendrical memorialization. Rituals
following death serve a very functional purpose of last offices and the disposal
of the corpse, but they also provide a framework of meaning, beliefs,
and behaviour that can enable the bereaved to make sense of their loss
(Davies 1997).

The faith traditions provide a rich source of ritual practice that people can
draw upon, and often those who have no connection with a faith community
may still seek ritual expression for their grief patterned upon faith practices.

Suffering

Terminal illness is an assault on the integrity of the person, which may result
in expressions of suffering. In addition to the bodily burdens resulting from
symptoms of the disease a patient can suffer through the many dimensions of
personhood. This is because a terminal illness is a threat to a person's existence
in the world and to the individual's life-course affecting such things as social
roles and identity, relatedness to self and others, and a sense of well being and
purpose. People can suffer therefore when the integrity of their personhood is
damaged or where there is some form of irrecoverable loss. When people
cannot make sense of what is happening to them, and particularly when they
can find no place for it within their framework of meaning, then suffering
may be related to the spiritual dimension (Van Hooft 1998). It is important
therefore that we can differentiate the spiritual factors that contribute to
suffering and pain from the physical and psychological (Mako *et al.* 2006).

Suffering has the potential to diminish people but many find a resilience to
respond to suffering. This enforced challenge may result in striving for a new
sense of wholeness in which the self that emerges incorporates or transcends
the illness. Transcendence enables connectedness and removes the isolation of
suffering by setting it within a larger landscape and through bringing people
close to sources of ultimate meaning and hope (Cassel 1982). The religious
traditions of the world have their own interpretations of suffering and many
have practices that enable people to transcend their immediate selves through
prayer, meditation, and ritual. While they acknowledge the reality of suffering,
they point towards an ultimate goodness of the universe and the fulfilment of
the human soul beyond suffering.

Existential doubt or spiritual disorientation may be unfathomable for some
people to the extent that it can overwhelm them. In these circumstance people
speak of injustice, hopelessness, darkness, and despair. Any faith a patient may
have had can become shattered, they can feel abandoned and hell can seem a
very present reality. Spiritual suffering can be related at this level to depression

and a psychiatric assessment may help in determining whether the patient has a mood disorder that may benefit from treatment or if the patient is at risk of suicide. This degree of suffering can be difficult to endure for carers and there are no quick remedies to lighten the troubled spirit. Patients may literally give up, become withdrawn, and become disconnected from people. The spiritual challenge for carers is to be able to contain this sense of dereliction and maintain a consistent presence that may bear witness to the possibility of relatedness and love.

Death

It can be difficult to grasp the fact of death from a personal perspective and people with a terminal illness may avoid anticipating the end of their lives. But for those who do contemplate it there can be significant spiritual issues that follow from a consideration of mortality. Some people hold that the result of death is simply nothing (Nagel 1986), or to be more accurate the permanent absence of the dead person from the world with its resultant losses for the bereaved. Many people with a religious commitment place death within the transcendent possibilities of the eternal and attempt to live their life in preparation for this reality. But what all these accounts have in common is the question of human destiny, and it is this that patients, out of self-interest alone, may wish to explore.

In a detailed study of the last months of nine terminally ill people, researchers reported that participants, regardless of their spiritual or religious orientation, searched for 'some tangible evidence of continuity with ongoing life after their own death.' (Staton *et al.* 2001) Transcending physical death for these people was in part about finding a connection with something that endured and this seemed to be related to accepting the finality of their existence. This was expressed both through a notion of a tangible legacy, such as passing on valued objects or property, and an intangible spiritual connection with others, creation, and the transcendent. Death can therefore be seen as something of a spiritual boundary that marks both the cessation of life and a reintegration of the self with the natural world or the infinite.

Exploring what death means to people can often betray their deepest fears and hopes, but paradoxically the anticipation of decay and death can also hold the expectation of liberation. Symbolic images and stories are often the means for contemplating death and many can be found in the religious traditions. However, contemporary culture also supplies plentiful examples that express ideas of death and destiny through fiction, songs, and films. These attempts to make sense of death and find meaning in it can provide the starting point for a patient and this is where the creative arts can provide a language and means of personal exploration. However, attempts to explore death by a patient can be overlooked or unintentionally blocked by healthcare professionals who have not considered their own mortality or are fearful of it. The result can be that patients are obstructed from engaging with a meaningful part of their dying.

Providing spiritual care

The philosophy of palliative care is premised on an understanding of person-hood that includes the spiritual dimension. However, this philosophy requires putting into action if it is to mean anything in terms of the care that is offered, and this raises questions about how we understand and respond to the spiritual needs of patients. It is clear that we will need to take a broad approach that allows for a wide spectrum of spiritual orientations: from those that can be highly differentiated as religious to those that have no reference to faith traditions and are markedly humanistic and personal. The benefit of this approach is that it is an attempt at being inclusive of the range of spiritualities that are found among patients. However, this should not be a fudge of the very real differences that exist between different spiritual orientations, nor an attempt at reaching the lowest common denominator, but a means of accommodating the breadth of spirituality that people present.

The variety of spiritual beliefs, experiences, and practices that coexist in the population served will depend on local demographic, cultural, and social factors. Religion will constitute an obvious part of the spiritual terrain. It is estimated that 60% of the population of Great Britain belong to a specific religion (Self and Zealey 2007) and socially and culturally significant forms of religious life will be evident in organizations, worship places, and the office-holders of the faith communities (Weller 2000). However, while people may hold beliefs associated with a particular religion they may not belong actively to a faith community, or they may only turn to it when faced with major life events (Davie 2000). Most healthcare services make some attempt to record the 'religion' of a patient, but beyond this cursory question there may be no further steps taken to enquire about the patient's spirituality. However, results of research among patients suggest that spiritual issues may be more prevalent and meaningful than professionals sometimes accept (Murray *et al.* 2004).

There are some patients who will disclose their spirituality directly to healthcare professionals or indirectly through their faith practices, rituals, and symbols. Many will not, and professionals may lack the interest, confidence, understanding, or skills to explore this area or identify concerns. Patients may also withhold their concerns in order to appear that they are coping or if they perceive staff would not cope (Heaven and Maguire 1997). The spiritual domain is one that can be subject to prejudice, presumption, and neglect, and consequently patients may feel isolated and unsupported. What this suggests is that a consistent approach should be taken by palliative care services to ensure patients are given the opportunity to express their spiritual beliefs and practices and for healthcare professionals to understand their needs. We shall consider three aspects of the care process: patient assessment, modes of spiritual care, and resources.

Assessment

Guidance on supportive and palliative care in the UK recommends that there should be opportunities for the assessment of the spiritual needs of patients and their carers along the patient pathway (National Institute for Clinical Excellence 2004) and a holistic common assessment framework has been proposed (Cancer Action team 2007). Assessments in palliative care typically focus on pathology, problematic symptoms, and disruptions to well being. Spirituality can be problematic, but there are also aspects of spirituality that are positive and fulfilling. A spiritual assessment therefore needs to incorporate this wider compass in order to capture faithfully the patient's understanding. However, as one of the early writers on spiritual assessment noted:

> [t]he values and beliefs elicited in these areas may or may not be expressed by the person through conventional religious language and rituals. Some people may find these content areas vague, verbally incongruent with their behaviour, or even threatening to discuss. It is important, therefore, to acknowledge each person's right to his own values and beliefs and to respect his right to remain silent about them.
>
> Stoll (1979)

Spirituality touches on profound and sacred aspects of people's lives and it is important that any form of assessment is approached within a robust ethical framework of trust, understanding, and respect. In addition, if an assessment is to be reliable and sensitive it must be informed, responsive to the particular patient and mindful of the potential for the subject area to be problematic. Proceeding with these caveats and cautions it is important that a palliative care service has a properly considered approach to assessing spirituality that takes account of:

- the context, circumstances, and environment of the assessment;
- the range of patients and carers using the service in terms of beliefs, culture, and language;
- the knowledge and skills of the healthcare professionals carrying out assessments and their ability to cope with the potential responses of a patient or carer;
- the availability of support and information relevant to the range of spiritual needs;

- the way in which the assessment process is incorporated into care planning and documented;
- the ongoing process of assessment.

The assessment process must begin by addressing the question of whether or not spirituality is important to a patient. Even this most basic stage in the process cannot proceed without good communication skills and an informed approach. Consideration must be given to the wording of questions and what may be known already about the patient (see Table 10.1). The patient's previous notes may contain data about religious affiliation and this may provide a starting point: 'I see from your notes that you describe your religion as Jewish, can you tell me about this?' If there is no data prior to meeting the patient then a broader and more open-ended type of question needs to be used: 'Do you have any spiritual or religious beliefs?' These questions are the first stage of the assessment process and should demonstrate to the patient that a positive awareness of spirituality and that it is taken as seriously as other aspects of patient care.

Table 10.1 Examples of helpful questions in an initial assessment

---

1 "I see from your notes that you describe your religion as Jewish, can you tell me about this?"

or if no data is available

"Do you have any spiritual or religious beliefs?"
"Can you tell me about them?"

---

2 "Is your faith/spirituality/religion helpful to you?"

or

"How important would you say this is to you?"

---

3 "Are they ways in which we can support you in your faith/spirituality/religion?"

or

"Can we help provide you with anything or any facilities to support you in your faith/spirituality/religion?"
"Are there things we need to know about your faith/spirituality/religion that would help us in caring for you?"

---

4 "Would you like to talk with someone about these matters?"

or

"We have a chaplain who is part of the team, would you like see him/her?"

or

"Would you like us to arrange a member of your faith community to visit you?"

Providing that the patient has indicated that this is a meaningful aspect of their life and that they are willing to talk about it, the assessment can move on to eliciting some outline description of the nature and significance of the patient's spirituality. Spirituality may have obvious form and content, or it may be more abstract, in which case the professional carrying out the assessment must ensure that the patient's description has been correctly understood, and where there is doubt, clarification sought. Patients are often more than willing to explain the nature of their spirituality and what it means to them, and it is one way for professionals to demonstrate their concern and respect.

Once an outline of a patient's spiritual orientation has been gained the next stage in the assessment is to ascertain how important and helpful it is. A simple question is often sufficient: 'Is your faith/spirituality/religion helpful to you?' or 'How important would you say this is to you?' Patients may indicate that while they hold certain beliefs they are not something, at this time, which concerns them, and the assessment can be concluded with reassurance that if the patient wants to talk about their spirituality a member of the team will be happy to do so. If a patient indicates that their spiritual orientation is significant then the assessment needs to continue to establish how the patient may be supported in this. Questions can be open: 'Are they ways in which we can support you in your faith/spirituality/religion?' and practical: 'Can we help provide you with anything or any facilities to support you in your faith/spirituality/religion?' Equally it is important for a palliative care service to know about aspects of a patient's spiritual orientation, which may promote or prohibit certain practices or which may be an important reference point in decision making: 'Are there things we need to know about your faith/spirituality/religion that would help us in caring for you?'

Finally, in an initial form of assessment the patient should be given the opportunity to speak further with someone: 'Would you like to talk with someone about these matters?' or 'We have a chaplain who is part of the team, would you like see him/her?' It may be, depending upon previous answers, that the patient is already involved with a faith community, and the more appropriate question might be: 'Would you like us to arrange a member of your faith community to visit you?'

This overview assessment is person-focused, sensitive to the responses of the individual and can proceed at their pace. A more objective and systematic approach may be gained by using some form of patient-completed questionnaire (King *et al.* 2001), which may provide the basis for a more personal follow-up discussion. Whatever form is taken the assessment should provide basic information to enable a palliative care team to support a patient's spiritual orientation and ensure the care plan is consistent with a patient's beliefs and practices. It should be recognized that an assessment interview may be therapeutically beneficent for a patient, in part because of the cathartic opportunity that it may present someone. As with other forms of assessment it is not a single event, but needs to be an ongoing process. Professionals should be alert to the patient who has initially declined any discussion of spirituality but who may seek some form of spiritual care in the future.

Any form of assessment needs to be incorporated into care planning and it must be properly documented. Information gained about a patient's spiritual beliefs and practices should be evaluated alongside other aspects of the person within the multidisciplinary team and used to inform decisions about care and interventions. However, there is a limitation in this exercise in that the spiritual can never be captured adequately by words and that the fullest understanding of a person's spirituality is usually only gained by sharing in some of their spiritual journey where metaphors, symbols, and silence may be the preferred language of the spirit (Stanworth 2004).

Modes of spiritual care

The form and type of spiritual care is best determined by the patient in consultation with a member of the care team. There will be patients who will have their spiritual care needs met by people from their own faith community or others external to the team. In this case supportive arrangements need to be put in place to allow access and provide necessary facilities. For patients who are not involved or do not wish to be referred to any external agency, or for those with access difficulties, then the team will need to facilitate spiritual care.

One of the principal modes of spiritual care is rooted in the Judeo-Christian tradition of pastoral care:

> Pastoral care involves the establishment of a relationship or relationships whose purpose may encompass support in time of trouble and personal and/or spiritual growth through deeper understanding of oneself, other and/or God. Pastoral care will have at its heart the affirmation of meaning and worth of persons and will endeavour to strengthen their ability to respond creatively to whatever life brings.

Lyall (2001)

Healthcare chaplains are trained and experienced practitioners of pastoral care, which takes seriously the uniqueness of an individual's spiritual journey. Pastoral care begins by listening to the narrative or life stories that a person is willing to share and to reflect upon these using the theological resources and the traditions of the faith community. This is a 'critical' conversation that respects beliefs, faith, and experience, and seeks to understand better the depths of humanity and the possibilities of the Holy (Lartey 2006).

Patients whose spirituality is not orientated around any particular faith tradition or related to any particular faith community may still benefit from a pastoral care approach. It will be important for both parties to have mutual respect and to maintain their own integrity. Beyond this mode spiritual care will operate within a more general therapeutic framework. This humanistic mode will be located in a patient's world view and their understanding. This is a supportive mode of spiritual care that aims at fostering positive coping and the enhancement of well-being. A humanistic approach to spiritual care will provide opportunities for patients to explore their spiritual beliefs and experience, to address concerns and to empower them in their own spiritual journey. This mode will draw upon counselling skills and the relational context, but it is not just problem focused and will involve sustaining positive aspects of spirituality.

Resources

The patient

It is not with the intention of objectifying the patient that we should consider him or her as a primary resource. It is in valuing the person's spiritual history, beliefs, and experiences that the resources within someone may emerge and be encouraged to develop. A patient may have much to teach the care team about his or her spiritual beliefs and practices. But the patient may require assistance in making use of his or her own resources. For example, a patient may have a developed a daily habit of prayer that seems difficult to sustain in an inpatient unit. Without regular prayer the patient may feel spiritually isolated and alone. Prayer requires attention and focus and with appropriate support, encouragement, and some practical rearrangements, the patient may be enabled to draw upon this deeply personal and transcendent aspect of their spirituality.

The patient's own resources may include spiritual practices and beliefs, and they may involve significant people. It may be helpful for palliative care teams to have in mind some form of spiritual genogram for those patients whose spirituality has transpersonal and social aspects. The involvement of other people may be correspond to significant personal relationships, such as those of a partner or family; it may relate to people who have died but are still active in the person's world view; or it may involve members of a faith community. This will need to be carefully and sensitively explored with the patient and could form part of an ongoing assessment.

The palliative care team

It is probable that the only member of the team with a specified responsibility will be that of the chaplain, but many team members have an expectation of being able to provide some level of spiritual care. Doctors may be attentive to the spiritual dimension as part of their overall concern for the wellbeing of patients and compassionate medical care (Brown *et al.* 2006). Nurses in particular consider this to be an aspect of their role. In a study of nurses almost half of them responded that they provided spiritual help and support for the terminally ill primarily by taking them to spiritual events on the ward, facilitating participation in Holy Communion, entering discussions about the meaning of life and God, and consulting with a chaplain. However, almost half of the nurses felt they had poor skills and knowledge in this area and over one-third of the nurses were not willing to provide spiritual support (Kuuppelomäki 2001).

If a team is functioning well then it will appreciate the complementary skills and knowledge of its members (Speck 2006). A chaplain who is properly integrated into a team should be an important resource to a team not only for direct patient care but also for advice and consultation. As part of the care planning a decision should be taken with the patient on who should be the lead person in facilitating and providing spiritual care. In this way spiritual care does not dissolve into some generic but marginal team function, nor does it exclude others members of the team from contributing.

Facilities

Palliative care services are hostages to architecture, competing demands on space and financial restraints. The facilities originally planned for a service may no longer meet the current needs of service users and new or additional facilities may be required. For community-based services access may be a real problem. Copies of sacred texts, prayer mats, and rosaries are all examples of small-scale equipment that may be easily obtained, but more permanent facilities, such as prayer rooms, require long-term planning and financial commitment. In developing facilities user involvement can ensure that what seems like a good idea 'on paper' is in reality useful and fulfils its intended purpose. In addition to specific facilities, spiritual care needs should be considered in all aspects of how a service operates and functions.

Faith communities

Local communities are important resources and should be involved in public services. In matters of spiritual care there is much that can be learnt from local faith communities and services need to develop effective mechanisms to allow this to happen. People are often very willing to be involved and it is important that hard to reach or minority groups are encouraged and supported in this. The involvement of faith communities may be strengthened by establishing a Faith Forum to be involved in service developments and in providing relevant advice. The Faith Forum may also be an effective route through which to establish associate chaplains from minority faith groups.

Education, training and professional development

Spirituality is a complex domain and one that requires different levels of skill, knowledge, and practice. If spirituality is an important dimension of palliative care then training programmes should be provided to resource staff with an adequate knowledge base and clinical skills. At present there are wide variations among disciplines and organization as to what is available, and a more systematic approach would suggest, including spiritual care within the educational strategy of a service (Johnson 1998) and teaching from a common syllabus, which includes a consistent evaluation of the knowledge, skills, behaviours, and practice of learners (Marr *et al.* 2007).

Spiritual care also requires more than the application of theory or knowledge because spirituality is necessarily a reflective and contemplative practice. Professionals who work in this domain need to be resourced with some form of supervision to enable them to: explore the impact of intimate personal encounters upon their own spirituality; develop skills; and face their own doubts, distress, prejudices, and defences (Hawkins and Shohet 2007). Reflective practice skills should support spiritual care as well as the use of creative arts.

Conclusions

If we are to treat patients as whole persons then spiritual care will not be something extraneous to palliative care. If we are to listen to patients and pay attention to their spiritual beliefs, experiences, and practices then professionals have a responsibility to integrate spiritual care into clinical practice. This can be a challenging aspect of care but it is one that can reveal the inspiring nature of the human spirit even in the face of death. Throughout this chapter we have been reminded that spirituality is not one thing and therefore spiritual care will be diverse. But whatever form it takes, spiritual care must be purposeful, properly resourced, and undertaken within a clear ethical framework. Inevitably professionals who develop skills and knowledge in this domain will need to address their own spirituality and mortality. In doing so they may deepen their own humanity and be more able to respond to the spiritual depths of others.

References

Argyle M (2000). *Psychology and religion*. London: Routledge.

Brown AE, Whitney SN, Duffey JD (2006). The physician's role in the assessment and treatment of spiritual distress at the end of life. *Palliat Support Care* 4:81–6.

Cancer Action Team (2007). *Holistic common assessment of supportive and palliative care needs for adults with cancer: assessment guidance*. London: Cancer Action Team.

Cassel EJ (1982). The nature of suffering and the goals of medicine. *N Engl J Med* 306(11):639–45.

Cobb M (2001). *The dying soul: spiritual care at the end of life*. Buckingham: Open University Press.

Cottingham J (2003). *On the meaning of life*. London: Routledge.

Davie G (2000). Religion in modern Britain: changing sociological assumptions. *Sociology* 34:113–28.

Davies DJ (1997). *Death, ritual and belief*. London: Cassell.

Gilliat-Ray S (2001). Sociological perspective on the pastoral care of minority faiths in hospital. In: Orchard H (ed.). *Spirituality in health care contexts*. London: Jessica Kingsley.

Hamel RP, Lysaught MT (1994). Choosing palliative care: do religious beliefs make a difference? *J Palliat Care* 10(3):61–6.

Hawkins P, Shohet R (2007). *Supervision in the Helping Professions*. Maidenhead: Open University Press.

Hay D, Nye R (2006). *The spirit of the child*. London: Jessica Kinglsey.

Heaven CM, Maguire P (1997). Disclosure of concerns by hospice patients and their identification by nurses. *Palliat Med* 11:283–90.

Hick J (1999). *The fifth dimension: an exploration of the spiritual realm*. Oxford: Oneworld.

Holland JC, Passik S, Kash KM *et al* (1999). The role of religious and spiritual beliefs in coping with malignant melanoma. *Pscho-Oncology* 8:14–26.

Johnson A (1998). The notion of spiritual care in professional practice. In: Cobb M, Robshaw V (ed.). *The spiritual challenge of health care*. Edinburgh: Churchill Livingstone.

King M, Speck P, Thomas A (2001). The Royal Free Interview for Spiritual and Religious Beliefs: development and validation of a self-report version. *Psychol Med* 31(6):1015–23.

Kuuppelomäki M (2001). Spiritual support for terminally ill patients: nursing staff assessments. *J Clin Nurs* 20:660–70.

Lartey E (2006). *Pastoral theology in an intercultural world*. Peterborough: Epworth

Lyall D (2001). *Integrity of pastoral care*. London: SPCK, p. 12.

Mako C, Galek K, Poppito SR (2006). Spiritual pain among patients with advanced cancer in palliative care. *J Palliat Med* 9(5):1106–13.

Marr L, Billings JA, Weissman DE (2007). Spirituality training for palliative care fellows. *J Palliat Med* 10:169–77.

Mayne M (2006). *The enduring melody*. London: Darton, Longman and Todd.

Murray SA *et al* (2004). Exploring the spiritual needs of people dying of lung cancer or heart failure: a prospective qualitative interview study of patients and their carers. *Palliat Med* 18:38–45.

Nagel T (1986). *The view from nowhere*. New York: Oxford University Press, pp. 223–31.

National Institute for Clinical Excellence (2004). *Guidance on cancer services: improving supportive and palliative care for adults with cancer. The manual*. London: National Institute for Clinical Excellence, p. 98.

Pargament KI, Zinnbauer BJ, Scott AB, Butter EM, Zerowin J, Stanik P (1998). Red flags and religious coping: identifying some religious warning signs among people in crisis. *J Clin Psychol* 54:77–89.

Puchalski C, Romer AL (2003). Taking a spiritual history allows clinicians to understand patients more fully. *J Palliat Med* 3:129–37.

Self A, Zealey L (eds) (2007). *Social trends*, No. 37. Basingstoke: Palgrave Macmillan.

Sheldrake P (2007). *A brief history of spirituality*. Oxford: Blackwell.

Smart N (1996). *Dimensions of the sacred*. London: HarperCollins.

Speck P (ed.) (2006). Teamwork in palliative care: fulfilling or frustrating? Oxford: Oxford University Press.

Stanworth R (2004). *Recognizing the spiritual needs in people who are dying*. Oxford: Oxford University Press.

Staton J, Shuy R, Byock I (2001). *A few months to live: different paths to life's end*. Washington DC: Georgetown University Press, p. 255.

Stoll RI (1979). Guidelines for spiritual assessment. *Am J Nurs* 19:1574–7.

Tarakeshwar N, Vanderwerker LC, Paulk E, Perrce MJ, Kesl SV, Prigerson HG (2006). Religious coping is associated with the quality of life of patients with advanced cancer. *J Palliat Med* 9(3):646–57.

Van Hooft S (1998). Suffering and the goals of medicine. *Med Health Care Philos* 1(2):125–31.

Weller P (ed) (2000). *Religions in the UK: directory 2001–2003*. Derby: University of Derby.

Wright MC (2001). Spirituality: a developing concept within palliative care? *Prog Palliat Care* 9(4):143–8.

Chapter 11

Bereavement care and hope

Sheila Payne, Mari Lloyd-Williams,
and Vida Kennedy

Academics, poets, and novelists have written many words about bereavement and loss, but in everyday life our most common experience is being at a 'loss for words' when these momentous events happen. The feeling of not being able to explain and describe our grief is common in the immediate aftermath of a death. Also many of us are at a loss to know what to say to those who are recently bereaved. Health professionals may worry about saying the 'wrong' thing or try to find the 'right' words to comfort bereaved relatives. Finding the words to offer support is perhaps even more difficult if the bereaved person is a child. Ironically, a fundamental and reassuring task of health professionals is to acknowledge the normality of distress and not to trivialize it or imply that the bereavement person has a medical condition.

This chapter is about the language and discourses of bereavement. We will trace the ways of talking and understanding bereavement back to some of the theoretical ideas, which emerged in the last century.

It is generally agreed that there are no single 'correct' or 'true' theories that explain the experience of loss or account for the emotions, experiences, and cultural practices that characterize grief and mourning (Payne *et al.* 1999; Hockey *et al.* 2001). A post-modern position suggests that individual diversity is paramount, and that within broad cultural constraints each of us develops our own ways of *doing* bereavement (Walter 1999). This accords well with many health professionals' experiences and awareness of the range of responses from their patients and clients. Although there may not appear to be agreed social rules on how to behave when bereaved in the UK, Hockey (2001) has highlighted that there are more subtle injunctions—'that the individual shall express their emotions, shall acknowledge the reality of their loss and shall share their thoughts and feelings with appropriate others'. Many bereavement support services operate with these basic requirements of their clients.

This chapter explores how dominant theories of loss have shaped our understanding of bereavement. We offer a brief introduction to psychiatric and psychological theories, followed by more recent models derived from theories of stress and coping. Latterly, theories have emphasized continuity and integration and we will review their implications. While we will endeavour to draw on theories and research, which extend understanding of loss beyond Western cultural norms, much of this chapter is grounded in our research and practice in Britain. We are aware of much diversity but cannot adequately reflect this in one short chapter. The chapter will show how theoretical ideas have been incorporated into notions of 'normal' bereavement and the roles health professionals play in facilitating what most regard as a 'process'. We will draw on research which has examined adult bereavement support provided by hospices in the UK. These organizations have pioneered bereavement support within healthcare and many hospices regard the provision of bereavement support as integral to their services. Yet there has been great diversity in how bereavement support services are organized and delivered. We will argue that this has been one of the most marginalized aspects of hospice development and will try to identify the reasons for this (Payne 2001a). The chapter concludes with a discussion about the role and function of childhood bereavement services.

Theories of grief and bereavement

Most cultures have ideas about what happens after death and how bereaved people should feel and behave. Historical and archaeological evidence provide plenty of examples, perhaps the best known being ancient Egyptian tombs with their embalmed bodies and memorials. In our own times the range of beliefs, practices, and rituals associated with death and mourning is impressively large (see Parkes *et al.* 1997). Most religions provide accounts for what happens after death, and may proscribe pre-death thoughts and behaviours such as the 'last rites' given by Roman Catholic priests or the mouthful of Ganges water for dying Hindus (Firth 2001). Most major religions also provide guidance on how bereaved people should respond after the death, although these behaviours and practices may be modified over time and due to changes such as migration and acculturation. For example, Firth (2001) describes how British Hindus have had to adapt cremation and associated death rituals to the constraints of British crematoria. In San Francisco, Chinese Americans have adapted burial rituals such as the traditionally use of firecrackers and loud music to ward off evil spirits to the contemporary inclusion of marching bands in the funeral possession to the cemetery (Chung and Wegars 2005). It is important to acknowledge that ideas derived from religious teaching have evolved and continue to do so. However, Britain has become an increasingly secular society and arguably, religious teaching provides less guidance than in the past.

It is appropriate at this point to consider the meaning of the terms that we will use in this chapter. The common root of the words bereavement and grief (reave) are derived from the Old English word 'reafian', to plunder, spoil, or rob (Oxford English Dictionary 1989). Two aspects of loss by death—the sense of personal violation and the heaviness of the soul, are thus embedded in the language itself (Payne *et al.* 1999). Bereavement is usually considered to be the process surrounding the loss of a loved object. In the context of this chapter, this is a person who has died, but it may also refer to loss of significant relationships, a way of life, a pet, a belief, or anything that has personal meaning for the individual. The reaction to this loss is grief. There is much debate as to whether grief is a universal human response to bereavement and loss. Mourning is generally described as the behavioural, emotional, and cognitive expression of grief. Mourning is heavily influenced by cultural and gender-specific norms. For example, in some cultures women do not attend funerals. While it appears simple and straightforward to separate out these aspects of loss into neat definitions, Small (2001) has argued that they are intimately linked to our theoretical understanding of loss. So the language we use to describe bereavement both reveals and shapes our understanding of this experience.

Developmental theories

The first group of theories that will be discussed are based on developmental notions of change and growth. They make the assumption that bereavement is a *process* in which there is an *outcome*. The idea of process is typically expressed as phases, stages, or tasks to be accomplished. Notions of change and process are fundamental and failure to 'move on' or 'progress' gives rise to ideas of being 'stuck'. The theories have largely concentrated their attention on the intra-psychic domain, the inner workings of the mind. They have emphasized how people think and especially how they feel—their emotions. There is also an assumption that people have some control over their feelings and thoughts, and these can be accessed through talk. Moreover, they suggest that successful grieving requires effortful mental processing called 'grief work' and that failure to do this is 'abnormal'. So where do these ideas come from?

The most influential and earliest theories of bereavement emerged from the psychoanalytic tradition, perhaps the most important being those of Freud (1917). Freud contributed much to twentieth century thought and his ideas have been very influential in shaping our ways of understanding people. In 1917, Freud first pointed out the similarities and differences between grief and depression in his classic text 'Mourning and melancholia'. His paper offered one of the first descriptions of normal and pathological grief. The thoughts discussed in it underpin psychoanalytic theory of depression and provide the basis for many current theories of grief and its resolution. In the light of the impact of Freud's theory of grief on subsequent theoretical developments, it is surprising to acknowledge that grief, as a psychological process, was never Freud's main focus of interest. In the paper, he argued that people became attached to others who are important for the satisfaction of their needs and to whom emotional expression is directed. Love is conceptualized as the attachment of emotional energy to the psychological representation of the loved person. It is assumed that the more important the relationship, the greater the degree of attachment. According to Freudian theory, grieving represents a dilemma because there is a simultaneous need to relinquish the relationship so that the person may regain the energy invested and a wish to maintain the bond with the love object. The individual needs to accept the reality of the loss so that the emotional energy can be released and redirected. The process of withdrawing energy from the lost object is called 'grief work'. He regarded this intra-psychic processing as essential to the breaking of relationship bonds with the deceased, to allow the reinvestment of emotional energy and the formation of new relationships with others. Arguably Freud's most important contributions to loss have been:

- introducing a developmental perspective (his personality theory emphasized early childhood development);
- introducing the 'grief work' hypothesis; and
- defining the difference between grief and depression.

His ideas were taken up and developed by many other people such as Lindemann (1944), Fenichel (1945), and Sullivan (1956), to just mention a few important theorists. In the second half of the twentieth century, Bowlby (1969, 1973, 1980) proposed a complex theory to account for the formation of close human relationships, especially between mothers and their babies, and for what happened when these bonds were broken. He suggested that human evolution resulted in mothers and infants needing to be in close proximity for survival and that this was achieved through an interactional process involving reciprocal behaviours and feelings between mothers and babies called attachment. Temporary separation was marked by characteristic behaviours and feelings such as distress, calling, and searching. Permanent loss, such as bereavement, also triggered these feelings of intense distress and behavioural responses. Bowlby's ideas have been taken up by health and social care services, for example, in encouraging early contact between mothers and babies after birth. Bowlby's ideas were also influential in the development of Parkes' theories of loss (1996). Both Bowlby and Parkes were psychiatrists and were in contact with patients struggling to understand the impact of their bereavements. Parkes (1971, 1993) suggested that bereavement should be considered as a major psychosocial transition, which challenged the taken-for-granted world of the bereaved person. He argued that most people think of their world as relatively stable, in which they make assumptions of perceived control. Death, especially sudden death, challenges this, as people have to adapt to changes in relationships and social status (for example, from being a wife to a widow), and economic circumstances (having less money). He, like Bowlby, proposed that people progress through phases in coming to terms with their loss.

Finally, there are two well-known models, which are widely applied in palliative care. Kubler Ross (1969), a psychiatrist heavily influenced by psychoanalytic ideas, proposed a stage model of loss in relation to dying which has been applied to bereavement. This model emphasized changing emotional expression throughout the final period of life. Worden (1982, 1991) based his therapeutic model on phases of grief and what he called 'tasks of mourning'. He suggested that grief was a process not a state, and that people needed to work through their reactions to loss to achieve a complete adjustment. Of course, Parkes, Kubler Ross, and Worden have modified and developed their ideas over time and this simple account does not do justice to the complexity of their thinking. All these theories have been critiqued and challenged, especially in relation to notions of a linear progression through phases or stages and the necessity of 'grief work' (for example, see Wortman and Silver (1989)). Contemporary evidence suggests that bereaved people may be more resilient and less distressed than previously thought (Bonanno 2004).

Stress and coping

Over the last 50 years, in the psychological and medical literature, have emerged ideas about stress (Selye 1956) and coping. These ideas are based on an assumption that if certain things, called stressors, are present in sufficient amounts, they trigger a stress response. This response is both physical and psychological. Most things in our environment are within our abilities to adapt to, but it is those things that challenge this adaptation process that are considered to be stressful (Bartlett 1998). There have been a number of models proposed about how stress can be conceptualized. The most important for the purposes of this chapter is the transactional model of stress and coping developed by Lazarus and Folkman (1984). They proposed that any event may be perceived as threatening by an individual, and cognitive appraisal is undertaken to estimate its degree of threat and to mobilize resources to cope with it. Coping may focus on dealing with the threat directly or may emphasize the emotional response.

These are called 'problem-focused' and 'emotion-focused' coping. Stroebe and Schut (1999) developed these ideas within the context of bereavement. They proposed that, following a death, people oscillate between 'restoration-focused' coping, for example, dealing with everyday life, and 'grief-focused' coping, for example, by expressing their distress. They suggest that people move between these two forms of coping with loss, although over time more coping responses become progressively more 'restoration focused'. This is called 'the dual processing model'. From these ideas they have developed therapeutic interventions to help people address both types of coping to achieve a balance.

Continuity theories

A third set of ideas have challenged notions that successful resolution of grief involves 'moving on' and 'letting go' of the deceased person. These theories are based on an assumption that people wish to maintain feelings of continuity and that, even though physical relationships, end at the time of death, these relationships become transformed but remain important within the memory of the individual and community. For example, memories of the large number of deaths that occurred during the First World War continues to haunt Britain and other countries almost 100 years after the event (Hockey 2001). Rituals to mark these losses continue to be common and some are even increasing in popularity and significance, yet few people remain alive who were present in the trenches and witnessed these events first hand. Walter (1996, 1999) has proposed a biographical model of loss in which he suggests bereaved people seek to create a narrative which describes both the person who has died and the part they play in their lives. He argues that these narratives are socially constructed. Klass *et al.* (1996) also proposed a similar idea and illustrated this in relation to different types of loss. The elicitation of narratives (stories) are a common therapeutic device and are believed to help establish a durable and tolerable memory of the deceased and how they died.

Bereavement support in specialist palliative care

Hospice philosophy encompasses the care of patients and their families, which continues after death into the bereavement period. It has been argued that, for a number of reasons, bereavement support has been the least well-developed aspect of hospices and specialist palliative care services (Payne and Relf 1994; Payne 2001a). Most services are based on an assumption that bereavement is a major stressful life event and that a minority of people experience substantial disruption to their physical, psychological, and social functioning

(Parkes 1996). Parkes (1993) has argued that offering support to people who have adequate internal and external resources can be disempowering and be detrimental to coping. Evidence suggests that bereavement support is of most benefit for individuals who recognize that they require support but there is little justification for providing proactive therapeutic intervention for bereaved people with no signs of poor bereavement outcome. Critical reviews of the literature have questioned the relevance of the 'grief work' notion that challenges the basis of much of counselling with its focus on getting clients to talk about the loss (Stroebe *et al.* 2005).

In this section, we will draw upon a recent UK study that examined the nature and role of adult bereavement support services provided by hospices (for further information see Field *et al* 2004, 2006, 2007; Reid *et al* 2006). A survey was distributed to all 300 hospices and specialist palliative care units with adult bereavement services in the UK in 2003 and this was followed by detailed organizational case studies in five hospice bereavement services (Payne *et al.* 2007). The research collected information about the nature and role of bereavement support from the perspectives of service providers, including bereavement co-ordinators, professional bereavement workers and volunteers, and bereaved people who used services and those who declined. This study represents one of the first study's to investigate hospice bereavement support from multiple perspectives.

Most (73%) bereavement services provided by hospices in the UK are associated with inpatient units and had been in existence for at least 10 years (Field *et al.* 2004). The services were predominantly provided by nurses (56%), social workers (46%), and counsellors (46%), with chaplains, psychologists, and medical staff less commonly involved. In many services (68%) volunteers played an important part in supporting bereaved people. Typically, bereavement services usually involved two to three paid staff assisted by 11–12 volunteers and about a quarter of them reported having insufficient staff to offer a full range of support. Volunteers may enhance the range of services offered and address the need to make services culturally appropriate by involving local people and those from different minority ethnic groups. However, there is controversy about the extent to which volunteer labour is valued and how the needs of volunteer workers are met (Payne 2001b). Volunteers require recruitment, selection, training, and supervision, and evidence suggests that only a small minority of services failed to provide supervision. Relf (1998) has pointed out that providing for the needs of volunteer workers in bereavement support is a demanding and skilled activity. Bereaved people appeared to value the input of trained volunteers, especially their approachability (Field *et al.* 2007).

The emotional demands placed on those who witness grief and support bereaved people requires skill, knowledge, and sensitivity. The paradoxical nature of bereavement support, which requires both professional standards of knowledge and skill, and the warmth of human understanding and sensitivity, represents a challenge for all. There is a dilemma in training volunteers and professionals that the compassion and empathy, which lead them into this work, becomes constrained by a framework imposed by models of bereavement. However, exposure to repeated distress needs to be acknowledged as potentially difficult to deal with. It is generally considered to be good practice to ensure that supervision is available to bereavement care workers, in which emotional off-loading and discussion of difficult situations can be dealt with on a regular basis (Payne *et al.* 1999).

Bereavement support may start before the death, when families are put in touch with volunteer workers who may maintain contact with them into the bereavement period. Such services offer the opportunity for relationships to be built up over time, and for newly bereaved people to be spared the difficulty of making new relationships when they are at their most vulnerable. Bereaved people also reported that the care received from community nurses and hospice staff during the final illness of their family member was perceived as helpful in preparing them for their loss and bereavement (Reid *et al.* 2006). 'I think all the support I was given you know, through the four months, saved my sanity afterwards. Erm, and although I was at, you know, a very low, desperate ebb, you know, if I hadn't had the support that I had, and in the latter sort of, shall we say month of it, you know … it was totally hospice support' (Bereaved Female, service user).

Bereavement support included a broad range of activities, the most common being: one-to-one support either face-to-face or via the telephone, written information, memorialization events, and group support (Field *et al.* 2004).

> I felt that I could talk about him and I could be as upset as I wanted to be. And all she did was listened. She didn't tell me 'Come on, you've got to be brave', and that was excellent. And she phoned me two or three times until she said 'Would you like me to phone you back?' and I said 'It's always lovely talking to you, but I know how busy you are and really you've done everything for me that you can.
>
> Bereaved Female, service user

Fewer services offered befriending and one-to-one counselling. It might be helpful to consider bereavement support in three broad categories, as shown in Table 11.1. Readers may be aware of other activities that are offered in their own services. Of course, there may be considerable overlap in the aims and delivery of some of these activities. For example, a drop-in centre might enable a bereaved person to talk one-to-one with a social worker, which may

Table 11.1 Types of hospice and specialist palliative care bereavement support for adults

Social activities	Supportive activities	Therapeutic activities
Condolence cards	'Drop in' centre/ Coffee mornings	One-to-one counselling with professional or trained volunteer
Anniversary (of death) cards	Self-help groups	
Bereavement information leaflets	Information support groups	Therapeutic support groups
Bereavement information resources (videos/books)	Volunteer visiting or befriending	Drama, music, or art therapy
Staff attending the funeral		Relaxation classes
Social evenings		Complementary therapies
Memorial services or other rituals		Psychotherapy

be perceived as therapeutic. Likewise, a bereaved person may agree to attend an art therapy programme because it enables him to get out of the house and meet new people, which is a predominantly social outcome.

The recognition of complicated (or abnormal) bereavement outcomes is important in identifying who might benefit from support services. While it is acknowledged that mental health problems, such as depression and anxiety are relatively more common in bereaved people than others, there remains debate about definitions of complicated bereavement. However, it is usually taken to mean unduly protracted or severe distress (Schut and Stroebe 2005). Just under half (43%) of UK hospice bereavement services reported using formal ways, such as using questionnaires and checklists, to assess how likely it is that a bereaved person will have an adverse outcome (Field *et al.* 2004). There are well-recognized attributes of the person, their environment and the nature of the death, which allow predictions to be made about which people need help (Saunders 1993). This is called risk assessment. For example, a person with previous mental health problems experiencing concurrent losses, such as their job or home, and witnessing a traumatic sudden death of their young child in a car accident, is likely to be more vulnerable than a person bereaved of their elderly grandmother after a chronic illness. Although risk assessment measures are available none are perfect. Hospice bereavement support services also need to be able to identify when clients present such difficult and complex problems that it exceeds their capacity to deal with them and to have well established mechanisms to refer on. Close and well established links with other services, such as psychiatric, clinical psychology, and specialist bereavement liaison support services (e.g. suicide support groups) are needed but evidence from our five case studies indicated that these were either lacking or inadequate because of concerns about long waiting lists (Field *et al.* 2007). Overall, evidence suggests that UK hospices were providing bereavement support that was well regarded by bereaved people and fulfilled national recommendations (National Institute for Clinical Excellence 2004) in respect of providing information on the types of support available and the nature of grief, and in providing a wide range of general support but not necessarily access to specialist support. This was largely due to inadequate staffing and resources. Arguably this also meant that the skills developed in hospices were not available more generally in hospitals and the wider community to develop bereavement care (Field *et al.* 2007).

Children and bereavement

Tom aged 8 and Jake aged 6, knew there was something wrong with their dad. They had noticed over the past year that he no longer took them out, that he stayed in bed for quite a lot of the time. One Saturday morning they were told that as a special treat (although it was not school holidays) they were going to stay for a week or two with their aunt and uncle some 50 miles away. When mum came to collect them nearly 2 weeks later, they were told that dad had died and that he had gone to a special place. The funeral had taken place the day before they returned home. Initially both children were surprised (and delighted!) by all the attention they were getting. They were always being invited to stay with friends or to go home with school friend for tea and had never had so many visits to the cinema or Mcdonalds. Six months later the invitations and treats had all but stopped. Jake was bedwetting and Tom's behaviour at school had changed from a little boy who worked hard to one who was rude, disruptive, and at times aggressive towards other children.

The above case history illustrates some of the difficulties that families face when a parent is diagnosed with a terminal illness. Should the children be told what is happening and if so how and when should they be told and who should tell them? Should they be present at the death and be involved in the funeral?

Support prior to the death

Each year, 2% of all children are bereaved of a parent before the age of 18 years—many of these deaths are sudden, e.g. due to accident or sudden cardiac death, but a significant number may be due to terminal illness. How can children be helped around the dying process and their bereavement? It is known that children whose parents die from cancer where there is often time to prepare the child and family, have less psychological difficulties than children whose parents die suddenly, e.g. suicide (Pfeffer *et al.* 2000).

Siegel *et al.* (1992) was one of the first to address the psychological adjustment of children with a terminally ill parent. They used a variety of standard rating scales with 62 school aged children with a terminally ill parent and compared the results with those of a community sample. They found that children with terminally ill parents had higher levels of self-reported depression and anxiety, and lower self-esteem. Siegel *et al.* (1992) suggest three possible ways to conceptualize the children's distress in their study: (1) that it is an important aspect of the mourning process and therefore temporary and ultimately helpful; (2) that it may lead to pathological mourning that may lead to depression and anxiety in later life; and/or (3) as a reflection of the 'upheavals' of the terminal stage of the illness.

In fact a later study by Siegel *et al.* (1996) reported that children's levels of depression and anxiety were higher pre-death than they were post-death (7–12 months post-death). This evidence suggests, therefore, that the terminal phase of a parent's illness may be a period of greater psychological vulnerability than the period following the loss (Siegel *et al.* 1995, 1996). This has also been described in siblings where one child in the family has terminal cancer (Birenbaum *et al.* 1989). Suggested reasons for these findings include the possibility that the terminal phase is the stage of greater suffering by a parent that may be connected to a decreased role in the family and diminished appearance that may distress the child. Or also that it may be that the severity of the illness can no longer be denied and that parents choose this time to tell their children that death will occur (Siegel *et al.* 1996).

Siegel *et al.* (2000) found that children facing the loss of a parent to cancer demonstrated low levels of self-esteem and that this was correlated to, for example, being younger, having high levels of anxiety, and to the perception of the child of the well parent's parenting. They feel that pre-death interventions focusing on helping children's self-esteem would help elevate their distress.

A more recent study by Beale *et al.* (2004) interviewed 29 children of patients with terminal cancer and their parents. This study found that children with dying parents experience considerable distress, and they also found that they have a greater understanding of parents illness than is usually suspected. They state that a child's increased anxiety is directly linked to lack of information about a parent's diagnosis and that anxiety increases when information is available but when there is no opportunity for discussion. As a result of their findings Beale *et al.* (2004) suggest that a timely intervention by a child psychologist/mental health professional may help children cope better with their parents dying.

It can be difficult to involve a child during the parents' illness. The surviving parent in a desperate bid to spare the children the pain they themselves are facing, may act similarly to the mother in the case history above and may be coerced into doing so by other family members in the belief that they are protecting and helping the child. However, these actual mechanisms may not be protective and while delaying the initial pain do not spare children from later distress or the reality of what has happened.

A recent study by Kennedy (2008), where children whose parents had advanced cancer were interviewed, found that children (aged 8–18) reported wanting to know what was going on with their parents. Knowing was important for children in order to feel prepared to cope with what was ahead and to be able to make the most of the time they had with their ill parent and other family members.

> it is a good thing [being informed] because I want to keep up with dad's illness I want to know what's going on with him, I want to know if he's ok, or if he's ill, getting better or even if he's getting worse I want to know even if it's going to upset me because I know what's going to happen ... just so I know what's going to happen to him, because I don't want anything bad to just happen straight away I want to keep up with everything so that I know what's going to happen ...
>
> Ffion (age 14)

Levels of information needed, however, varied between children, highlighting the importance of individualized needs. Children in this study also highlighted the need for and lack of access to formal services where they could seek objective, age appropriate, and confidential information and support. Barriers to formal services reported by children included not knowing what was available as well as not wanting to let their parents know they had concerns in fear of upsetting them.

The study also interviewed health professionals (from a hospice and cancer centre) working with families where a parent with dependant children had a diagnosis of advanced cancer. They identified children's issues as the most challenging aspect of care. They recognized that children had needs (particularly informational needs) and wanted to help them but felt frustrated by barriers that prevented access to such children. Barriers described by health professionals included parental barriers (where parents acted as gate-keepers to children, not wanting them to know the truth); working hours that conflicted with children's schedules (e.g. school hours); and lack of resources (including financial, time, training, and lack of information, e.g. family situation).

> Yes it's difficult from the point of view of recognizing that the parents have to give consent for the work you do with the children but then actually the children's protection

laws say that if you suspect a child is in some kind of danger then you can intervene and ehm it's a very fine balance isn't it? not wanting to upset the parents but if you can see that the children's needs are being neglected not from any wilfully intention to damage the children but because the parents genuinely believe that's the best thing for them, and it's very difficult to know when to come in and say, and override the parents wishes.

Health professional (Hospice setting)

The data suggest a need to encourage parents to give children permission to seek support outside the family, and inform them of the services available to children. It also suggests that children need to be able to access support independently from parents (such as at school or health professionals).

Some studies, have looked at the support available to children whose parents have a terminal illness. Berman *et al.* (1988) interviewed children who had lost a parent to cancer and found that there was disagreement in terms of sources of support available to the adolescents. Family friends, relatives, and peers were described by the adolescents as important sources of support while parents identified doctors and school personnel. Furthermore, they describe little support from healthcare professionals and feelings of isolation when parents were terminally ill.

Support available before, during, and after death have been identified as being a contributing factor in the outcome of the grieving process (Elizur and Kaffman 1983), and therefore it will be crucial to gain further information regarding what and who children find supportive in the period before death in order to help children not only at this time but also in the longer term grieving process.

The UK NICE Guidelines on cancer services: Improving supportive and Palliative care for Adults with cancer (2004) recommended that psychological care be available to families. To date, however, development of such services particularly focusing on children has been very limited (Watson *et al.* 2006).

Additionally, the sick parent may be so unwell as to be unable to tolerate the child for any length of time and sometime parents may withdraw from the family during the latter stages of the illness again making it difficult for children to have any meaningful interaction. Encouraging children to visit for short periods and to write stories or draw pictures may be one method of keeping them involved. Older children will have more real understanding of what is happening. All children, however, need to be reassured that whatever happened they would be loved and cared for. This can be difficult, as often the partner is so involved in caring for the dying parent that they may not have the emotional capacity or the time to give to the children. Increasing numbers of children grow up in single parents families and for them, the prospect of losing their only parent is enormous. The mobilization of extended family resources is necessary to help in the future and support the child who may be the care-giver to the dying parent (Segal and Simkins 1993).

In some circumstances children in the family may take on the primary role of caring for their ill parent. An increased recognition of children's caring role has resulted in the development of the term 'Young Carers'. The Department of Health defines young carers as children who are providing, or are intending to provide, a 'substantial amount of care on a regular basis' (Department of Health 1996). The 2001 census estimated that there are 175 000 young carers in the UK but some researchers have suggested that the true figure could be even higher (Bibby and Becker 2000). There are currently, however, no figures regarding the number of young carers caring for someone with a terminal illness.

It has been recognized that caring for an ill parent/relative can impact a child in many ways, including: physically, socially, educationally, emotionally, and behaviourally (Aldridge and Becker 1999; Thomas et al. 2003). Recognition of such impacts on the quality of a young carers childhood has led to the call for improved support for children in these situations. A recent Help the Hospices young carers guide has been developed to help provide support and information for young people who provide practical and/or emotional support to someone with a terminal illness (Help the Hospices 2006). This guide gives details regarding where to find help and information as well as providing advice about feelings and specific illnesses. In addition it also provides a section for professionals working with young carers providing help in how to identify as well as support young carers.

Christ (2000) studied the experiences of 88 families and their 157 children throughout the 6 months of a parent's terminal illness due to cancer and for 14 months after their death. Her analysis indicates that children reacted in ways that were heavily influenced by their developmental stage at the time of their loss. She also proposed that childhood loss should not be conceptualized as a single event, because it tended to precipitate a cascade of events brought about by the experience of illness on family functioning, the transition from dual to single parenting, and the possible subsequent remarriage of their remaining parent and the formation of a new family. Each of these events are challenging in their own right but bereaved children are often faced with a multitude of changes that may challenge their coping resources. Therefore, psychological and other responses to bereavement may be triggered by any one or a combination of these challenges as children grow to adulthood.

Support after death

Although the above study by Siegel et al. (1996) suggests that children experience greater psychological distress pre-bereavement than post-bereavement, this does not imply that children do not experience psychological symptoms post-bereavement. Children, for example, who have lost a parent or sibling are considered to be more at risk of emotional, social and behavioural problems (e.g. anxiety, depression, and aggression) (Worden 1996; Thompson *et al.* 1998).

Children who experience sudden, unexpected bereavement are thought to be at a higher risk of developing problems. For those who have witnessed traumatic events, such as accidents or suicide, there may be residual horrific images to contend with and for a minority, post traumatic stress disorder may occur (Cerel *et al.* 1999).

A review by Dowdney (2000), however, described psychological outcomes in children who have experienced the death of a patent as 'heterogeneous'. This variation in outcomes have suggested an increased importance of mediating and moderating factors in the risk of psychological problems after the death of a parent (Dowdney 2000; Christ and Christ 2006). The more common mediating and moderating factors described include the quality of parental care and the presence of other stressful events in the children's lives (Harris *et al.* 1986; Kwok *et al.* 2005; Christ and Christ 2006). In particular, the quality of the relationship between a child and their surviving parent has been identified as an important mediator. When a surviving parent demonstrated more active coping, less depression, and greater family cohesion, children are considered less likely to be at risk for psychological problems (Kwok *et al.* 2005). In addition to this where more open communication and a greater degree of information sharing regarding the parents death exists children have also been considered less likely to be at risk for psychological problems (Siegel *et al.* 1996; Raveis *et al.* 1999).

A study by Cerel *et al.* (2006) interviewed 360 parent-bereaved children (aged 6–17) and their surviving parents four times in the 2 years following a parent's death. They compared the psychiatric symptomology with that of community control and depressed children and their parent. They found there was an association between bereavement and increased psychiatric symptomology. Additionally they found that children whose surviving parent had higher levels of depression, who had other stressful life events in the family occurring and who were of a lower socio-economic status were of higher risk for psychiatric symptomology. Such findings support the implications of the importance of moderating and mediating factors described previously. In light of these findings Cerel *et al.* (2006) suggests that children who have these additional risk factors should be targeted for more careful monitoring. Furthermore, they suggest that providing help for the surviving parent will also indirectly help children's recovery.

It is widely believed that where possible it is helpful if children are able to attend the funeral if they so wish and also if they wish to be involved in the actual service itself. It is important, however, for a child to have an accompanying adult and to be reassured that they can leave at any time they wish—the surviving parent may be so overcome by their own grief as to be unable to support the children during the funeral. Encouraging children to draw pictures, write a story or letter that can be placed in the coffin can also help the child in the process of saying goodbye. There is still a belief that children do not understand the meaning of death but research has suggested that children as young as 5 or 6 years old have a clear concept of what death means (Lansdown and Benjamin 1985). Following a longitudinal study of bereaved children in the USA and Israel, Silverman (2000) has argued that even very young children can be helped by being given a clear explanation about what is happening when a family member dies. Children need to be told about what has happened in a language that they can understand (Black 1998). Euphemisms such as 'passed away' or 'gone to sleep' should be avoided. Children often have many questions regarding the terminal illness, e.g. what is cancer, what is chemotherapy, etc.—again these questions need to be answered in a language that children can understand and the support of a doctor who is willing to discuss such question with children is invaluable (Monroe and Kraus 1996; Thompson and Payne 2000).

Do all bereaved children need support? Harrington and Harrison (1999) describes a plethora of counselling services and at present no evidence to suggest which, if any, are of value for the bereaved child and their family. Although it remains that there is little evidence to support the benefits of bereavement support for children due predominantly to methodological issues (Curtis and Newman 2001; Nabors et al. 2004), the research that does exist suggests a positive result (Nabors et al. 2004; Kirwin and Hamrin 2005; Schmiege et al. 2006).

Sandler et al. (2003) for example evaluated a Family Bereavement Programme (FBP) by randomly assigning 156 families to either the FBP or a self-study condition. This programme was an intervention for bereaved children (aged 8–16) and caregivers, where positive coping, stress appraisals, control beliefs, and self-esteem skills were addressed with children, and mental health, life stressors, and improved discipline in the home were addressed with caregivers. They found that the FBP improved parenting, coping, and caregiver mental health, and led to a decrease in internalizing and externalizing problems (in girls and those with a higher problem score at the beginning). These findings have later been supported by Schmiege et al. (2006).

In addition to the above, Nabors et al. (2004) evaluated children's perceptions of the effectiveness of a hospice-sponsored grief camp in the USA.

They found a positive response where children reported that the camp helped them in expressing their feelings. In addition they said that it helped to be in groups with peers that had also lost a family member.

Evaluating the effectiveness of such services is difficult especially as outcomes, e.g. reduction of psychiatric morbidity can only be assessed several years later (Stokes *et al.* 1997). Most professionals would agree that all bereaved children should be given the opportunity to talk about the death and to explore and share their feelings (Carroll and Griffin 1977; Blanche and Smith 2000). Variations in children's responses, however, can make it difficult for parents and professionals to support children before, during, and after the death of a family member. In response to such variations some (Christ and Christ 2006) have developed recommendations on how to help bereaved children across variable developmental levels; such recommendations, however, need further research prior to being universally adopted.

Children do not grieve constantly and may dip in and out of intense grief for very short time periods. This can be difficult for family members to deal with alongside their own grief. Our case history illustrated how problems can be minimized during the first few months following a death when family and friends rally round and provide support. Lloyd-Williams *et al.* (1998) found that the peak time for children to present to the general practitioner following the death of a parent was 4.8 months and these presentations were frequently for somatic symptoms for which no organic causes could be found. This probably reflects the time when the attention of others is decreasing and when the reality of the loss may overwhelm the surviving parent causing strained relationships within the family.

Several models of bereavement support groups for children have been suggested (Zambelli *et al.* 1988; Christ *et al.* 1991; Mulcahey and Young 1995). A recent survey of 107 childhood bereavement services in the UK identified that 85% of childhood bereavement services were located within the voluntary sector; 14% were dedicated childhood bereavement services while 86% were located within another organization, 44% of these being hospices (Rolls and Payne 2003). The majority of services (71%) took referral for any child, the remaining 27% only offered services if the family members had died in their care. Most services (72.5%) relied on both paid and unpaid staff with 115 relying entirely on paid staff and 14.3% relying entirely on unpaid staff. The interventions offered ranged from individual family work (85.7%), individual child work (61.5%), group work with families (52.7%), and group work with children (45.1%). In addition services offered pre-bereavement support (63.7%), a 'drop-in' service (16.5%), information and advice (94.5%), training (31.9%), and the provision resources (87.9%). In addition to offering a service to children and their families, 75% of childhood bereavement services provided a service to secondary user's, for example, school (70%), emergency service (27.5%), and other professionals (63%).

Following the above, a related paper by Rolls and Payne (2003) reported that although many bereavement services had a 'shared objective of helping bereaved children', these services were very diverse. Much variation in location, type of service, organization, management, funding, and type of staff, for example, were described as seen above. In addition to this they suggest that as many of the services are accommodated within host services, they may not be easily identified. They highlight the publication of a 'Directory of Childhood Bereavement Services' by the Childhood bereavement Network, which may begin to make the available services more visible.

Winston's Wish is an example of a child bereavement programme in the UK that focuses on providing support and informing those closest to the child, for example, teachers, nursing, and care staff as to how to help a child through their grief (Stokes *et al.* 1999). Children who are bereaved may feel very isolated—they may be the only children who have been bereaved within their school, for example, causing them to feel stigmatized and very alone. The weekend camps are aimed at bringing bereaved children together to meet others in a similar situation and to give them an opportunity to tell their story, to ask questions and also to have fun and also to encourage them to think of life in the future, which for many children bereaved of a parent, may include a step-parent. One of the key aims of the programme is to help parents to support their children, for example, encouraging children to talk about the deceased parent and sharing memories, 'do you remember when' ... (Nickman *et al.* 1998).

The Child Bereavement Trust is another organization that is aimed specifically at providing resources for children and families who are grieving, and for the professionals who support them. Their document 'Understanding bereaved children and young people' is a helpful summary of what reactions to expect from children and ways in which parents, professionals, teachers, and/or others may help grieving children (http://www.childbereavement. org.uk/documents/Bereaved_Children_6pp.pdf).

Although as we have seen above, literature supports service provision for bereaved children, it also describes the service as variable. Dowdney *et al.* (1999), for example, found that service provision related to both the child's age and the nature of parental death. Children under 5 were found to be less likely to be offered services than older children, and children whose parents had committed suicide or whose death was expected were also more likely to be offered services. In addition they found that children who were already (pre-death) in contact with services (e.g. hospice) were more likely to be offered services than those who were not.

A bereaved child may experience the grieving process at several different time points many years after the death at major milestones in their lives (Baker *et al.* 1992; Lohnes and Kalter 1994). This chapter has aimed to discuss some of the issues that are important for those working within palliative care. The last words should go to those we are trying to help:

> In the days after she had gone, I had mixed emotions ... at times I felt pathetic like if only I hadn't hidden all those sandwiches, if only I hadn't answered back all those times ... At other times I would think she hadn't gone, it's only we can't touch her or see her and we'll always, always love her and as my Gran told me, the sadness will go eventually and I believe her.
>
> Izzie

Acknowledgements

Data for this chapter are drawn from a study funded by The Health Foundation and the Clara Burgess Trust. We wish to acknowledge the contribution of the bereavement co-ordinators, bereavement workers, and bereaved people and other members of the research team: Professor David Field, Dr Marilyn Relf, and David Reid to this study. We also wish to acknowledge Izzie for allowing us to share her feelings at her mum's death.

References

Aldridge J, Becker S (1999). Children as carers: the impact of parental illness and disability on the children's caring role. *J Fam Ther* 21:303–20.

Baker J, Sedney M, Gross E (1992). Psychological tasks for beraved children. *Am J Orthopsychiatry* 62:105–16.

Bartlett D (1998) *Stress.* Buckingham: Open University Press.

Beale EA, Sivesind D, Bruera E (2004). Parents dying of cancer and their children. *Palliat Support Care* 2:387–93.

Berman H, Cragg CE, Kuenzig L (1988). Having a parent die of cancer: adolescents' reactions. *Oncol Nurs Forum* 15(2):159–63.

Bibby A, Becker S (2000). *Young carers in their own words.* London: Calouste Gulbenkian Foundation.

Birenbaum LK, Robinson MA, Phillips DS, Stewart BJ, McCown DE (1989). The response of children to the dying and death of a sibling. *Omega* 20:213–28.

Black D (1998) Bereavement in childhood. *BMJ* 316:931–3.

Blanche M, Smith S (2000). Bereaved children's support groups: where are we now? *Eur J Palliat Care* 7:142–4.

Bonanno GA (2004). Loss, trauma and human resilience: have we underestimated the human capacity to thrive after extremely aversive events? *Am Psychol* 59:20–8.

Bowlby J (1969). *Attachment and loss.* Vol. 1. *Attachment.* London: The Hogarth Press.

Bowlby J (1973). *Attachment and loss.* Vol. 2. *Separation.* London: The Hogarth Press.

Bowlby J (1980). Attachment and Loss Vol. 3. Loss: Sadness and Depression. London: The Hogarth Press.

Carroll M, Griffin R (1997). Reaffirming life's puzzle: support for bereaved children. *Am J Hospice Palliat Med* 14:231–5.

Cerel J, Fristed M, Weller E, Weller R (1999). Suicide-bereaved children and adolescents: a controlled longitudinal examination. *J Am Acad Child Adoles Psychiatry* 38:672–9.

Cerel J, Fristad MA, Verducci J, Weller RA, Weller EB (2006). Childhood bereavement: Psychopathology in the 2 years postparental death. *J Am Acad Child Adoles Psychiatry* 45(6):681–90.

Christ G (2000). *Healing children's grief; surviving a parent's death from cancer.* New York: Oxford University Press.

Christ GH, Christ AE (2006). Current approaches to helping children cope with a parent's terminal illness. *CA Cancer J Clin* 56:197–212.

Christ G, Siegel K, Mesagno F, Langosch D (1991). A preventative intervention program for bereaved children: problems of implementation. *Am J Orthopsychiatry* 61:168–78.

Chung SF, Wegars P (2005). Chinese American Death Rituals: respecting the ancestors. Lanham: Altamira Press.

Curtis K, Newman T (2001). Do community-based support services benefit bereaved children? A review of empirical evidence. *Child Care Health Dev* 27(6):487–95.

Department of Health (1996). *Carers (Recognition and Services) Act 1995: policy guidance and practice guide.* London: Department of Health.

Dowdney L (2000). Annotation: childhood bereavement following parental death. *J Child Psychol Psychiatry* 41(7):819–30.

Dowdney L, Wilson R, Maughan B, Allerton M, Schofield P, Skuse D (1999). Psychological disturbance and service provision in parently bereaved children: prospective case-control study. *BMJ* 319:354–7.

Elizur E, Kaffman M (1983). Factors influencing the severity of childhood bereavement reactions. *Am J Orthopsychiatry* 53(4):668–76.

Fenichel O (1945). *The psychoanalytic theory of neurosis.* New York: Norton.

Field D, Reid D, Payne S, Relf M (2004). A national postal survey of adult bereavement support in hospice and specialist palliative care services in the UK. *Int J Palliat Nurs* 2004, 10(12):569–76.

Field D, Reid D, Payne S, Relf M (2006). Evaluating adult bereavement support services provided by hospices: a comparative perspective on service provision. *Int J Palliat Nurs* 12(7):320–7.

Field D, Payne S, Relf M, Reid D (2007). An overview of adult bereavement support in the United Kingdom: issues for policy and practice. *Soc Sci Med* 64(2):428–38.

Firth S (2001). Hindu death and mourning rituals: the impact of geographic mobility. In: Hockey J, Katz J, Small N (ed.). *Grief, mourning and death ritual.* Buckingham: Open University Press, pp. 237–46.

Freud S (1917). *Mourning and melancholia.* London: Hogarth Press.

Harrington R, Harrison L (1999). Unproven assumptions about the impact of bereavement on children. *J R Soc Med* 92:230–3.

Harris T, Brown GW, Bifulco A (1986). Loss of parent in childhood and adult psychiatric disorder: the role of lack of adequate parental care. *Psychol Med* 16:641–59.

Help the Hospices (2006). *Young carers guide.* Available at http://www.timetocare.org.uk/pack/ycguide.asp (last accessed 1/4/2007).

Hockey J (2001). Changing death rituals. In: Hockey J, Katz J, Small N (ed.). *Grief, mourning and death ritual.* Buckingham: Open University Press, pp. 185–211.

Hockey J, Katz J, Small N (2001). *Grief, mourning and death ritual.* Buckingham: Open University Press.

Kennedy V (2008). 'I don't know what to say' PhD thesis University of Liverpool.

Kirwin KM, Hamrin V (2005). Decreasing the risk of complicated bereavement and future psychiatric disorders in children. *J Child Adoles Psychiatr Nurs* 18(2):62–78.

Klass D, Silverman PR, Nickman SL (1996). *Continuing bonds.* Philadephia, PA: Taylor and Francis.

Kubler-Ross E (1969). *On death and dying.* New York: Macmillan.

Kwok OM, Haine R, Sandler I, Ayers TS, Wolchik SA, Tein JY (2005). Positive parenting as a mediator of the relations between parental psychological distress and mental health problems of parently bereaved children. *J Clin Child Adoles Psychol* 34:260–271.

Lansdown R, Benjamin C (1985). The development of the concept of death in children aged 5–9. *Child Care Health Dev* 11:13–20.

Lazarus RS, Folkman S (1984). *Stress, appraisal and coping.* New York: Springer-Verlag.

Lindemann E (1944). Symptomatology and management of acute grief. *Am J Psychiatry* 101:141–8.

Lloyd-Williams M, Wilkinson C, Lloyd-Williams F. (1998). Do bereaved children consult the primary care team more frequently? *Eur J Cancer Care* 7:120–4.

Lohnes K, Kalter N (1994). Preventative intervention groups for parentally bereaved children. *Am J Orthopsychiatry* 64:594–603.

Monroe B and Kraus C (1996). Children and loss. *Br J Hosp Med* 56:260–4.

Mulchaey A, Young M (1995). A bereavement support group for children. *Cancer Pract* 3:150–6.

Nabors L, Ohms M, Buchanan N, Kirsh KL, Nash T, Passik SD, Johnson JL, Snapp J Brown G (2004). A pilot study of the impact of a grief camp for children. *Palliat Support Care* 2:403–8.

National Institute for Clinical Excellence (2004). Services for families and carers, including bereavement care. *Improving supportive and palliative care for adults with cancer. The manual.* London: National Institute for Clinical Excellence.

Nickman S, Silverman P, Normand C (1998). Children's construction of a deceased parent: the surviving parent's contribution. *Am J Orthopsychiatry* 68:126–34.

Oxford English Dictionary (2nd edn) (1989). Oxford: Oxford University Press.

Parkes CM (1971). Psychosocial transitions: a field for study. *Soc Sci Med* 5(2):101–14.

Parkes CM (1993). Bereavement as a psychosocial transition: processes of adaptation to change. In: Stroebe MS, Stroebe W, Hansson RO (ed.). *Handbook of bereavement.* Cambridge: Cambridge University Press, pp. 91–101.

Parkes CM (1996). *Bereavement,* (3rd edn). London: Routledge.

Parkes CM, Laungani P, Young B (1997). *Death and bereavement across cultures.* London: Routledge.

Payne S (2001a). Bereavement support: something for everyone? *Int J Palliat Nurs* 7(3):108.

Payne S (2001b). The role of volunteers in hospice bereavement support in New Zealand. *Palliat Med* 15:107–15.

Payne S, Relf M (1994). The assessment of need for bereavement follow-up in palliative and hospice care. *Palliat Med* 8:291–7.

Payne S, Horn S, Relf M (1999). *Loss and bereavement*. Buckingham: Open University Press.

Payne S, Field D, Rolls L, Kerr C, Hawker S (2007). Evaluating case study methods research for use in end of life care practice: reflections on three studies. *J Adv Nurs* 58:236–245.

Pfeffer C, Karus D, Siegel K (2000). Child survivors of parental death from cancer or suicide:depressive behavioural outcomes. *Psycho-Oncology* 9:1–10.

Raveis VH, Siegel K, Karus D (1999). Children's psychological distress following the death of a parent. *J Youth Adolesc* 28(2):165–80.

Reid D, Payne S, Field D, Relf M (2006). Adult bereavement support in five English hospices: research methods and methodological reflections. *Int J Palliat Nurs* 12(9):430–7.

Relf M (1998). Involving volunteers in bereavement counselling. *Eur J Palliat Care* 5(2):61–5.

Rolls E, Payne S (2003). Childhood bereavement services: a survey of UK provision. *Palliat Med* 17:423–32.

Sandler IN, Ayers TS, Wolchik SA, Tein JY, Kwok OM, Haine RA, Twohey-Jacobs J, Suter J, Lin K, Padgett-Jones S, Weyer, JL, Cole E, Griffin WA, Kriege G (2003). The family bereavement program: efficacy evaluation of a theory-based prevention program for parently bereaved children and adolescents. *J Consult Clin Psychol* 71(3):587–600.

Saunders CM (1993). Risk factors in bereavement outcome. In: Stroebe MS, Stroebe W, Hansson RO (ed.). *Handbook of bereavement*. Cambridge: Cambridge University Press, pp. 255–70.

Schmiege SJ, Khoo ST, Sandler IN, Ayers TS, Wolchik SA (2006). Symptoms of internalizing and externalizing problems. *Am J Prev Med* 31(6S1):S152–60.

Schut H, Stroebe MS (2005). Interventions to enhance adaptation to bereavement. *J Palliat Med* 8:140–7.

Siegel K, Mesagno FP, Karus D, Christ G, Banks K, Moynihan R (1992). Psychosocial adjustment of children with a terminally ill parent. *J Am Acad Child Adoles Psychiatry* 31(2):327–33.

Siegel K, Karus D, Raveis V (1995). Adjustment of children facing the death of a parent due to cancer. *J Am Acad Child Adoles Psychiatry* 35(4):442–50.

Seigel K, Raveis VH, Karus D (1996). Pattern of communication with children when a parent has cancer. In: Baider L, Cooper CL, De-Nour AK (ed.). *Cancer and the family*. Chichester: John Wiley and Sons, pp. 109–28.

Siegel K, Raveis VH, Karus D (2000). Correlates of self-esteem among children facing the loss of a parent to cancer. In: Baider L, Cooper CL, De-Nour AK (ed.). *Cancer and the family*, (2nd edn). Chichester: John Wiley and Sons, pp. 223–37.

Segal J, Simkins J (1993). *My mum needs me: helping children with ill or disabled parents*. London: Penguin.

Selye H (1956). *The stress of life*. New York: McGraw-Hill.

Silverman P (2000). *Never too young to know*. New York: Oxford University Press.

Small N (2001). Theories of grief: a critical review. In: Hockey J, Katz J, Small N (ed.). *Grief, mourning and death ritual.* Buckingham: Open University Press, pp. 19–48.

Stokes J, Wyer S, Crossley D (1997). The challenge of evaluating a child bereavement programme. *Palliat Med* 11:179–90.

Stokes J, Pennington J, Monroe B, Papadatou D, Relf M (1999). Developing services for bereved children: a discussion of the theoretical and practical issues involved. *Mortality* 4:291–307.

Sullivan HL (1956). The dynamics of emotion. In Sullivan HL (ed.). *Clinical studies in psychiatry.* New York: Norton.

Stroebe M, Schut H (1999). The dual process model of coping with bereavement: rationale and description. *Death Stud* 23:197–224.

Stroebe W, Schut H, Stroebe M (2005). Grief work, disclosure and counselling: Do they help the bereaved? *Clin Psychol Rev* 25:395–414.

Thomas N, Stainton T, Jackson S, Cheung WY, Doubtfire S Webb A (2003). 'Your friends don't understand': invisibility and unmet need in the lives of 'young carers'. *Child Fam Soc Work* 8:35–46.

Thompson F, Payne S (2000). Bereaved children's questions to a doctor. *Mortality* 5:74–96.

Thompson MP, Kaslow NJ, Kingree JB, King M, Bryant L, Rey M (1998). Psychological symptomatology following parental death in a predominantly minority sample of children and adolescents. *J Clin Child Psychol* 27:434–41.

Walter T (1996). A new model of grief: bereavement and biography. *Mortality* 1:1–29.

Walter T (1999). *On bereavement.* Buckingham: Open University Press.

Watson M, St James-Roberts I, Ashley S, Tilney C, Brougham B, Edwards L, Baldus C, Romer G (2006). Factors associated with emotional and behavioural problems among school age children of breast cancer patients. *Br J Cancer* 94:43–50.

Worden JW (1982). *Grief counselling and grief therapy: a handbook for the mental health practitioner.* New York: Springer.

Worden JW (1991). *Grief counselling and grief therapy,* (2nd ed). New York: Springer Publishing.

Worden JW (1996). *Children and grief: when a parent dies.* New York: Guilford Press.

Wortman CB, Silver RC (1989). The myths of coping with loss. *J Consult Clin Psychol* 57(3):349–57.

Zambelli G, Lcark E, Barile L, de Jong A (1988). An interdisciplinary appraoch to clinical intervention for childhood bereavement. *Death Stud* 12:41–50.

Chapter 12

Staff support

Malcolm Payne

Introduction

Why staff support is a psychosocial issue in palliative care

Staff support is an issue in psychosocial palliative care for three reasons: (1) employers have a legal and moral responsibility to ensure the well-being of the people they employ, so therefore palliative care services have a concern for staff well-being; (2) staff well-being at work has an impact on quality of service, including psychological and social interventions, for patients and service users; and (3) health and social care services, such as palliative care, are a resource to the population served. They contribute to the community, through both service and staff, and through expertise, commitment, energy, and a fund of knowledge and skill. Therefore, staff support also contributes to the social capital generated by the staff of a palliative care service for the community it serves. It is a valid psychosocial contribution to any aspect of health and social care.

Death and bereavement, the main focus of palliative care, are major social transitions that bring social and psychological strains and opportunities, because a death changes all the relationships within a family and social network. Social and psychological strains in families and networks may be transferred to the workplace and the staff within it. One reason why staff support is an important issue for palliative care is the 'accumulated loss phenomenon' (Adams *et al.* 1991). That is, palliative care staff may experience one loss through death after another over an extended period of time. However, such experienced commentators as Parkes (1986) and Worden (2003, p. 178) suggest that in a well-run supportive agency, experience will strengthen rather than weaken people's capacity to deal with loss.

The existence of stress and its impact on people's health and well-being is widely accepted, but it is a varying human response to a social situation. Most people are self-caring most of the time, dealing with their stress through everyday social interaction and family and community support. Many health and social care staff deal with equally stressful issues, such as child abuse or severe mental ill-health, and the satisfactions and patient and family appreciation of facilitating a good death balance the stress that may arise from a constant involvement with death and dying. Dying is a natural human process that we must all incorporate into our social experience, and it should not be represented too negatively as a stressor. Palliative care, after all, aims to ensure a satisfactory social experience of death, and if it is successful this should apply to staff just as much of patients, their families and social networks. Therefore, an agency needs to be supportive and its staff need to be prepared to deal with their stress, but our concern to ensure adequate staff support should be proportionate, recognizing that self-care will usually be sufficient to deal with difficulties.

In reviewing some recent work on staff support in this chapter, I concentrate on empirical studies of staff dealing with what they experience as stressful and support for them. Public health research showing that workplace stress is an important contributor to early mortality among lower socio-economic groups in the population and legal and management information are also important. Most of the research in palliative care consists of small-scale surveys relying strongly on self-report by staff, mainly female nurses, the largest staff group. Therefore much of the research is about the perceptions of a particular staff group, which may be affected by gendered behaviour and social relationships.

What is staff support?

Human beings are *social* animals. Therefore, relationships are a crucial part of being human. Most people value relationships that are supportive. Staff support is, of course, about relationships in the workplace, but the same is true, and workplace relationships usually include elements of support. However, where staff experience stresses in their workplace, particularly if the consequent distress leads to psychological and physical ill-health, the natural support of social relationships may need to be enhanced. Discussing staff support in palliative care means looking at both specialist and generalist services Non-specialist staff, who deal with death and dying less frequently than their specialist colleagues, will have different but equally important support needs. Medical, nursing, social work, and allied health professionals, chaplains may all have different support needs; so also may administrative, domestic and manual staff and volunteers. In some palliative care settings, volunteers may not be regarded as staff at all, but the employer will still have responsibility for their well-being.

Finally, it is not obvious what different people might find supportive. The concept implies helpful ways of sustaining or restoring an individual's sense of wholeness and their capacity to manage life events. Human beings will vary in what they find supportive, and so their psychological perceptions and reactions are important.

Workplace stress

Stress is a psychological reaction to social situations, which may lead to physical consequences, and if sustained possibly ill-health. It may present itself in a range of physical symptoms. These may include tiredness, headaches, high blood pressure, sleep problems, stomach upsets, anxiety, hyperventilation, and memory loss. There are also behavioural consequences, which may include: excessive alcohol or drug use, irritability, loss of concentration, heavy smoking, aggression, moodiness, or overeating (Buchanan and Huczynski 2004, p. 159). In extreme cases, stress may lead to clinically identifiable anxiety and depression.

Demands and difficulties are universal in life and in work. How do such universal difficulties create stress? Connections between social psychological and physical and ill-health are not fully understood. In palliative care, Vachon's (1987) groundbreaking study of hospice workers proposed that stress arises when stressors in the work environment are such that staff cannot use coping mechanisms that balance their personal needs and values against the pressures of the work. This emphasizes the importance of the individual's self-management or self-caring balancing of stress with challenge. The individual's reaction to events that are potential stressors in their work and home environment is, therefore, a crucial starting point. Some stressors may be insignificant to particular individuals; others may be powerful. Sometimes, people react to stressors as a challenge and are stimulated to work hard to overcome their effects. Other stressors, or the same stressors at a different time, may lead to a different reaction.

Workplace issues may not be the most important source of stress in people's lives. The Schedule of Recent Experiences (Holmes and Rahe 1967) developed in the 1960s, identified important life events that raised anxiety and stress, such as the death of a friend or moving house. This has been recently re-scaled as a Life Events Inventory based on a UK population and examining age and gender differences (Spurgeon *et al.* 2001). However, workplace events were not rated as high in either scale as events such as the death of a spouse, loss of a job, a jail sentence, debt, or homelessness. Therefore, although stress presents itself in a workplace, it may not be generated by the workplace, or workplace stresses may interact with stresses from elsewhere in an employee's life.

When people refer to stress they may several aspects of a social situation. Kristenson (2006) disentangles the elements as follows:

- a stressor or a stimulus that staff may be exposed to
- the self-perception or self-report of the person's experience of the situation
- the stress response, a psycho-physiological activation or wakening to the stressor
- the self-perception or self-report of the experience of the somatic response to the psychophysiological response.

Cognitive activation theory suggests that people whose minds and bodies are activated, as the result of experiencing a stressor or stimulus, experience a psychoneuroimmunological response. The body maintains itself in a functioning balance (allostasis). However, if these physical processes are overtaxed for a long period, the body loses this balance. The physical processes are described by Ursin and Eriksen (2004). A useful summary of recent studies related to public health analysis of socio-economic status, psychobiology, and coping mechanisms is contained in Kristenson (2006). Broadly, the position is that lower status individuals have a double burden of greater exposure to stressors and fewer socio-economic resources for coping. Therefore, in addition to intervention by providing personal support, Kristenson (2006) argues for public health interventions to increase coping abilities in at-risk populations. Staff support for people at risk of stress in their workplace is one of those public health interventions.

Bringing together the present discussion, to understand how stress develops we need to keep three contributory factors in mind:

- the individual's personality and coping mechanisms
- life and work conditions and aspects of them that may be experienced as stressful
- organizational factors in the workplace that may be stressful or helpful (Buchanan and Huczynski 2004).

These are moderated by the individual's physical and mental health, their social environment outside the workplace, their cognitive appraisal of stressors, their hardiness or resilience in the face of adversity, and whether the stress is episodic or continues over a long period (Buchanan and Huczynski 2004, p. 160). Hardiness is a capacity for positive performance in complex tasks and emotional stability, where people see problems as challenges, expect to be able to perform successfully and expect to have energy and excitement rather than tension and difficulty in their lives (Kristenson 2006, p. 133).

There are two approaches to understanding job stress: demand–control and effort–reward imbalances. Demand–control imbalances are like Vachon's (1987) analysis of palliative care stress, mentioned above. They refer to jobs that are stressful because they make heavy psychological and other demands of an employee but do not promote self-efficacy, the feeling that the employee has control over the conditions that would enable them to meet the demands (Siegrist and Theorell 2006). This analysis suggests that staff support can seek both to reduce demands and also to improve self-efficacy. Studies of socio-economic factors in mortality suggest that over the life course, poor control over job activity leads to increased mortality (Davey Smith and Harding 1997). Generally, people in lower socio-economic groups for various reasons, have less control over their work and work conditions, and so are more likely to experience stress and consequent stress-related ill-health than people in higher socio-economic groups. This has consequences for palliative care services, as they employ many people in lower socio-economic positions who have contact with the stressful features of palliative care services. While professional staff, such as doctors and nurses, are often the most vocal about the need for support, and the most researched, they usually have more control over stressful aspects of their work and the environment than a domestic worker or healthcare assistant.

Effort–reward imbalances arise where the employee feels a strong commitment to the work, but does not receive psychological or material rewards consistent with the degree of commitment that they give. This means that, although employment contracts balance requirements to perform duties with financial and other social rewards, some jobs offer unsatisfactory social reciprocity for the effort put in. The position is affected by three factors. Dependency occurs where the employee is particularly dependent on the work for some reason, for example, where a person has limited choice because their mobility is restricted by the need to remain in the same geographical area as their spouse. The employer is able to exploit this dependency. Strategic choice means that people accept high cost/low gain employment for a period in order to improve their life chances. An example is younger professionals such as doctors working long hours as the basis of a future career. Overcommitment also occurs. Some people overcommit themselves out of ambition, or because of the need for esteem or reward. However, the extent of their commitment may not be recognized by the employer (Siegrist and Theorell 2006), perhaps legitimately, because it is not a requirement of the job, but a self-imposed requirement.

Fillion *et al.* (2007) studied the issues raised by these models of stress in 209 palliative care nurses. They found that the best predictors of job satisfaction were job demand, effort, reward, and a people-oriented culture, whereas best predictors of emotional distress were reward, professional and emotional demands, and self-efficacy. This suggests that the demanding aspects of palliative care are rewarding, where the work culture is supportive, but that stress will arise where demands are unrewarding and the job is experienced as out of the practitioner's control.

Burnout and compassion fatigue

Burnout and compassion fatigue are two important ideas that have developed from looking at how stress may affect people. They refer to long-term effects, and should be viewed with caution. Their striking terminology may emphasize negative perceptions and hyper-awareness of stress, rather than a measured consideration of evidence of problems arising from everyday events.

Burnout derives from the work of Maslach (1982). The Maslach Burnout Inventory (MBI), introduced in the 1980s (Maslach and Jackson 1981) has been validated in various versions among widely varying Western populations (for example, Schutte *et al.* 2000) and is often used in palliative care studies as a rating scale, although it refers to long-term exposure to the effects of stress, rather than occasional or potentially stressful events. MBI builds upon the concept of burnout: '... a syndrome of emotional exhaustion, depersonalisation and reduced personal accomplishment that can occur among individuals who do "people work" of some kind' (Maslach and Jackson 1981). It assesses employees' perceptions of their exhaustion, indifference, and cynicism towards work and expectations that they will not continue to be effective. The MBI has recently been used with HIV/AIDS specialist community nurses, in one of the few community-based studies, showing that burnout among this group (Hayter 2000) is high. A Japanese study of 782 nurses working in 72 different palliative care units (Wada and Sasaki 2006) found that nurses with higher burnout scores had more unstable interpersonal relationships, were more concerned with outward appearances and more susceptible to emotion. This shows how different personality types may be more susceptible to both long- and short-term effects of stress. It also indicates the importance of interpersonal relationships for mediating stress and burnout.

Compassion stress is a feeling of helplessness, confusion, and isolation said to result from knowing about and closeness to repeated difficult illness experiences and deaths, as distinct from burnout, where staff personally experience them. Compassion fatigue is 'a state of exhaustion and dysfunction, biologically, physiologically, and emotionally, as a result of prolonged exposure to compassion stress' (Figley 1995, p. 1).

Research on compassion fatigue has appeared referring to palliative care, although much of this work also includes broader ideas of stress. Garfield (1995), referring to compassion fatigue among AIDS/HIV caregivers comments that, in contrast to caregivers heading for burnout who unconsciously begin to wall off increasingly strong feelings associated with their work, people with compassion fatigue are able to monitor their decrease in empathy and feeling and remain emotionally accessible. However, their difficulty in processing their emotions increases, anxiety or distress also rises, distressing images and painful memories of work situations intrude on their days and nights outside the care-giving arena. An American self-report study of compassion fatigue among 217 nurses from 22 hospices revealed 78% of the sample at moderate to high risk of compassion fatigue, the key stressors being trauma, anxiety, life demands, and excessive empathy with patients. More research is needed in this area in palliative care to assess whether the phenomenon actually exists, how it might be differentiated from other conceptualization of workers' stress and if it may be alleviated.

Sources and mediators of stress

Studies of stress in palliative care and related areas of work identify a wide range of sources of stress. However, they cluster around two crucial areas: distress arising from constant association with dying and bereaved people and workplace organization and relationship issues. Research about sources and mediators of stress may be generic, deriving from work experience of all employees, or more specialized, deriving from health and social care or specifically palliative care sources. Moreover, there may be differences between different sorts of palliative care settings and different sorts of staff, in particular different professional groups and these are researched in different ways. Much of the research about sources of stress derives from self-report surveys, and should therefore be approached with caution as they reflect personal attitudes and experiences in particular social situations rather than behaviour or events assessed externally according to identified criteria.

Generalist studies

A systematic literature review of workplace stress in nursing indicates the type of stress experienced by healthcare professionals, with which palliative care experience may be compared. Covering the period 1985 to 2003, McVicar (2003) concluded that studies found that workload, leadership style, professional conflict, and the emotional cost of caring were the main sources of distress. Lack of reward and shift working had more recently become important. Organizational interventions to respond to these difficulties were ineffective in the short to medium term and better individual support was an important intervention. However, efforts at providing personal support were hampered because there was little understanding of how workplace factors affected nurses in different specialist areas, assessment tools appeared to have little predictive power and there was little understanding of how personal and workplace factors interacted.

Some other stress self-report studies describe healthcare services that provide generalist end of life care, Stress arises for staff where a general healthcare service does not support palliative care interventions. For example, Llamas *et al.* (2001) surveyed, with a high response rate, the staff stress caused by the absence of a palliative care service in a major Australian teaching hospital. While 79% of staff expressed a need for more support, mainly education, medical staff were significantly less likely to report this need. Concerns here were about the adequacy of services, such as grief and bereavement support and spiritual care and the poor environment for caring for dying people. Kirchhoff *et al.*'s (2000) US focus group study of critical care nurses identified similar issues. Disagreement among family members, uncertainty about prognosis and communication problems among staff as the main difficulties in end of life care. A survey of self-reported stress among 350 Australian nurses (Bryant *et al.* 2000) found that workload was the main source of stress but that nurses were likely to bring their personal stress with them into the workplace. Regular exercise was correlated with reduced workplace stress. An Australian survey of stress among a range of allied healthcare professionals, social workers, and psychologists (Harris *et al.* 2006) found that levels of psychological distress were similar across all groups, and workplace stressors were also similar, so that generic support interventions were likely to be appropriate. Not all staff involved in end of life care work in specialist palliative care settings. A qualitative interview study of residential care and nursing homes for the Department of Health (Katz *et al.* 2001) found that mainly young female staff had little experience of death. They were thought to need emotional and practical support in dealing with the needs of dying people. However, organizational and budgetary pressures meant that few homes had the flexibility to provide for intensive caring or time off for staff under stress because of feelings of grief. Most support was *ad hoc* and consisted of sympathetic listening. Similar outcomes emerged from a US study (Ersek and Wilson 2003).

Specialist studies

A number of qualitative studies explore the situation of relatively small groups of staff in palliative care settings, which may be compared with the general position, discussed above, and provide a basis for considering staff support actions. In these studies, the extent of distress arising from the accumulated loss phenomenon is ambiguous. It is sometimes reported, particularly in relation to work with children, but appears often to be compensated by the satisfactions of providing a good service and, particularly for nurses, by the satisfactions of a close relationship with patients. This may be important because James's (1993) research on emotional labour in cancer care has shown that there is a division of labour in emotional work, with high-status staff, and men, carrying out work that often requires less emotional intensity and able to separate their roles from emotional work. Lower status staff and women often carry a higher burden of emotionally intense work. Therefore, a mainly female nursing workforce might be expected both to undertake a higher burden of the emotionally intense and also to gain satisfaction from it. Stress is sometimes reported around family conflicts, as in the generalist studies. However, a greater source of stress is various workplace difficulties, including conflicts with other staff, in particular nurse–physician conflicts and communication difficulties. High workloads leading to poor service can also be stressful, possibly because this reduces the rewards gained from relationships and satisfaction about achievement. Uncertainty about diagnosis, prognosis, and ability to control symptoms is also experienced consistently as stressful. Staff in specialist palliative care services, as in the generalist studies, find that supportive team environments are important mediators of stress, especially for nurses; this was true in Vachon's (1987) study.

A number of surveys deal with paediatric palliative care; perhaps this is because the stress of seeing children die before their time has been supposed to be more distressing than the death of adults, many of whom are from older population groups, whose death is more likely to be expected and accepted more readily. A literature review on staff stress in children's hospices (Barnes 2001) concluded that the main sources of stress lay in conflict within the staff group, communication problems, and role conflict rather than the work itself. A survey of staff in Irish paediatric palliative care (O'Leary *et al.* 2006) identified stress as arising from the fact that the death of a child is an unnatural event and from the distress of parents and siblings. There was anticipatory apprehension at referral, but this anxiety declined as the people involved became personally known to the staff. McCluggage's (2006) UK survey of 10 doctors and 18 nurses from children's hospices found more anxiety about identifying symptoms correctly than responding once they were identified. Papadatou and Bellili (2002) compared grief reactions of Greek doctors and nurses at the death of a child. They found that doctors were emotionally distressed to be present, while nurses derived satisfaction from the relationship with the child and parents, and saw presence at the death and caring tasks associated with it as integral to that relationship. The doctors saw their grief as a private process while nurses shared experiences with colleagues and sought group support.

Studies of palliative care for adults discloses many of the same features. Payne's (2001) study of 89 nurses for nine hospices found low levels of burnout mainly caused by work stressors rather than their private lives.

The most important stressors were dealing with death and dying, staff conflict, and higher responsibility and grade contributed most to stress. Kulbe's (2001) self-report study of 97 US nurses in New Jersey provided some comparative data by using a questionnaire similar to that used by Duffy and Jackson (1996) almost a decade earlier. The stresses rated most difficult were the same in both studies: managing physical complications and pain and symptom control. The next three items rated less difficult were emotional support to the patient, the family, and co-ordinating community resources. Paperwork is also perceived as stressful, but this refers to US insurance documentation. A study of 38 workers in a New York hospice (Di Tullio and MacDonald 1999) identified the view of hospice workers on the differences between hospice work and other similar work, rewards, and stresses. The themes of relationship and 'being there' or present alongside patients in their illness rather than simply organizing services for patients reflected an interpersonal rather than medicalized problem-solving role for hospice workers. Rewards derived from team support, appreciation by patients and families, and opportunities for personal growth, autonomy, and achievement. Stresses derived from 'cramping' of time, limitations on emotional involvement and service policy, volume, diversity and complexity of demands and difficulties in the work and organization. For these workers, what was stressful was the inability to achieve their satisfactions because of difficulties within the organization. Australian community study of 12 nurses, comparing rural and urban situations identified role conflict, family dynamics, time, and workload as the main issues. Newton and Waters's (2001) UK study of 21 community palliative care nurses identified workload and relationships with healthcare professionals, particularly a small number of general practitioners as the main stressors. Sadness about death, while important, was only found in particular circumstances.

Most studies in palliative care are of nurses, the largest staff group, and little information is available about other groups. However, Lloyd-Williams et al.'s (2004) survey of chaplains in UK hospices had a good response rate and found that 23% scored at or above the threshold on the GHQ-12 (General Health Questionnaire) for identifiable psychological morbidity. Clear role definitions were associated with less stress, while being involved in bereavement work led to levels of stress that were greater. Hammons's (2000) survey of 192 social workers found that the level of burnout was low, and workplace relationships provided most support; family and general social support was less important. Good coping skills and spiritual or religious commitment were important mitigators of stress. Tedium was associated with a higher level of burnout.

Spirituality appears to be an important mediator of stress. A sense of spirituality can be helpful to caregivers as they struggle to find meaning in the work they are doing (Vachon 2000; Holland and Neimeyer 2005). Nurses attracted to hospice work have been found to be more religious than others (Vachon 1995). Compared with oncology nurses, hospice nurses reported a greater sense of personal spirituality, more frequent spiritual care-giving, and more positive perspectives regarding spiritual care-giving (Taylor *et al.* 1999). A US study found that nurses were more religious than other groups. Those who described being extremely religious had significantly lower scores on diminished empathy or depersonalization and lower emotional exhaustion on the MBI (Kash *et al.* 2000).

Dealing with stress

Kristenson (2006), identifies research supporting the importance of three kinds of resources useful in dealing with stress:

- Social resources available to the person, through the organization or in their lives. These include interpersonal networks with both superiors and peers at work, to be beneficial in promoting good health. Good personal support and wide interpersonal networks in private life are also beneficial, and are less prevalent in people with low socio-economic status (Mickelson and Kubzansky 2003), provided they are intimate, nurturing, and support-ive, rather than conflicted (Berkman and Melchior 2006).

- Psychological resources, their inherent or learned coping ability. These include self-esteem or negative attitudes towards oneself, and 'mastery' the belief that our life chances are under our control. This is connected with self-efficacy, the belief that in general a person has the capacity to manage their life chances. People with a 'sense of coherence' (Antonovsky 1979) have the capacity to define life events as less stressful, manage life events, and maintain their motivation and desire to cope. These ideas correspond closely to the palliative care use of the term 'spirituality', and expand how we understand the finding that spirituality protects against stress.

- Specific coping responses to the particular situation, or coping strategies. These may be concerned either with changing the situation by, for exam-ple, problem-solving or alternatively, neutralizing or managing the experi-ence of stress when it occurs.

Recent studies show significant efforts in palliative care to get to grips with staff support where stress is experienced. For example, Baverstock and Finlay's

(2006) survey of staff support mechanisms in UK children's hospices, which achieved a good response rate, identified widespread use of team meetings, team debriefing after significant events, availability of a bereavement counsellor for staff and in-house training as staff support mechanisms. Blomberg and Sahlberg-Blom's (2007) Swedish focus group study of the way 77 oncology nurses handled difficult situations identified the importance of balancing closeness and distance in relationships with patients and informal carers. Strategies included reflection on personal and professional identity, the personal meaning attributed to events and relationships, setting limits to involvement and touching, setting priorities, and gaining the support of the team and workplace organization.

How can we understand such a range of interventions? Three broad approaches to dealing with staff stress in organizations are:

- Organization adjustments, such as management, organizational, or personnel changes, which seek to prevent, reduce, or remove the effect of stressors in organizations.
- Development actions, such as training in personal skills and coping mechanisms.
- Individual emotion-focused actions, which aim to improve individuals' resilience and coping mechanisms (Williams and Cooper 2002; Buchanan and Huczynski 2004).

Organizational approaches

Williams and Cooper (2002) suggest that the main role of organization-focused strategies is to 'shift the mean', that is to reduce the average level of feelings of stress in an organization. This would not necessarily help someone directly who was experiencing feelings of stress.

Employers have a legal duty of care for their employees, including avoiding work or action that may cause stress-related injury and carrying out risk assessments to prevent or reduce hazards, including psychological hazards (Spiers 2003). Concern was raised by the case of a senior social worker who had two 'nervous breakdowns' and received compensation for stress due to pressure of work when the employer, knowing of his illness, did nothing to help him (Walker v Northumberland County Council 1 All ER 737 at 749). This led employers to fear that they may be liable for a breach of their duty of care where workplace stress affects employees psychologically as well as physically. However, Earnshaw and Morrison (1999) show that for the employer to be liable the injury has to be reasonably foreseeable, and workplace circumstances have to be shown to be the cause of it. Moreover, there are practical difficulties in bringing a case: it may be difficult to finance a claim, the plain-tiff may not be aware of the possibility of bringing a case within the required time limits and the plaintiff's psychological well-being may not be robust enough to pursue a claim. However, according to Earnshaw and Morrison (1999) there are signs that where stress is due to bullying and harassment it is easier to show the employer's liability, and demonstrate if the employer has not taken simple measures to remedy the problem behaviour.

As a result of these concerns, the UK Health and Safety Executive publish guidance (ISMA 2005) on reducing stress at work and advice on management standards required, taking a risk-assessment approach. The main points are: identifying the demands of the job, increasing staff's control over or say in their work, developing support among managers and colleagues, strengthen-ing relationships at work, being clear about workers' roles in the organization and being careful about how change is managed. A common approach in large employers is to run a stress survey to identify particular locations of stress and groups of personnel affected (Williams and Cooper 2002). However, this may not discriminate between groups well enough to identify stress within small staff groups associated with palliative care where they are in larger non-specialist organization, and may be too resource-intensive for small voluntary organizations, such as many hospices to contemplate.

As support is integral to any human and workplace relationship, employers as part of their ordinary management arrangements will provide a range of supports appropriate to particular staff and their professional roles and devel-opment needs. This might include well-defined job descriptions, appraisal, professional updating and staff development opportunities, effective policies and procedures and clear occupational health arrangements for dealing with problems in staff's private lives. In addition, a range of ordinary organiza-tional structures may prove helpful. For example, Hopkinson's (2002) phenomenological study of the experiences of 28 qualified nurses caring for dying people in hospital settings found that handover meetings as shifts changed on wards were helpful in reducing stress by providing a forum in which staff could discuss opinions and express feelings. They could also obtain information and advice to guide their nursing decisions; this reduced anxiety and uncertainty. Raising awareness of the role of such structures in stress management should lead to managers ensuring that they can be used for this purpose.

Multiprofessional teamwork

An organizational approach that links with development actions is the promotion and development of multiprofessional teamwork. Studies of the sources of stress discussed above suggest that conflict within teams of workers, physician–nurse conflict, and communication problems are common sources of stress, and that many staff, particularly nurses, valued team support in managing emotionally difficult tasks, reducing uncertainty about diagnosis, prognosis, and treatment strategies and in 'debriefing' after a particularly stressful event. Multiprofessional teams are commonly advocated as a way of dealing with the complexity of palliative care work, although there is no evidence of any particular model of teamwork that is most effective in delivering good services (Gysels and Higginson 2004). Teamwork literature (Payne 2000, 2001, 2006) focuses on clarifying work objectives and roles, developing a shared sense of purpose and learning, creativity, and good leadership. A large study of 500 UK mainly community-based healthcare (but not palliative care) teams, found four factors relevant to successful outcomes:

- clear team objectives
- participation, through frequent meetings
- commitment to quality, through always seeking improved care rather than accepting current practices
- support for innovation, through always seeking improved ways of doing things.

In the context of staff support, it is important to note that achieving this pattern of work enhanced the mental health of the team members.

Development actions

The main development actions reported are:

- training and information provision
- group work, associated with a range of activities
- professional supervision.

Training and information provision may be both general, as people appreciate opportunities to develop skills in areas of difficulty, and related to stress. Most studies that referred to training were concerned with generalist staff who needed training and development opportunities in coping with dying people. An example is Yam et al.'s (2001) study of nurses in a Hong Kong neonatal intensive care unit, who recommend culture-specific death education. However, skills in problem-solving with difficulties, such as team and counselling training are also recommended (Payne 2001) and semi-therapeutic techniques, such as stress inoculation training are also recommended (Payne 2001).

Professional supervision is a relationship in which professionals come together to develop learning from shared reflection and discussion on a particular professional experience, usually critical incidents or case discussions. Jones's (2003a) qualitative study of five hospice nurses in a group supervision format showed that they felt it enabled them to calm, regulate, and plan interactions with themselves and others, both patients and colleagues. In a broader discussion, Jones (2003b) argues that supervision helps in the management of self, addressing strong feelings and avoiding repetition of unhelpful behaviours. More broadly, different forms of supervision by managers, external consultants and in peer groups are accepted practice as a way of dealing with emotional responses to practice experiences that may raise difficulties for staff in doing their work (Hawkins and Shohet 2006).

In a useful and critical review of literature on supervision and support strategies responding to burnout in community-based AIDS/HIV nurse specialists, Hayter (2000) suggests that:

♦ Supervision is adapted to emphasize restorative tasks, which enable professionals to deal with feelings that arise from working with people in distress and formative tasks, an educative approach teaching new methods and insights.

♦ Teaching coping skills in relation to stress and providing mechanisms to express concerns and anxieties related to practice have been found effective.

♦ Informal and less structured support from colleagues has been found effective.

Short-term and long-term staff support groups have been valued where they have been tried, although evidence of effectiveness is weak. Trust-building, time focused on giving individual support and building team mechanisms of support have been suggested as a useful programme (Hunsberger 1989). Small group support using educational materials has been shown to be more effective in reducing self-reported stress and doctor attendances than educational information alone (Rahe et al. 2002). In an evidence-based literature review of workplace stress management programmes in the nursing profession (Mimura and Griffiths 2003), one approach using cognitive techniques was found effective, three approaches using exercise, music, and relaxation were potentially effective and one approach using social support was possibly effective. Such supportive treatments of the stress response were more effective in reducing stress than environmental changes, such as changing workplace practices. Fillion et al. (2006) described a psycho-educational groups for nurses designed to focus on giving meaning to events experienced in professional practice, thus enhancing spirituality as a supportive element of their work.

Personal, emotion-based approaches to support

Support may be gained in two broad ways: through having opportunities for social participation, thus reducing a sense of isolation, and through interpersonal support directed particularly at a person who is stressed. The studies of sources of stress discussed above often refer to debriefing opportunities to discuss particularly stressful events, and sometimes indicate effective multiprofessional teams as a location for debriefing. West (2004) outlines four kinds of support that psychological research has demonstrated to be helpful to people in organizational settings:

- Emotional support, by being a receptive, open, non-critical but thoughtful listener, and being careful to look out for occasions when people need to be listened to
- Informational support, by being prepared to offer information and consultation to deal with a problem
- Instrumental support, by routinely being prepared to do things that benefit the other person rather than yourself
- Appraisal support, by giving feedback on how things have gone and helping to plan how to learn and improve functioning.

Conclusions

I have argued in this chapter that for people to experience human relationships as positive, support has to be a part of them, and therefore, staff support is integral to employment relationships. Employers have a legal and moral duty to ensure the well-being of their staff, and to organize work in such a way that it does not adversely affect staff well-being. In law and in good management practice, therefore, staff support is a natural part of the relationships in any employment and of any workplace. The employer's responsibilities for staff also contribute to the quality of the service, its contribution to the community and the professional development and security of staff. Where there are stressful demands in the employment that cause ill-health, including psychological ill-health, the employer and the employee need to manage the demands of work and the psychological reactions to enhance self-efficacy in responding to stresses.

Stress arises as a psychoneuroimmunological reaction in which the demands of a social situation are out of balance with the capacities of an individual to manage their contribution to work ad other aspects of their lives. Sustained experience of stress leads to physical and behavioural consequences and potential ill-health. People experience a range of factors as stressful in their home, family and work lives. The individual's personality and coping mechanisms, their life and work and organizational factors in the workplace interact with people's experience of stress. Throughout the life course, cumulative stress, including workplace stress, is an important contributor to socio-economic inequality in early mortality: generally the lower the socio-economic position of an employee, the greater the risk of an early death.

Therefore, interventions to prevent and respond to stress in work are important contributions to staff well-being and the quality of the service. Two ways of understanding the effect of stress in the workplace, demand–control and effort–reward imbalances, are relevant. Demand–control imbalances arise when demands prevent employees from remaining in control of their work and lives. Effort–reward imbalances occur when the effort required for the work are not balanced by its social and financial rewards. Burnout and compassion fatigue may result from long-term stress.

The demands of, and effort required in palliative care work may be experienced as stressful in two ways: because of accumulated losses in staff lives, through the experience of repeated death and bereavement and because of difficulties in the workplace. Evidence from palliative care settings suggests that staff experience stress for both reasons. However, stress because of loss is often balanced by the satisfactions of the work, especially where there is a supportive work environment. Staff may deal with grief in different ways, with higher status staff and men managing grief in different ways. Lower status and female nursing staff may carry a greater proportion of emotionally demanding work, be more satisfied by it and value a sharing, mutually supportive emotional environment at work to enable them to do so. Nursing staff often found work with patients less stressful and more satisfying than work with families, particularly where there were family or social network conflicts; whether this factor affects other staff such as social workers whose work often focuses on families is unclear. This may raise questions about the capacity of different groups of staff to engage with and implement the holistic conceptualization of palliative care work. Another area of difficulty for nursing staff is uncertainty about diagnosis, prognosis, and treatment.

Resources to respond to stress may be divided into general social resources, both personal and organizational, personal psychological resources and specific coping strategies to deal with particular situations. Organizational responses mostly affect the general level of stress in an organization. These include effective management and organizational structures and practices and use of existing devices such as handover meetings and multiprofessional team meetings to include emotional as well as practical matters. Multiprofessional teamwork practice improves staff mental health if it encourages clarification of objectives and participation together with active commitment to and support for consistent quality improvement and innovation in practice. Personal supports include training and information provision about stress and in skills in responding to difficult situations, group work and activities such as relaxation, exercise, and use of music and spiritual resources, such as meditation and effective professional supervision.

Several areas of discussion above suggest important future directions for work on staff support:

- Concern about negative aspects of stress in palliative care needs to be proportionate to the evidence of difficulties, recognizing that support is integral to all human relationships and that people are to a large extent self-caring. It may be appropriate to focus on successful self-management and self-care in research, management and professional work, rather than the negative consequences of stress. Public health research and employers' legal and moral responsibilities suggests that risk assessment for stress in different groups of staff is important. Employers' liability may arise more in relation to staff conflict, bullying, and harassment than over stress from working constantly with death and bereavement.

- Another useful strategy may be to identify how commonplace structures, such as handover meetings and other team events, help to respond to stressful situations and encourage managers to incorporate concern for handling stress explicitly in such events. This, in effect, gives staff permission to use suitable occasions for stress reduction.

- It is important to be clear in research, in management, and in professional work what we mean when we talk about stress: is it an event that people perceive as potentially stressful, or is it experience of stressful feelings or ill-health or adverse reactions? Some studies have shown the possibility of looking at rates of consultation with doctors or other helpers or sickness rates as proxies for ill-effects, rather than using self-reported concerns, which may have been successfully managed.

- Research and management approaches is needed to cover all staff groups as so far most research has been concerned with the largest staff group, nurses. There are indications that other staff groups may have similar experiences. However, there are also differences in the way that some groups deal with grief, stress, self-care, and care within organizational structures. Employers and professionals should develop appropriate differentiated responses.

- In particular, much of the research is on inpatient nurses, and suggests the importance of group- or team-based mutual support as a response to experiences of stress. However, inpatient staff are a self-selecting population, who may prefer such group interventions, while community staff prefer other forms of support within their social network. More research is needed to differentiate stress experiences and support needs and appropriate responses among specialist and non-specialist palliative care staff, volunteers and in different settings for palliative care work.

♦ Research and management approaches also need to move beyond self-report and avoid disproportionately negative social representations of stress, which also has benefits in challenging and motivating staff to deal with social difficulties. It is also important to examine precisely what is giving difficulty, for example, O'Leary *et al*'s (2006) finding that it is the apprehension of difficulty rather than the difficulty itself that was sometimes the problem.

♦ Research on workplace stress over the life course suggests that people in lower socio-economic groups are at higher risk of long-term health problems as a result of workplace stress. We should therefore be particularly concerned with lower status staff especially where they have less autonomy, less meaningful and interesting work and less respect from the people that they work with. Little research has been carried out to identify the stresses of palliative care work for this staff group. A useful general intervention that employers might make is to advise and train professional staff to maintain the participation of and respect by professional colleagues for domestic, administrative, and lower grades of staff and volunteers.

Acknowledgements

The author acknowledges with appreciation the help received in preparing this chapter, as follows: a systematic search of healthcare databases provided for the NHS through Dialog Datastar, carried out by Denise Brady, Librarian, St Christopher's Hospice, and material from the related chapter in the first edition of the book by Mary L. S. Vachon and Ruth Benor.

References

Adams J, Hershatter MJ, Moritz A (1991). Accumulated loss phenomenon among hospice caregivers. *Am J Hospice Palliat Care* 8(3):29–37.

Antonovsky A (1979). *Health, stress and coping: new perspectives on mental and physical wellbeing*. San Francisco, CA: Jossy-Bass.

Barnes K (2001). Staff stress in the children's hospice: causes, effects and coping strategies. *Int J Palliat Nurs* 7(5):248–54.

Baverstock AC, Finlay FO (2006). A study of staff support mechanisms within children's hospices. *Int J Palliat Nurs* 12(11):506–8.

Berkman LF, Melchior M (2006). The shape of things to come: how social policy impacts social integration and family structure to produce population health. In: Siegrist J, Marmot M (ed.). *Social inequalities in health: new evidence and policy implications*. Oxford University Press, pp. 55–72.

Blomberg K, Sahlberg-Blom E (2007). Closeness and distance: a way of handling difficult situations in daily care. *J Clin Nurs* 16(2):244–54.

Bryant C, Fairbrother G, Fenton P (2000). The relative influence of personal and workplace descriptors of stress. *Br J Nurs* 9(13):876–80.

Buchanan D, Huczynski A (2004). *Organizational behaviour: an introductory text*, (5th edn). Harlow: Prentice-Hall.

Davey Smith G, Harding S (1997). Is control at work the key to socio-economic gradients in mortality? *Lancet* 350:1369–70.

DiTullio M, MacDonald D (1999). The struggle for the soul of hospice: stress, coping, and changes amog hospice workers *Am J Hospice Palliat Care* 16(5):641–55.

Duffy S, Jackson F (1996). Stressors affecting hospice nurses. *Home Healthcare Nurse* 14:54–60.

Earnshaw J, Morrison L (1999). Should employers worry? Workplace stress claims following the John Walker decision. *Personnel Rev* 30(4):468–87.

Ersek M, Wilson SA (2003). The challenges and opportunities in providing end-of-life care in nursing homes. *J Palliat Med* 6:7–9.

Figley CR (1995). Compassion fatigue as a secondary traumatic stress disorder: an overview. In: Figley CR (ed.). *Compassion fatigue*. New York: Brunner/Mazel, pp. 1–20.

Fillion L, Dupuis R, Tremblay I, de Grâce GR, Beitbart W (2006). Enhancing meaning in palliative care practice: a meaning-centered intervention to promote job satisfaction. *Support Palliat Care* 4(4):333–44.

Fillion L, Tremblay I, Truchon M, Côté D, Struthers CW, Dupuis R (2007). Job satisfaction and emotional distress among nurses providing palliative empirical evidence for an integrative occupational stress-model. *Int J Stress Manage* 14:1–25.

Garfield C with Spring C, Ober D (1995). *Sometimes my heart goes numb: love and caring in a time of AIDS*. San Francisco, CA: Jossey-Bass.

Gysels M, Higginson I (2004). *Improving supportive and palliative care for adults with cancer: research evidence*. London: National Institute for Clinical Excellence.

Hammons KH (2000). An analysis of social factors which mitigate burnout in hospital social workers who work with terminally ill inpatient populations. *Dissertation Abstr Int A Humanities Soc Sci* 60(9-A):3527.

Harris LM, Cumming SR, Campbell AJ (2006). Stress and psychological well-being among allied health professionals. *J Allied Health* 35(4):198–207.

Hawkins P, Shohet R (2006). *Supervision in the helping professions*, (3rd edn). Buckingham: Open University Press.

Hayter M (2000). Utilizing the Maslach Burnout Inventory to measure burnout in HIV/AIDS specialist community nurses: the implications for clinical supervision and support. *Prim Health Care Res Dev* 1:243–53.

Holland JM, Neimeyer RA (2005). Reducing the risk of burnout in end-of-life care settings: the role of daily spiritual experiences and training. *Support Palliat Care* 3(3):173–81.

Holmes TH, Rahe RH (1967). The social readjustment rating scale. *J Psychsom Res* 11:213.

Hopkinson JB (2002). The hidden benefit: the supportive function of the nursing handover for qualified nurses caring for dying people in hospital. *J Clin Nurs* 11(2):168–75.

Hunsberger P (1989). Creation and evolution of the hospice staff support group: lessons from four long-term groups. *Am J Hospice Palliat Care* 5:37–41.

ISMA (2005). *Making the stress management standards work: how to apply the standards in your workplace*. London: International Stress Management Association/Advisory and Arbitration Service/Health and Safety Executive.

James N (1993). Divisions of emotional labour: disclosure and cancer. In: Robb M, Barrett S, Komaromy C, Rogers A (2004). *Communication, relationships and care: A Reader*. London: Routledge, pp. 259–69.

Jones A (2003a). Some benefits experienced by hospice nurses from group clinical supervision. *Eur J Cancer Care* 13(3):224–32.

Jones A (2003b). Clinical supervision in promoting a balanced delivery of palliative nursing care. *J Hospice Palliat Nurs* 5(3):168–75.

Kash KM, Holland JC, Breitbart W, Brenson S, Dougherty J, Ouellette-Kobasa S (2000). Stress and burnout in oncology. *Oncology* 14:1621–9.

Katz JS, Sidell M, Komaromy C (2001). Dying in long-term care facilities: support needs of other residents, relatives and staff. *Am J Hospice Palliat Care* 18(5):321–6.

Kirchhoff KT, Spuhler V, Walker L, Hutton A, Cole BV, Clemmer T (2000). Intensive care nurses' experiences with end-of-lfe care. *Am J Crit Care* 9:36–42.

Kristenson M (2006). Socio-economic position and health: the role of coping. In: Siegrist J, Marmot M (ed.). *Social inequalities in health: new evidence and policy implications*. Oxford University Press, pp. 127–51.

Kulbe J (2001). Stressors and coping measures of hospice nurses. *Home Healthcare Nurse* 19(11):707–11.

Llamas KJ, Llamas M, Pickhaver AM, Piller NB (2001). Provider perspective on palliative care needs at a major teaching hospital. *Palliat Med* 15(6):461–70.

Lloyd-Williams M, Wright M, Cobb M, Shiels C (2004). A prospective study of the roles, responsibilities and stresses of chaplains working within a hospice. *Palliat Med* 18(7):638–46.

McCluggage HL (2006). Symptoms suffered y life-limited children that cause anxiety to UK children's hospice staff. *Int J Palliat Nurs* 12(6):254–8.

McVicar A (2003). Workplace stress in nursing: a literature review. *J Adv Nurs* 44(6):633–42.

Maslach C (1982). *Burnout: the cost of caring*. Englewood Cliffs, NJ: Prentice-Hall.

Maslach C, Jackson SE (1981). The measurement of experienced burnout. *J Occupat Behav* 2:99–113.

Mickelson KD, Kubzansky LD (2003). Social distribution of social support: the mediating role of life events. *Am J Community Psychol* 32:265–81.

Mimura C, Griffiths P (2003). The effectiveness of current approaches to workplace stress management in the nursing profession: an evidence based literature review. *Occup Environ Med* 60:10–16.

Newton J, Waters V (2001). Community palliative care clinical nurse specialists descriptions of stress in their work. *Int J Palliat Nurs* 7(11):531–40.

O'Leary N, Flynn J, MacCallion A, Walsh E, McQuillan R (2006). Paediatric palliative care delivered by an adult palliative care service. *Palliat Med* 20:433–7.

Papdatou D, Bellali T (2002). Greek nurse and physician grief as a result of caring for children dying of cancer. *Pediatr Nurs* 28(4):345–53.

Parkes CM (1986). Orienteering the caregiver's grief. *J Palliat Care* 1:7.

Payne M (2000). *Teamwork in multiprofessional care*. Basingstoke: Palgrave.

Payne M (2006). Teambuilding: how, why and where? In: Speck P (ed.). *Teamwork in palliative care: fulfilling or frustrating?* Oxford: Oxford University Press, pp. 117–36.

Payne N (2001). Occupational stressors and coping as determinants of burnout in female hospice nurses. *J Adv Nurs* 33(3):396–405.

Rahe RH, Taylor CB, Tolles RL, Newhall LM, Veach TL, Bryson S (2002). A novel stress and coping workplace program reduces illness and healthcare utilization. *Psychosom Med* 64:278–86.

Schutte N, Oppinen S, Kalimo R, Schaiufeli W (2000). The factorial validity of the Maslach Burnout Inventory–General Survey (MBI_GS) across occupational groups and nations. *J Occup Organ Psychol* 73:53–66.

Siegrist J, Theorell T (2006). Socio-economic position and health: the role of work and employment. In: Siegrist J, Marmot M (ed.). *Social inequalities i health: new evidence and policy implications*. Oxford University Press, pp. 73–100.

Spiers C (2003). Tools to tackle workplace stress. *Occup Health* 55(12):22–5.

Spurgeon A, Jackson CA, Beach JR (2001). The Life Events Inventory: re-scaling based on an occupational sample. *Occup Med* 51(4):287–93.

Taylor EJ, Highfield MF, Amenta M (1999). Predictors of oncology and hospice nurses' spiritual care perspectives and practices. *Appl Nurs Res* 12:30–7.

Ursin H, Eriksen HR (2004). The cognitive activation theory of stress. *Psychoneuroendocrinology* 29:567–92.

Vachon MLS (1987). *Occupational stress in the care of the critically ill, dying, and the bereaved*. New York: Hemisphere.

Vachon MLS (1995). Staff stress in palliative/hospice care: a review. *Palliat Med* 9:91–122.

Vachon MLS (2000). Burnout and symptoms of stress in staff working in palliative care. In: Chochinov HM, Breitbart W (ed.). *Handbook of psychiatry in palliative medicine*. New York: Oxford University Press, pp. 303–19.

Wada Y, Sasaki Y (2006). Characterization of burnout and interpersonal relationships—overall and age-stratified analyses of nurses working in palliative care units. *J Jpn Acad Nurs Sci* 26(2):76–86.

West MA (2004). *Effective teamwork*. Oxford: BPS Blackwell.

Williams S, Cooper C (2002). *Managing workplace stress: a best practice blueprint*. Chichester: Wiley.

Worden JW (2003). *Grief counselling and grief therapy: a handbook for the mental health practitioner*. Hove: Brunner-Routledge.

Yam BMC, Rossiter JC, Cheung KYS (2001). Caring for dying infants: experiences of neonatal intensive care nurses in Hong Kong. *J Clin Nurs* 10(5):651–9.

Index